Injury & Trauma Sourcebook

Learning Disabilities Sourcebook, 3rd Edition

Leukemia Sourcebook

Liver Disorders Sourcebook

Medical Tests Sourcebook, 4th Edition

Men's Health Concerns Sourcebook, 3rd Edition

Mental Health Disorders Sourcebook, 4th Edition

Mental Retardation Sourcebook

Movement Disorders Sourcebook, 2nd Edition

Multiple Sclerosis Sourcebook

Muscular Dystrophy Sourcebook

Obesity Sourcebook

Osteoporosis Sourcebook

Pain Sourcebook, 3rd Edition

Pediatric Cancer Sourcebook

Physical & Mental Issues in Aging Sourcebook

Podiatry Sourcebook, 2nd Edition

Pregnancy & Birth Sourcebook, 3rd Edition

Prostate & Urological Disorders Sourcebook

Prostate Cancer Sourcebook

Rehabilitation Sourcebook

Respiratory Disorders Sourcebook, 2nd Edition

Sexually Transmitted Diseases Sourcebook, 4th Edition

Sleep Disorders Sourcebook, 3rd Edition

Smoking Concerns Sourcebook

Sports Injuries Sourcebook, 4th Edition

Stress-Related Disorders Sourcebook, 2nd Edition

Stroke Sourcebook, 2nd Edition

Surgery Sourcebook, 2nd Edition

Thyroid Disorders Sourcebook

Transplantation Sourcebook

Traveler's Health Sourcebook

Urinary Tract & Kidney Diseases & Disorders Sourcebook, 2nd Edition

Vegetarian Sourcebook

Women's Health Concerns Sourcebook, 3rd Edition

Workplace Health & Safety Sourcebook

Worldwide Health Sourcebook

Teen Health Series

Abuse & Violence Information for Teens

Accident & Safety Information for Teens

Alcohol Information for Teens, 2nd Edition

Allergy Information for Teens

Asthma Information for Teens, 2nd Edition

Body Information for Teens

Cancer Information for Teens, 2nd Edition

Complementary & Alternative Medicine Information for Teens

Diabetes Information for Teens, 2nd Edition

Diet Information for Teens, 3rd Edition

Drug Information for Teens, 3rd Edition

Eating Disorders Information for Teens, 2nd Edition

Fitness Information for Teens, 2nd Edition

Learning Disabilities Information for Teens

Mental Health Information for Teens, 3rd Edition

Pregnancy Information for Teens, 2nd Edition

Sexual Health Information for Teens, 3rd Edition

Skin Health Information for Teens, 2nd Edition

Sleep Information for Teens

Sports Injuries Information for Teens, 2nd Edition

Stress Information for Teens

Suicide Information for Teens, 2nd Edition

Tobacco Information for Teens, 2nd Edition

Diabetes
SOURCEBOOK

Fifth Edition

Health Reference Series

Fifth Edition

Diabetes
SOURCEBOOK

Basic Consumer Health Information about Type 1 and Type 2 Diabetes, Gestational Diabetes, and Other Types of Diabetes and Prediabetes, with Details about Medical, Dietary, and Lifestyle Disease Management Issues, Including Blood Glucose Monitoring, Meal Planning, Weight Control, Oral Diabetes Medications, and Insulin

Along with Facts about the Most Common Complications of Diabetes and Their Prevention, Current Research in Diabetes Care, Tips for People following a Diabetic Diet, a Glossary of Related Terms, and a Directory of Resources for Further Help and Information

Edited by
Sandra J. Judd

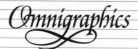

Omnigraphics

P.O. Box 31-1640, Detroit, MI 48231

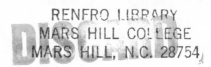
Bibliographic Note

Because this page cannot legibly accommodate all the copyright notices, the Bibliographic Note portion of the Preface constitutes an extension of the copyright notice.

Edited by Sandra J. Judd

Health Reference Series

Karen Bellenir, *Managing Editor*
David A. Cooke, MD, FACP, *Medical Consultant*
Elizabeth Collins, *Research and Permissions Coordinator*
Cherry Edwards, *Permissions Assistant*
EdIndex, Services for Publishers, *Indexers*

* * *

Omnigraphics, Inc.

Matthew P. Barbour, *Senior Vice President*
Kevin M. Hayes, *Operations Manager*

* * *

Peter E. Ruffner, *Publisher*

Copyright © 2011 Omnigraphics, Inc.

ISBN 978-0-7808-1149-2

Library of Congress Cataloging-in-Publication Data

Diabetes sourcebook : basic consumer health information about type 1 and type 2 diabetes, gestational diabetes, and other types of diabetes and prediabetes, with details about medical, dietary, and lifestyle disease management issues, including blood glucose monitoring, meal planning, weight control, oral diabetes medications, and insulin; along with facts about the most common complications of diabetes and their prevention, current research in diabetes care, tips for people following a diabetic diet ... / edited by Sandra J. Judd. -- 5th ed.
        p. cm.
  Includes bibliographical references and index.
  Summary: "Provides basic consumer health information about diagnosis, treatment, and management of type 1 and type 2 diabetes, along with facts about lifestyle issues and preventing complications. Includes index, glossary of related terms, and other resources"-- Provided by publisher.
  ISBN 978-0-7808-1149-2 (hardcover : alk. paper) 1. Diabetes--Popular works. I. Judd, Sandra J.
  RC660.4.D56 2011
  616.4'62--dc23
                                                                        2011018919

SEP 0 3 2012 ∞

This book is printed on acid-free paper meeting the ANSI Z39.48 Standard. The infinity symbol that appears above indicates that the paper in this book meets that standard.

Printed in the United States

Table of Contents

Visit www.healthreferenceseries.com to view *A Contents Guide to the Health Reference Series*, a listing of more than 15,000 topics and the volumes in which they are covered.

Part II: Identifying and Managing Diabetes

Part IV: Dietary and Other Lifestyle Issues Important for Diabetes Control

Part V: Complications of Diabetes and Co-Occurring Disorders

Part VIII: Additional Help and Information

Preface

About This Book

Diabetes is a chronic disorder characterized by high levels of blood sugar. It can lead to a host of complications, including heart disease, stroke, high blood pressure, blindness, kidney disease, nervous system disease, and limb amputation. Although many of the complications of diabetes occur over long periods of time, poorly controlled blood glucose levels can also result in acute medical emergencies, such as seizures or coma or even death.

The number of people with diabetes in the United States is growing. According to the American Diabetes Association, 25.8 million children and adults in the United States are living with diabetes—8.3 percent of the total population. Among people aged twenty and older, almost two million new cases were diagnosed in 2010. Furthermore, an estimated 79 million Americans have prediabetes, and another estimated seven million have the disease but have not yet been diagnosed.

Despite its prevalence, many Americans are unaware of the basic facts about diabetes and the progress being made in the fight against it. For example, new forms of treatment are being developed making it easier to manage, and work on pancreatic islet transplantation and an artificial pancreas offer hope for an eventual cure.

Diabetes Sourcebook, Fifth Edition, provides basic consumer information about the different types of diabetes and how they are diagnosed. It discusses strategies for controlling diabetes and managing daily life challenges. It includes information about the complications of diabetes and their prevention and offers guidelines for recognizing and treating diabetic emergencies. The book concludes with updated information regarding the most recent research in diabetes care, a glossary of related terms, and a list of resources for additional help and information.

How to Use This Book

This book is divided into parts and chapters. Parts focus on broad areas of interest. Chapters are devoted to single topics within a part.

Part I: Understanding Diabetes explains how the body processes glucose and what can go wrong. It describes different types of diabetes and provides statistics on the prevalence of diabetes and diabetes-related complications.

Part II: Identifying and Managing Diabetes describes metabolic syndrome and other risk factors for developing diabetes. It gives details about the tests most commonly used to diagnose diabetes and monitor blood glucose levels. It also explains the importance of achieving good diabetes control. The part concludes with a description of the tests, check-ups, and vaccinations doctors recommend for people with diabetes.

Part III: Medications and Diabetes Care discusses the medications used to manage diabetes. It describes different types of insulin and the methods used to administer insulin, including injections, external insulin pumps, and other new and emerging insulin delivery systems. It also describes oral and non-insulin injectable medications, new diabetes medications, and alternative and complementary diabetes treatments.

Part IV: Dietary and Other Lifestyle Issues Important for Diabetes Control describes the components of the diabetic diet and the types of meal planning that can be used to control blood glucose levels. It explains the importance of physical activity and weight management and offers tips for handling the challenges diabetics face in daily life. The part concludes with information about identifying and dealing with emergency situations.

Part V: Complications of Diabetes and Co-Occurring Disorders provides facts about the impact diabetes can have on the eyes, feet, skin, cardiovascular system, kidneys, mouth, and elsewhere in the body. It describes the symptoms of these complications and discusses ways to prevent their occurrence. It also describes disorders that often accompany diabetes and offers suggestions for their prevention and treatment.

Part VI: Diabetes in Specific Populations discusses the particular challenges of managing diabetes among pregnant women, the elderly, and children. It offers suggestions for overcoming such challenges as managing diabetes at school, coping with sick days, and celebrating special occasions.

Part VII: New Research in Diabetes Care describes the most current research into the management and prevention of diabetes. It explains the results of recent research studies and details the most current advances in stem cell research, pancreatic islet transplantation, and efforts toward developing an artificial pancreas. It concludes with a discussion of clinical trials currently being conducted.

Part VIII: Additional Help and Information includes a glossary of terms related to diabetes, recipes for diabetics and their families, information about sources of financial assistance, and a directory of other resources for additional help and support.

Bibliographic Note

This volume contains documents and excerpts from the following U.S. government agencies: Centers for Disease Control and Prevention; Clinicaltrials.gov; National Center for Complementary and Alternative Medicine; National Diabetes Education Program; National Institute for Diabetes and Digestive and Kidney Diseases; National Institute of Arthritis and Musculoskeletal and Skin Diseases; National Institutes of Health; *NIH News*; National Women's Health Information Center; U.S. Equal Employment Opportunity Commission; and the U.S. Food and Drug Administration.

In addition, this volume contains copyrighted documents from the following organizations: A.D.A,M., Inc.; American Association for Clinical Chemistry; American Heart Association; Baylor College of Medicine, Office of Public Affairs; Canadian Diabetes Association; Diabetes Services, Inc.; Diabetes Teaching Center, University of California, San Francisco; HealthDay/ScoutNews LLC; Joslin Diabetes Center; LifeMed Media; MyDR.com.au; Nemours Foundation; Ohio State University Medical Center; R. A. Rapaport Publishing; *Technology Review*

(MIT); University of Idaho Cooperative Extension Service, Franklin County Extension; University of Illinois Urban Extension; University of Manchester; University of Michigan Health System; Virginia Department of Health; and Yale University Office of Public Affairs.

Acknowledgements

Thanks go to the many organizations, agencies, and individuals who have contributed materials for this *Sourcebook* and to medical consultant Dr. David Cooke and prepress services provider WhimsyInk. Special thanks go to managing editor Karen Bellenir and permissions coordinator Liz Collins for their help and support.

About the Health Reference Series

The *Health Reference Series* is designed to provide basic medical information for patients, families, caregivers, and the general public. Each volume takes a particular topic and provides comprehensive coverage. This is especially important for people who may be dealing with a newly diagnosed disease or a chronic disorder in themselves or in a family member. People looking for preventive guidance, information about disease warning signs, medical statistics, and risk factors for health problems will also find answers to their questions in the *Health Reference Series*. The *Series*, however, is not intended to serve as a tool for diagnosing illness, in prescribing treatments, or as a substitute for the physician/patient relationship. All people concerned about medical symptoms or the possibility of disease are encouraged to seek professional care from an appropriate healthcare provider.

A Note about Spelling and Style

Health Reference Series editors use *Stedman's Medical Dictionary* as an authority for questions related to the spelling of medical terms and the *Chicago Manual of Style* for questions related to grammatical structures, punctuation, and other editorial concerns. Consistent adherence is not always possible, however, because the individual volumes within the *Series* include many documents from a wide variety of different producers and copyright holders, and the editor's primary goal is to present material from each source as accurately as is possible following the terms specified by each document's producer. This sometimes means that information in different chapters or sections may follow other guidelines and alternate spelling authorities. For example, occasionally a copyright holder may require that eponymous terms be shown in possessive forms (Crohn's disease *vs.* Crohn disease) or that British spelling norms be retained (leukaemia *vs.* leukemia).

Locating Information within the Health Reference Series

The *Health Reference Series* contains a wealth of information about a wide variety of medical topics. Ensuring easy access to all the fact sheets, research reports, in-depth discussions, and other material contained within the individual books of the series remains one of our highest priorities. As the *Series* continues to grow in size and scope, however, locating the precise information needed by a reader may become more challenging.

A *Contents Guide to the Health Reference Series* was developed to direct readers to the specific volumes that address their concerns. It presents an extensive list of diseases, treatments, and other topics of general interest compiled from the Tables of Contents and major index headings. To access A *Contents Guide to the Health Reference Series*, visit www.healthreferenceseries.com.

Medical Consultant

Medical consultation services are provided to the *Health Reference Series* editors by David A. Cooke, MD, FACP. Dr. Cooke is a graduate of Brandeis University, and he received his M.D. degree from the University of Michigan. He completed residency training at the University of Wisconsin Hospital and Clinics. He is board-certified in Internal Medicine. Dr. Cooke currently works as part of the University of Michigan Health System and practices in Ann Arbor, MI. In his free time, he enjoys writing, science fiction, and spending time with his family.

Our Advisory Board

We would like to thank the following board members for providing guidance to the development of this series:

Dr. Lynda Baker, Associate Professor of Library and Information Science, Wayne State University, Detroit, MI

Nancy Bulgarelli, William Beaumont Hospital Library, Royal Oak, MI

Karen Imarisio, Bloomfield Township Public Library, Bloomfield Township, MI

Karen Morgan, Mardigian Library,
University of Michigan-Dearborn, Dearborn, MI

Rosemary Orlando, St. Clair Shores Public Library,
St. Clair Shores, MI

Health Reference Series Update Policy

The inaugural book in the *Health Reference Series* was the first edition of *Cancer Sourcebook* published in 1989. Since then, the *Series* has been enthusiastically received by librarians and in the medical community. In order to maintain the standard of providing high-quality health information for the layperson the editorial staff at Omnigraphics felt it was necessary to implement a policy of updating volumes when warranted.

Medical researchers have been making tremendous strides, and it is the purpose of the *Health Reference Series* to stay current with the most recent advances. Each decision to update a volume is made on an individual basis. Some of the considerations include how much new information is available and the feedback we receive from people who use the books. If there is a topic you would like to see added to the update list, or an area of medical concern you feel has not been adequately addressed, please write to:

Editor
Health Reference Series
Omnigraphics, Inc.
P.O. Box 31-1640
Detroit, MI 48231
E-mail: editorial@omnigraphics.com

Part One

Understanding Diabetes

Chapter 1

What Is Diabetes?

What is diabetes?

Diabetes is a disease in which blood glucose levels are above normal. Most of the food we eat is turned into glucose, or sugar, for our bodies to use for energy. The pancreas, an organ that lies near the stomach, makes a hormone called insulin to help glucose get into the cells of our bodies. When you have diabetes, your body either doesn't make enough insulin or can't use its own insulin as well as it should. This causes sugar to build up in your blood.

Diabetes can cause serious health complications including heart disease, blindness, kidney failure, and lower-extremity amputations. Diabetes is the sixth leading cause of death in the United States.

What are the symptoms of diabetes?

People who think they might have diabetes must visit a physician for diagnosis. They might have some or none of the following symptoms:

- Frequent urination

- Excessive thirst

- Unexplained weight loss

Excerpted from "Basics About Diabetes," Centers for Disease Control and Prevention, June 4, 2010.

- Extreme hunger

- Sudden vision changes

- Tingling or numbness in hands or feet

- Feeling very tired much of the time

- Very dry skin

- Sores that are slow to heal

- More infections than usual

Nausea, vomiting, or stomach pains may accompany some of these symptoms in the abrupt onset of insulin-dependent diabetes, now called type 1 diabetes.

What are the types of diabetes?

Type 1 diabetes, which was previously called insulin-dependent diabetes mellitus (IDDM) or juvenile-onset diabetes, may account for 5 to 10 percent of all diagnosed cases of diabetes. Type 2 diabetes, which was previously called non-insulin-dependent diabetes mellitus (NIDDM) or adult-onset diabetes, may account for about 90 to 95 percent of all diagnosed cases of diabetes. Gestational diabetes is a type of diabetes that only pregnant women get. If not treated, it can cause problems for mothers and babies. Gestational diabetes develops in 2 to 5 percent of all pregnancies but usually disappears when a pregnancy is over. Other specific types of diabetes resulting from specific genetic syndromes, surgery, drugs, malnutrition, infections, and other illnesses may account for 1 to 2 percent of all diagnosed cases of diabetes.

What are the risk factors for diabetes?

Risk factors for type 2 diabetes include older age, obesity, family history of diabetes, prior history of gestational diabetes, impaired glucose tolerance, physical inactivity, and race/ethnicity. African Americans, Hispanic/Latino Americans, American Indians, and some Asian Americans and Pacific Islanders are at particularly high risk for type 2 diabetes.

Risk factors are less well defined for type 1 diabetes than for type 2 diabetes, but autoimmune, genetic, and environmental factors are involved in developing this type of diabetes.

Gestational diabetes occurs more frequently in African Americans, Hispanic/Latino Americans, American Indians, and people with a family history of diabetes than in other groups. Obesity is also associated with higher risk. Women who have had gestational diabetes are at increased risk for later developing type 2 diabetes. In some studies, nearly 40 percent of women with a history of gestational diabetes developed diabetes in the future.

Other specific types of diabetes, which may account for 1 to 2 percent of all diagnosed cases, result from specific genetic syndromes, surgery, drugs, malnutrition, infections, and other illnesses.

What is the treatment for diabetes?

Healthy eating, physical activity, and insulin injections are the basic therapies for type 1 diabetes. The amount of insulin taken must be balanced with food intake and daily activities. Blood glucose levels must be closely monitored through frequent blood glucose testing.

Healthy eating, physical activity, and blood glucose testing are the basic therapies for type 2 diabetes. In addition, many people with type 2 diabetes require oral medication, insulin, or both to control their blood glucose levels.

People with diabetes must take responsibility for their day-to-day care, and keep blood glucose levels from going too low or too high.

People with diabetes should see a healthcare provider who will monitor their diabetes control and help them learn to manage their diabetes. In addition, people with diabetes may see endocrinologists, who may specialize in diabetes care; ophthalmologists for eye examinations; podiatrists for routine foot care; and dietitians and diabetes educators who teach the skills needed for daily diabetes management.

What causes type 1 diabetes?

The causes of type 1 diabetes appear to be much different than those for type 2 diabetes, though the exact mechanisms for developing both diseases are unknown. The appearance of type 1 diabetes is suspected to follow exposure to an "environmental trigger," such as an unidentified virus, stimulating an immune attack against the beta cells of the pancreas (that produce insulin) in some genetically predisposed people.

Can diabetes be prevented?

A number of studies have shown that regular physical activity can significantly reduce the risk of developing type 2 diabetes. Type 2 diabetes is associated with obesity.

Researchers are making progress in identifying the exact genetics and "triggers" that predispose some individuals to develop type 1 diabetes, but prevention remains elusive.

Is there a cure for diabetes?

In response to the growing health burden of diabetes, the diabetes community has three choices: prevent diabetes; cure diabetes; and improve the quality of care of people with diabetes to prevent devastating complications. All three approaches are actively being pursued by the U.S. Department of Health and Human Services.

Both the National Institutes of Health (NIH) and the Centers for Disease Control and Prevention (CDC) are involved in prevention activities. The NIH is involved in research to cure both type 1 and type 2 diabetes, especially type 1. CDC focuses most of its programs on making sure that the proven science to prevent complications is put into daily practice for people with diabetes. The basic idea is that if all the important research and science are not applied meaningfully in the daily lives of people with diabetes, then the research is, in essence, wasted.

Several approaches to "cure" diabetes are currently under investigation:

- Pancreas transplantation

- Islet cell transplantation (islet cells produce insulin)

- Artificial pancreas development

- Genetic manipulation (fat or muscle cells that don't normally make insulin have a human insulin gene inserted — then these "pseudo" islet cells are transplanted into people with type 1 diabetes)

Each of these approaches still has a lot of challenges, such as preventing immune rejection, finding an adequate number of insulin cells, keeping cells alive, and others, but progress is being made in all areas.

Chapter 2

How the Body Processes Glucose

Chapter Contents

Section 2.1

The Pancreas and Insulin

Your pancreas is one of the organs of your digestive system. It lies in your abdomen, behind your stomach. It is a long thin structure with two main functions:

- producing digestive enzymes to break down food; and
- producing the hormones insulin and glucagon to control sugar levels in your body.

Production of Digestive Enzymes

The pancreas produces secretions necessary for you to digest food. The enzymes in these secretions allow your body to digest protein, fat, and starch from your food. The enzymes are produced in the acinar cells, which make up most of the pancreas. From the acinar cells the enzymes flow down various channels into the pancreatic duct and then out into the duodenum. The secretions are alkaline to balance the acidic juices and partially digested food coming into the duodenum from the stomach.

Production of Hormones to Control Blood Sugar Levels

A small proportion (1 to 2 percent) of the pancreas is made up of other types of cells called islets of Langerhans. These cells sit in tiny groups, like small islands, scattered throughout the tissue of the pancreas. The islets of Langerhans contain alpha cells, which secrete glucagons, and beta cells, which secrete insulin.

Insulin and glucagon are hormones that work to regulate the level of sugar (glucose) in the body to keep it within a healthy range. Unlike the acinar cells, the islets of Langerhans do not have ducts and secrete insulin and glucagon directly into the bloodstream.

Depending on what you've eaten, how much exercise your muscles are doing, and how active your body cells are, the amount of glucose in your bloodstream and cells varies. These two hormones have the job of keeping tight control of the amount of glucose in your blood so that it doesn't rise or fall outside of healthy limits.

How Insulin Works

Insulin is released from the beta cells in your pancreas in response to rising glucose in your bloodstream. After you eat a meal, any carbohydrates you've eaten are broken down into glucose and passed into the bloodstream. The pancreas detects this rise in blood glucose and starts to secrete insulin.

Insulin works by improving the uptake of glucose from the blood across cell membranes and into the cells of the body, and so takes glucose out of the bloodstream. Once in the cells, the glucose is used as the energy to fuel the cells doing their different jobs or is stored in the liver or muscle cells as glycogen. This results in the glucose level of the blood dropping, which then triggers the pancreas to switch off the release of insulin.

The problem in people with diabetes is that either they don't produce enough insulin, or the insulin they do produce doesn't work properly, or their cells don't respond properly to insulin. The net result is that glucose isn't cleared from their bloodstream and they have high blood glucose levels, which the body tries to clear by various compensatory methods, such as increased urination.

How Glucagon Works

Glucagon has an opposite (antagonistic) effect to insulin. When your blood glucose level falls, for example during exercise when your muscles are using glucose for fuel, your pancreas detects the drop in blood glucose. This prompts the pancreas to slow down the secretion of insulin, but increase the output of glucagon.

The role of glucagon is to break down glycogen (the stored form of glucose) in the liver. Then the liver releases glucose into the bloodstream. This results in a rise in the blood glucose level to bring it back to a healthy level, which in turn signals the pancreas to switch off glucagon release.

The control of blood glucose levels operates by what is known as a negative feedback mechanism. Here is a summary of the two control loops.

When the blood glucose level goes up:

- blood sugar (glucose) rises;

9

- the pancreas detects the rise;

- the pancreas pumps out insulin into the blood;

- insulin helps the uptake of glucose into muscles and other cells;

- this causes the blood glucose level to fall to its normal set point; and

- the pancreas detects the fall and switches off insulin production.

When the blood glucose level goes down:

- blood sugar (glucose) drops;

- the pancreas detects the drop in blood sugar;

- the pancreas switches on the output of glucagon into the blood;

- glucagon signals the liver to break down glycogen into glucose;

- the liver releases glucose into the bloodstream;

- blood glucose goes up to its normal set point; and

- the pancreas detects the rise in blood sugar and switches off glucagon release.

Section 2.2

The Liver, Ketones, and Blood Sugar

The Liver and Blood Sugar

The Liver Both Stores and Produces Sugar

The liver acts as the body's glucose (or fuel) reservoir, and helps to keep your circulating blood sugar levels and other body fuels steady and constant. The liver both stores and manufactures glucose depending upon the body's need. The need to store or release glucose is primarily signaled by the hormones insulin and glucagon.

During a meal, your liver will store sugar, or glucose, as glycogen for a later time when your body needs it. The high levels of insulin and suppressed levels of glucagon during a meal promote the storage of glucose as glycogen.

The Liver Makes Sugar When You Need It

When you're not eating—especially overnight or between meals, the body has to make its own sugar. The liver supplies sugar or glucose by turning glycogen into glucose in a process called glycogenolysis. The liver also can manufacture necessary sugar or glucose by harvesting amino acids, waste products, and fat byproducts. This process is called gluconeogenesis.

The Liver Also Makes Another Fuel, Ketones, When Sugar Is in Short Supply

When your body's glycogen storage is running low, the body starts to conserve the sugar supplies for the organs that always require sugar. These include: the brain, red blood cells, and parts of the kidney. To supplement the limited sugar supply, the liver makes alternative fuels

11

called ketones from fats. This process is called ketogenesis. The hormone signal for ketogenesis to begin is a low level of insulin. Ketones are burned as fuel by muscle and other body organs. And the sugar is saved for the organs that need it.

Ketones

In a person without diabetes, ketone production is the body's normal adaptation to starvation. Blood sugar levels never get too high or too low, because the production is regulated by just the right balance of insulin, glucagons, and other hormones. However, in an individual with diabetes, dangerous and life-threatening levels of ketones can develop.

What Are Ketones and Why Do I Need to Know about Them?

Ketones and ketoacids are alternative fuels for the body that are made when glucose is in short supply. They are made in the liver from the breakdown of fats.

Ketones are formed when there is not enough sugar or glucose to supply the body's fuel needs. This occurs overnight, and during dieting or fasting. During these periods, insulin levels are low, but glucagon and epinephrine levels are relatively normal. This combination of low insulin and relatively normal glucagon and epinephrine levels causes fat to be released from the fat cells.

The fats travel through the blood circulation to reach the liver where they are processed into ketone units. The ketone units then circulate back into the bloodstream and are picked up by the muscle and other tissues to fuel your body's metabolism.

However, the situation is very different in type 1 diabetes, where the presence of excess ketones can be dangerous and life threatening. In type 1 diabetes, when there is not enough insulin, the fat cells keep dumping fat into the circulation, and the liver keeps making more and more ketones and ketoacids. The problem is too many ketones! The rising ketoacid levels make the blood pH too low (acidotic/diabetic ketoacidosis), which is an emergency medical situation and requires immediate care.

Chapter 3

Who Gets Diabetes?

Chapter Contents

Section 3.1

Diabetes Prevalence in America

Excerpted from "The Facts about Diabetes: America's Seventh
Leading Cause of Death," National Diabetes Education Program,
U.S. Department of Health and Human Services, July 2008.

What Is Diabetes?[1]

Diabetes is a group of diseases marked by high levels of blood glucose resulting from defects in insulin production, insulin action, or both. Diabetes can lead to serious complications and premature death, but people with diabetes can take steps to manage the disease and lower the risk of complications.

How Many Americans Have Diabetes and Pre-Diabetes?[1]

- 23.6 million Americans have diabetes—7.8 percent of the U.S. population. Of these, 5.7 million do not know they have the disease.

- Each year, about 1.6 million people aged twenty or older are diagnosed with diabetes.

- The number of people diagnosed with diabetes has risen from 1.5 million in 1958 to 17.9 million in 2007, an increase of epidemic proportions.

- It is estimated that 57 million adults aged twenty and older have pre-diabetes. Pre-diabetes is a condition where blood glucose levels are higher than normal but not high enough to be called diabetes. Studies have shown that by losing weight and increasing physical activity people can prevent or delay prediabetes from progressing to diabetes.

What Is the Prevalence of Diabetes by Type?

- Type 1 (previously called insulin-dependent or juvenile-onset) diabetes accounts for 5 to 10 percent of all diagnosed cases of diabetes.

- Type 2 (previously called non-insulin-dependent or adult-onset) diabetes accounts for 90 to 95 percent of all diagnosed cases of diabetes. Type 2 diabetes is increasingly being diagnosed in children and adolescents.

What Is the Prevalence of Diabetes by Race/Ethnicity?[1]

Non-Hispanic Whites:

- 14.9 million; 9.8 percent of all non-Hispanic whites aged twenty and older have diagnosed and undiagnosed diabetes

African Americans:

- 3.7 million; 14.7 percent of all non-Hispanic blacks aged twenty and older have diagnosed and undiagnosed diabetes.

- Non-Hispanic blacks are about 1.8 times more likely to have diabetes as non-Hispanic whites aged twenty and older.

Hispanics/Latinos:

- 10.4 percent of Hispanics/Latinos aged twenty or older have diagnosed diabetes.

- Among Hispanics/Latinos, diabetes prevalence rates are 8.2 percent for Cubans, 11.9 percent for Mexican Americans, and 12.6 percent for Puerto Ricans.

American Indians and Alaska Natives:

- About 16.5 percent of American Indians and Alaska Natives aged twenty years and older who are served by the Indian Health Service have diagnosed diabetes.

- Diabetes rates vary—among Alaska Native adults (6.0 percent) to American Indians in southern Arizona (29.3 percent).

Asian Americans and Pacific Islanders:

- The rate of diagnosed diabetes in Asian Americans is 7.5 percent. However, prevalence data for diabetes among Pacific Islanders is limited.

How Many Deaths Are Linked to Diabetes?[1]

- Diabetes is the seventh leading cause of death listed on U.S. death certificates.

- Cardiovascular disease is the leading cause of death among people with diabetes—about 68 percent die of heart disease or stroke.

- The overall risk for death among people with diabetes is about double that of people without diabetes.

Treating Diabetes[1]

Diabetes can lead to serious complications, such as blindness, kidney damage, cardiovascular disease, and lower-limb amputations, but people with diabetes can lower the occurrence of these and other diabetes complications by controlling blood glucose, blood pressure, and blood lipids.

Many people with type 2 diabetes can manage their blood glucose by following a healthy meal plan and exercise program, losing excess weight, and taking oral medication. Some people with type 2 diabetes may also need insulin to manage their blood glucose.

United Kingdom Prospective Diabetes Study (UKPDS) and UKPDS Follow-Up Study[2]

The United Kingdom Prospective Diabetes Study (UKPDS) was a groundbreaking study in people with newly diagnosed type 2 diabetes that ended in 1997. This study established that blood glucose control could reduce the risk of microvascular complications (eye disease, kidney disease, and the neuropathy that can lead to limb amputation) in type 2 diabetes. Unlike patients with diabetes of longer duration, in these patients, there was no increase in cardiovascular disease (CVD)–related deaths during the early treatment period.

Ten years later, the UKPDS Follow-Up Study found participants in the intervention group who achieved blood glucose control as close to normal as possible during the original UKPDS had a lower risk of heart attack than those in the control group who had less well controlled blood glucose. The intervention group also showed continued risk reduction in microvascular disease:

- This "legacy effect" indicates that the benefits of blood glucose control that is as close to normal as possible in the early years after diagnosis can lead to a lasting impact on health risks over a long period of time.

- Furthermore, a 27 percent reduction in the risk of heart attacks was seen in those who were overweight and managed their diabetes with blood glucose goals as close to normal as possible when using the common drug metformin.

This "legacy effect" underscores the importance of early detection of diabetes. If diabetes is diagnosed, working toward early blood glucose control as close to normal as possible can result in long-term benefits.

How Much Does Diabetes Cost the Nation?[1]

- Total healthcare and related costs for the treatment of diabetes run about $174 billion annually.

- Of this total, direct medical costs (e.g., hospitalizations, medical care, treatment supplies) account for about $116 billion.

- The other $58 billion covers indirect costs such as disability payments, time lost from work, and premature death.

Notes

1. The National Institute of Diabetes and Digestive and Kidney Diseases. *National Diabetes Statistics, 2007.* Bethesda, MD: U.S. Department of Health and Human Services.

2. 10-Year Follow-up of Intensive Glucose Control in Type 2 Diabetes *N Engl J Med* 2008; 359.

Section 3.2

Groups Especially Affected by Diabetes

Excerpted from "Groups Especially Affected," Centers for
Disease Control and Prevention, June 4, 2010.

How are women especially affected by diabetes?

Of the 20.8 million people with diabetes in the United States,
9.7 million are women. The risk of heart disease, the most common
complication of diabetes, is more serious among women than men.
Among people with diabetes who have had a heart attack, women
have lower survival rates and a poorer quality of life than men.
Women with diabetes have a shorter life expectancy than women
without diabetes, and women are at greater risk of blindness from
diabetes than men. Death rates for women aged twenty-five to forty-
four years with diabetes are more than three times the rate for
women without diabetes.

Women with diabetes must also plan childbearing carefully. It is
especially important to keep blood glucose levels as near to normal as
possible before and during pregnancy, to protect both mother and baby.
Pregnancy itself may affect insulin levels, as well as diabetes-related
eye and kidney problems.

What is gestational diabetes?

Gestational diabetes is a type of diabetes, or high blood sugar, that
only pregnant women get. If a woman gets high blood sugar when
she's pregnant, but she never had high blood sugar before, she has
gestational diabetes.

Managing gestational diabetes is very important in order to protect
the baby. Babies born to mothers with uncontrolled gestational diabetes can be overly large at birth, making delivery more dangerous. These
babies can also have breathing problems. Moreover, children exposed to
diabetes in the womb are more likely to become obese during childhood
and adolescence, and develop type 2 diabetes later in life.

Usually, gestational diabetes goes away after the baby is born. However, women who have had gestational diabetes are at higher risk for developing type 2 diabetes later in life, so healthy eating, physical activity, and weight maintenance are important steps to prevention.

What racial and ethnic groups are especially affected by diabetes?

African Americans, Hispanic/Latino Americans, American Indians, Asian Americans, and Pacific Islander Americans are at particularly high risk for type 2 diabetes. In addition, gestational diabetes occurs more frequently in African Americans, Hispanic/Latino Americans, and American Indians than in other groups.

Why do some racial and ethnic groups have higher rates of diabetes?

Diabetes can indeed "run in families," meaning that heredity often makes someone more likely to develop diabetes. Researchers believe that certain genes affecting immune response can play a role in the development of type 1 diabetes, while genes affecting insulin function can contribute to the development of type 2 diabetes. While African Americans, Hispanic/Latino Americans, American Indians, Asian Americans, and Pacific Islander Americans have a slightly lower rate of type 1 diabetes, they are at a higher risk for type 2 diabetes than the rest of the population.

Many researchers think that some African Americans, Hispanic/Latino Americans, American Indians, Asian Americans, and Pacific Islander Americans inherited a "thrifty gene" which helped their ancestors store food energy better during times when food was plentiful, to survive during times when food was scarce. Now that "feast or famine" situations rarely occur for most people in the United States, the gene which was once helpful may now put these groups at a higher risk for type 2 diabetes.

In addition, poverty, lack of access to healthcare, and cultural attitudes and behaviors are barriers to preventive and diabetes management care for some minority Americans.

How are children especially affected by diabetes?

Type 1 diabetes, which used to be called juvenile diabetes, is usually first diagnosed in children, teens, or young adults. In type 1 diabetes, the body's immune system attacks and destroys beta cells in the pancreas, so that they no longer make insulin. People with type 1 diabetes must take insulin every day. Approximately one of every four hundred to five hundred children and adolescents has type 1 diabetes.

Type 2 diabetes, a disease usually diagnosed in adults aged forty years or older, is now becoming more common among children and adolescents, particularly in American Indians, African Americans, and Hispanic/Latinos.

Among youth, obesity, physical inactivity, and prenatal exposure to diabetes in the mother have become widespread, and may contribute to the increased development of type 2 diabetes during childhood and adolescence.

How are older adults especially affected by diabetes?

As we age, our risk for developing diabetes increases. Approximately half of all diabetes cases occur in people aged sixty years or older. Approximately 20.9 percent (10.3 million) of people in the United States aged sixty years or older have diabetes. Diabetes often leads to chronic conditions that eventually result in death, such as heart disease and kidney disease. Thus, diabetes is often responsible for, but not listed as, the cause of many deaths.

How are some veterans affected by diabetes?

Vietnam veterans exposed to the herbicide Agent Orange may be at increased risk for developing type 2 diabetes. In the year 2000, the Veterans Administration announced that it would recognize diabetes as a Vietnam service-related disease.

Section 3.3

Prevalence of Diabetes Complications

Excerpted from "Prevalence of Diabetes Complications," National Institute of Diabetes and Digestive and Kidney Diseases, National Institutes of Health, NIH Publication No. 08-3892, June 2008.

Complications of Diabetes in the United States

Heart Disease and Stroke

- In 2004, heart disease was noted on 68 percent of diabetes-related death certificates among people ages sixty-five years or older.

- In 2004, stroke was noted on 16 percent of diabetes-related death certificates among people ages sixty-five years or older.

- Adults with diabetes have heart disease death rates about two to four times higher than adults without diabetes.

- The risk for stroke is two to four times higher among people with diabetes.

High Blood Pressure

- In 2003 to 2004, 75 percent of adults with self-reported diabetes had blood pressure greater than or equal to 130/80 millimeters of mercury (mm Hg) or used prescription medications for hypertension.

Blindness

- Diabetes is the leading cause of new cases of blindness among adults ages twenty to seventy-four years.

- Diabetic retinopathy causes twelve thousand to twenty-four thousand new cases of blindness each year.

Kidney Disease

- Diabetes is the leading cause of kidney failure, accounting for 44 percent of new cases in 2005.

- In 2005, 46,739 people with diabetes began treatment for end-stage kidney disease in the United States and Puerto Rico.

- In 2005, a total of 178,689 people with end-stage kidney disease due to diabetes were living on chronic dialysis or with a kidney transplant in the United States and Puerto Rico.

Nervous System Disease

- About 60 to 70 percent of people with diabetes have mild to severe forms of nervous system damage. The results of such damage include impaired sensation or pain in the feet or hands, slowed digestion of food in the stomach, carpal tunnel syndrome, erectile dysfunction, or other nerve problems.

- Almost 30 percent of people with diabetes ages forty years or older have impaired sensation in the feet—for example, at least one area that lacks feeling.

- Severe forms of diabetic nerve disease are a major contributing cause of lower-extremity amputations.

Amputations

- More than 60 percent of nontraumatic lower-limb amputations occur in people with diabetes.

- In 2004, about seventy-one thousand nontraumatic lower-limb amputations were performed in people with diabetes.

Dental Disease

- Periodontal, or gum, disease is more common in people with diabetes. Among young adults, those with diabetes have about twice the risk of those without diabetes.

- People with poorly controlled diabetes—A1C greater than 9 percent—were nearly three times more likely to have severe periodontitis than those without diabetes.

- Almost one-third of people with diabetes have severe periodontal disease with loss of attachment of the gums to the teeth measuring 5 millimeters or more.

Complications of Pregnancy

- Poorly controlled diabetes before conception and during the first trimester of pregnancy among women with type 1 diabetes can cause major birth defects in 5 to 10 percent of pregnancies and spontaneous abortions in 15 to 20 percent of pregnancies.

- Poorly controlled diabetes during the second and third trimesters of pregnancy can result in excessively large babies, posing a risk to both mother and child.

Other Complications

- Uncontrolled diabetes often leads to biochemical imbalances that can cause acute life-threatening events, such as diabetic ketoacidosis and hyperosmolar, or nonketotic, coma.

- People with diabetes are more susceptible to many other illnesses and, once they acquire these illnesses, often have worse prognoses. For example, they are more likely to die with pneumonia or influenza than people who do not have diabetes.

- People with diabetes ages sixty years or older are two to three times more likely to report an inability to walk a quarter of a mile, climb stairs, do housework, or use a mobility aid compared with people without diabetes in the same age group.

Chapter 4

Type 1 Diabetes

Type 1 diabetes is a chronic (lifelong) disease that occurs when the pancreas does not produce enough insulin to properly control blood sugar levels.

Causes

There are several forms of diabetes. Type 1 diabetes used to be called juvenile or insulin-dependent diabetes. Type 1 diabetes can occur at any age, but it is most often diagnosed in children, adolescents, or young adults.

Insulin is a hormone produced by special cells, called beta cells, in the pancreas, an organ located in the area behind your stomach. Insulin is needed to move blood sugar (glucose) into cells, where it is stored and later used for energy. In type 1 diabetes, these cells produce little or no insulin.

Without enough insulin, glucose builds up in the bloodstream instead of going into the cells. The body is unable to use this glucose for energy. This leads to the symptoms of type 1 diabetes.

Within five to ten years, the insulin-producing beta cells of the pancreas are completely destroyed and the body can no longer produce insulin.

The exact cause is unknown, but most likely there is a viral or environmental trigger in genetically susceptible people that causes an immune reaction. The body's white blood cells mistakenly attack the insulin-producing pancreatic beta cells.

Symptoms

Some people will have no symptoms before they are diagnosed with diabetes.

Others may notice these symptoms as the first signs of type 1 diabetes, or when the blood sugar is high:

- Feeling tired or fatigued
- Feeling hungry
- Being very thirsty
- Urinating more often
- Losing weight without trying
- Having blurry eyesight
- Losing the feeling or feeling tingling in your feet

For others, warning symptoms that they are becoming very sick may be the first signs of type 1 diabetes, or may happen when the blood sugar is very high:

- Deep, rapid breathing
- Dry skin and mouth
- Flushed face
- Fruity breath odor
- Nausea or vomiting, unable to keep down fluids
- Stomach pain

Low blood sugar (hypoglycemia) can develop quickly in people with diabetes who are taking insulin. Symptoms typically appear when the blood sugar level falls below 70 mg/dL. Watch for:

- headache;
- hunger;
- nervousness;
- rapid heartbeat (palpitations);
- shaking;
- sweating;
- weakness.

Exams and Tests

Diabetes is diagnosed with the following blood tests:

- **Fasting blood glucose level:** Diabetes is diagnosed if it is higher than 126 mg/dL on two occasions.

- **Random (nonfasting) blood glucose level:** Diabetes is suspected if it is higher than 200 mg/dL and the patient has symptoms such as increased thirst, urination, and fatigue (this must be confirmed with a fasting test).

- **Oral glucose tolerance test:** Diabetes is diagnosed if the glucose level is higher than 200 mg/dL after two hours.

- **Hemoglobin A1c test:** This test has been used in the past to help patients monitor how well they are controlling their blood glucose levels. In 2010, the American Diabetes Association recommended that the test be used as another option for diagnosing diabetes and identifying pre-diabetes. Levels indicate:

  - Normal: Less than 5.7 percent

  - Pre-diabetes: Between 5.7 and 6.4 percent

  - Diabetes: 6.5 percent or higher

Ketone testing is also used in type 1 diabetes. Ketones are produced by the breakdown of fat and muscle. They are harmful at high levels. The ketone test is done using a urine sample. Ketone testing is usually done at the following times:

- When the blood sugar is higher than 240 mg/dL

- During an illness such as pneumonia, heart attack, or stroke

- When nausea or vomiting occur

- During pregnancy

The following tests will help you and your doctor monitor your diabetes and prevent complications of diabetes:

- Check the skin and bones on your feet and legs.

- Check the sensation in your feet.

- Have your blood pressure checked at least every year (blood pressure goal should be 130/80 mm/Hg or lower).

- Have your glycosylated hemoglobin (HbA1c) checked every six months if your diabetes is well controlled; otherwise, every three months.

- Have your cholesterol and triglyceride levels checked yearly (aim for LDL cholesterol levels below 70–100 mg/dL).

- Get yearly tests to make sure your kidneys are working well (microalbuminuria and serum creatinine).

- Visit your ophthalmologist at least once a year, or more often if you have signs of diabetic retinopathy.

- See the dentist every six months for a thorough dental cleaning and exam. Make sure your dentist and hygienist know that you have diabetes.

Treatment

The immediate goals of treatment are to treat diabetic ketoacidosis and high blood glucose levels. Because type 1 diabetes can come on suddenly and the symptoms can be severe, newly diagnosed people may need to stay in the hospital.

The long-term goals of treatment are to:

- reduce symptoms;

- prevent diabetes-related complications such as blindness, kidney failure, nerve damage, amputation of limbs, and heart disease.

Insulin

Insulin lowers blood sugar by allowing it to leave the bloodstream and enter cells. Everyone needs insulin. People with type 1 diabetes can't make their own insulin. They must take insulin every day.

Insulin is usually injected under the skin. In some cases, a pump delivers the insulin continuously. Insulin does not come in pill form.

Insulin preparations differ in how fast they start to work and how long they last. The healthcare professional will review your blood glucose levels to determine the appropriate type of insulin you should use. More than one type of insulin may be mixed together in an injection to achieve the best blood glucose control.

The injections are needed, in general, from one to four times a day. People are taught how to give insulin injections by their healthcare provider or a diabetes nurse educator. At first, a child's injections may be given by a parent or other adult. By age fourteen, most children can be expected (but should not be required) to give their own injections.

People with diabetes need to know how to adjust the amount of insulin they are taking in the following situations:

- When they exercise

- When they are sick

- When they will be eating more or less food and calories

- When they are traveling

Diet

People with type 1 diabetes should eat at about the same times each day and try to be consistent with the types of food they choose. This helps to prevent blood sugar from becoming extremely high or low.

The American Diabetes Association and the American Dietetic Association have information for planning healthy, balanced meals. It can help to talk with a registered dietitian or nutrition counselor.

Physical Activity

Regular exercise helps control the amount of sugar in the blood. It also helps burn excess calories and fat to achieve a healthy weight.

Ask your healthcare provider before starting any exercise program. Those with type 1 diabetes must take special precautions before, during, and after intense physical activity or exercise:

- Always check with your doctor before starting a new exercise program.

- Ask your doctor or nurse if you have the right footwear.

- Choose an enjoyable physical activity that is appropriate for your current fitness level.

- Exercise every day and at the same time of day, if possible.

- Monitor your blood glucose levels at home before and after exercising.

- Carry food that contains a fast-acting carbohydrate in case your blood glucose levels get too low during or after exercise.

- Wear a diabetes identification bracelet and carry a cell phone to use in case of emergency.

- Drink extra fluids that do not contain sugar before, during, and after exercise.

- As you change the intensity or duration of your exercise, you may need to modify your diet or medication to keep your blood glucose levels in an appropriate range.

Self-Testing

Self-testing refers to being able to check your blood sugar at home yourself. Regular self-testing of your blood sugar tells you and your healthcare provider how well your diet, exercise, and diabetes medications are working. This is also called self-monitoring of blood glucose, or SMBG.

A healthcare provider or diabetes educator will help set up a testing schedule for you at home:

- Your doctor will help you set a goal for what level your blood sugar should be during the day.

- The results can be used to adjust meals, activity, or medications to keep blood sugar levels within an appropriate range. Tests are usually done before meals and at bedtime. More frequent testing may be needed when you are sick, under stress, or adjusting your insulin dosing.

Testing will provide valuable information so the healthcare provider can suggest improvements to your care and treatment. Testing will identify high and low blood sugar levels before serious problems develop.

A device called a glucometer can provide a blood sugar reading. There are different types of devices. Usually, you prick your finger with a small needle called a lancet to get a tiny drop of blood. You place the blood on a test strip and put the strip into the device. You should have results within thirty to forty-five seconds.

Keeping accurate records of your test results will help you and your healthcare provider plan how to best control your diabetes.

The American Diabetes Association recommends keeping blood sugar levels in a range that is based on your age. Discuss these goals with your physician and diabetes educator.

Before meals:

- 70–130 mg/dL for adults

- 100–180 mg/dL for children under age six

- 90–180 mg/dL for children six to twelve years old

- 90–130 mg/dL for children thirteen to nineteen years old

At bedtime:

- Less than 180 mg/dL for adults

- 110–200 mg/dL for children under age six

- 100–180 mg/dL for children six to twelve years old

- 90–150 mg/dL for children thirteen to nineteen years old

Foot Care

Diabetes causes damage to the blood vessels and nerves. This can reduce your ability to feel injury to or pressure on the foot. You may not notice a foot injury until severe infection develops. Diabetes can also damage blood vessels. Small sores or breaks in the skin may progress to deeper skin ulcers. Amputation of the affected limb may be needed when these skin ulcers do not improve or become larger or deeper.

To prevent problems with your feet, you should:

- Stop smoking if you smoke.

- Improve control of your blood sugar.

- Get a foot exam by your healthcare provider at least twice a year and learn whether you have nerve damage.

- Check and care for your feet *every day*, especially if you already have known nerve or blood vessel damage or current foot problems.

- Make sure you are wearing the right kind of shoes.

Treating Low Blood Sugar

Hypoglycemia can develop quickly in people with diabetes. Symptoms typically appear when the blood sugar level falls below 70 mg/dL. If you have symptoms:

- Do a blood sugar check.

- If the level is low or you have symptoms of hypoglycemia, eat something with sugar: four ounces of fruit juice, three to four Lifesavers candies, or four ounces of regular soda. Overtreating a mild low blood sugar reaction can lead to problems with high blood sugar and difficult blood sugar control overall.

- Symptoms should go away within fifteen minutes. If the symptoms don't go away, repeat the sugar-containing food as above, and test the sugar level again. When your blood sugar is in a safer range (over 70 mg/dL), you may need to eat a snack with carbohydrates and protein, such as cheese and crackers or a glass of milk.

Ask your doctor if you need a glucagon injection kit to raise blood sugar quickly in an emergency.

Medications to Prevent Complications

Your doctor may prescribe medications to reduce your chances of developing eye disease, kidney disease, and other conditions that are more common in people with diabetes.

An angiotensin-converting enzyme (ACE) inhibitor (or angiotensin receptor blocker, or ARB) is often recommended as the first choice for those with high blood pressure and those with signs of kidney disease. ACE inhibitors include:

- benazepril (Lotensin®);
- captopril (Capoten®);
- enalapril (Vasotec®);
- quinapril (Accupril®);
- lisinopril (Prinivil®, Zestril®);
- perindopril (Aceon®);
- ramipril (Altace®).

Statin drugs are usually the first choice to treat an abnormal cholesterol level. Aim for an low-density lipoprotein (LDL) cholesterol level of less than 100 mg/dL (less than 70 mg/dL in high-risk patients).

Aspirin to prevent heart disease is most often recommended for people with diabetes who:

- are older than forty;
- have a personal or family history of heart problems;
- have high blood pressure or high cholesterol;
- smoke.

Outlook (Prognosis)

Diabetes is a lifelong disease for which there is not yet a cure. However, the outcome for people with diabetes varies. Studies show that tight control of blood glucose can prevent or delay complications to the eyes, kidneys, nervous system, and heart in type 1 diabetes. However, complications may occur even in those with good diabetes control.

Possible Complications

After many years, diabetes can lead to serious problems with your eyes, kidneys, nerves, heart, blood vessels, and other areas in your body.

If you have diabetes, your risk of a heart attack is the same as someone who has already had a heart attack. Both women and men with diabetes are at risk. You may not even have the typical signs of a heart attack.

In general, complications include:

- cataracts;
- damage to the blood vessels that supply the legs and feet (peripheral vascular disease);
- foot sores or ulcers, which can result in amputation;
- glaucoma;
- high blood pressure;
- high cholesterol;
- kidney disease and kidney failure (diabetic nephropathy);
- macular edema;
- nerve damage, which causes pain and numbness in the feet, as well as a number of other problems with the stomach and intestines, heart, and other body organs (diabetic neuropathy);
- stroke;
- worsening of eyesight or blindness due to diabetic retinopathy (eye disease).

Other complications include:

- erection problems;
- infections of the skin, female genital tract, and urinary tract.

When to Contact a Medical Professional

If you are newly diagnosed with type 1 diabetes, you should probably have medical follow-up weekly until you have good control of blood glucose. Your healthcare provider will review the results of home glucose monitoring and urine testing. The provider will also look at your diary of meals, snacks, and insulin injections.

As the disease becomes more stable, follow-up visits will be less often. Visiting your healthcare provider is very important for monitoring possible long-term complications from diabetes.

Call 911 if you have:

- chest pain or pressure, shortness of breath, or other signs of angina;

- loss of consciousness;

- seizures.

Call your healthcare provider or go to the emergency room if you have these symptoms of ketoacidosis:

- Confusion

- Deep and rapid breathing

- Extreme thirst and drinking and frequent urination

- High glucose or ketone levels in your urine

- Severe abdominal pain

- Severe nausea and vomiting, and inability to drink liquids or eat

- Shortness of breath

- Sweet-smelling breath

- Very high blood sugar

Also call your doctor if you have:

- blood sugar levels that are running higher than the goals you and your doctor have set;

- numbness, tingling, pain in your feet or legs;

- problems with your eyesight;

- sores or infections on your feet;

- symptoms that your blood sugar is getting too low (weakness or fatigue, trembling, sweating, feeling irritable, unclear thinking, fast heartbeat, double or blurry vision, uneasy feeling);

- symptoms that your blood sugar is going too high (being very thirsty, having blurry vision, having dry skin, feeling weak or tired, needing to urinate a lot);

- blood sugar readings below 70 mg/dL.

You can treat early signs of hypoglycemia at home by eating sugar or candy or taking glucose tablets. If your signs of hypoglycemia continue or your blood glucose levels stay below 60 mg/dL, go to the emergency room.

Prevention

Currently, there is no way to prevent type 1 diabetes. There is no effective screening test for type 1 diabetes in people with no symptoms.

To prevent complications of diabetes, visit your healthcare provider or diabetes educator at least four times a year. Talk about any problems you are having.

Stay up-to-date with all of your vaccinations and get a flu shot every year in the fall.

References

Alemzadeh R, Wyatt DT. Diabetes Mellitus. In: Kliegman RM, ed. Kliegman: *Nelson Textbook of Pediatrics. 18th ed*. Philadelphia, Pa: Saunders; 2007:chap 590.

American Diabetes Association. Diagnosis and classification of diabetes mellitus. *Diabetes Care*. 2010. 33 Suppl 1:S62–S69.

American Diabetes Association. Standards of medical care in diabetes—2010. *Diabetes Care*. 2010. 33 Suppl 1:S11–S61.

Eisenbarth GS, Polonsky KS, Buse JB. Type 1 diabetes mellitus. In: Kronenberg HM, Melmed S, Polonsky KS, Larsen PR. Kronenberg: *Williams Textbook of Endocrinology. 11th ed*. Philadelphia, Pa: Saunders Elsevier;2008:chap 31.

Chapter 5

Insulin Resistance and Prediabetes

What Is Insulin Resistance?

Insulin resistance is a condition in which the body produces insulin but does not use it properly. Insulin, a hormone made by the pancreas, helps the body use glucose for energy. Glucose is a form of sugar that is the body's main source of energy.

The body's digestive system breaks food down into glucose, which then travels in the bloodstream to cells throughout the body. Glucose in the blood is called blood glucose, also known as blood sugar. As the blood glucose level rises after a meal, the pancreas releases insulin to help cells take in and use the glucose.

When people are insulin resistant, their muscle, fat, and liver cells do not respond properly to insulin. As a result, their bodies need more insulin to help glucose enter cells. The pancreas tries to keep up with this increased demand for insulin by producing more. Eventually, the pancreas fails to keep up with the body's need for insulin. Excess glucose builds up in the bloodstream, setting the stage for diabetes. Many people with insulin resistance have high levels of both glucose and insulin circulating in their blood at the same time.

Insulin resistance increases the chance of developing type 2 diabetes and heart disease. Learning about insulin resistance is the first

Excerpted from "Insulin Resistance and Pre-Diabetes," National Institute of Diabetes and Digestive and Kidney Diseases, National Institutes of Health, NIH Publication No. 09-4893, October 2008.

step toward making lifestyle changes that can help prevent diabetes and other health problems.

What Causes Insulin Resistance?

Scientists have identified specific genes that make people more likely to develop insulin resistance and diabetes. Excess weight and lack of physical activity also contribute to insulin resistance.

Many people with insulin resistance and high blood glucose have other conditions that increase the risk of developing type 2 diabetes and damage to the heart and blood vessels, also called cardiovascular disease. These conditions include having excess weight around the waist, high blood pressure, and abnormal levels of cholesterol and triglycerides in the blood. Having several of these problems is called metabolic syndrome or insulin resistance syndrome, formerly called syndrome X.

Metabolic Syndrome

Metabolic syndrome is defined as the presence of any three of the following conditions:

- Waist measurement of forty inches or more for men and thirty-five inches or more for women

- Triglyceride levels of 150 milligrams per deciliter (mg/dL) or above, or taking medication for elevated triglyceride levels

- High-density lipoprotein (HDL), or "good," cholesterol level below 40 mg/dL for men and below 50 mg/dL for women, or taking medication for low HDL levels

- Blood pressure levels of 130/85 or above, or taking medication for elevated blood pressure levels

- Fasting blood glucose levels of 100 mg/dL or above, or taking medication for elevated blood glucose levels

What Is Pre-Diabetes?

Pre-diabetes is a condition in which blood glucose levels are higher than normal but not high enough for a diagnosis of diabetes. This condition is sometimes called impaired fasting glucose (IFG) or impaired glucose tolerance (IGT), depending on the test used to diagnose it. The U.S. Department of Health and Human Services estimates that about one in four U.S. adults aged twenty years or older—or fifty-seven million people—had pre-diabetes in 2007.

People with pre-diabetes are at increased risk of developing type 2 diabetes, formerly called adult-onset diabetes or non-insulin-dependent diabetes. Type 2 diabetes is sometimes defined as the form of diabetes that develops when the body does not respond properly to insulin, as opposed to type 1 diabetes, in which the pancreas makes little or no insulin.

Studies have shown that most people with pre-diabetes develop type 2 diabetes within ten years, unless they lose 5 to 7 percent of their body weight—about ten to fifteen pounds for someone who weighs two hundred pounds—by making changes in their diet and level of physical activity. People with pre-diabetes also are at increased risk of developing cardiovascular disease.

What Are the Symptoms of Insulin Resistance and Pre-Diabetes?

Insulin resistance and pre-diabetes usually have no symptoms. People may have one or both conditions for several years without noticing anything. People with a severe form of insulin resistance may have dark patches of skin, usually on the back of the neck. Sometimes people have a dark ring around their neck. Other possible sites for dark patches include elbows, knees, knuckles, and armpits. This condition is called acanthosis nigricans.

How Are Insulin Resistance and Pre-Diabetes Diagnosed?

Healthcare providers use blood tests to determine whether a person has pre-diabetes but do not usually test for insulin resistance. Insulin resistance can be assessed by measuring the level of insulin in the blood. However, the test that most accurately measures insulin resistance, called the euglycemic clamp, is too costly and complicated to be used in most doctors' offices. The clamp is a research tool used by scientists to learn more about glucose metabolism. If tests indicate pre-diabetes or metabolic syndrome, insulin resistance most likely is present.

Diabetes and pre-diabetes can be detected with one of the following tests.

Fasting glucose test. This test measures blood glucose in people who have not eaten anything for at least eight hours. This test is most reliable when done in the morning. Fasting glucose levels of 100 to 125 mg/dL are above normal but not high enough to be called diabetes. This condition is called pre-diabetes or IFG. People with IFG often have had insulin resistance for some time. They are much more likely to develop diabetes than people with normal blood glucose levels.

Glucose tolerance test. This test measures blood glucose after people fast for at least eight hours, and two hours after they drink a sweet liquid provided by a doctor or laboratory. A blood glucose level between 140 and 199 mg/dL means glucose tolerance is not normal but is not high enough for a diagnosis of diabetes. This form of pre-diabetes is called IGT and, like IFG, it points toward a history of insulin resistance and a risk for developing diabetes.

People whose test results indicate they have pre-diabetes should have their blood glucose levels checked again in one to two years.

Risk Factors for Pre-Diabetes and Type 2 Diabetes

The American Diabetes Association recommends that testing to detect pre-diabetes and type 2 diabetes be considered in adults without symptoms who are overweight or obese and have one or more additional risk factors for diabetes. In those without these risk factors, testing should begin at age forty-five.

Risk factors for pre-diabetes and diabetes—in addition to being overweight or obese or being age forty-five or older—include the following:

• Being physically inactive

• Having a parent or sibling with diabetes

• Having a family background that is African American, Alaska Native, American Indian, Asian American, Hispanic/Latino, or Pacific Islander

• Giving birth to a baby weighing more than nine pounds or being diagnosed with gestational diabetes—diabetes first found during pregnancy

• Having high blood pressure—140/90 or above—or being treated for high blood pressure

• Having an HDL, or "good," cholesterol level below 35 mg/dL or a triglyceride level above 250 mg/dL

• Having polycystic ovary syndrome, also called PCOS

• Having impaired fasting glucose (IFG) or impaired glucose tolerance (IGT) on previous testing

- Having other conditions associated with insulin resistance, such as severe obesity or acanthosis nigricans

- Having a history of cardiovascular disease

If test results are normal, testing should be repeated at least every three years. Healthcare providers may recommend more frequent testing depending on initial results and risk status.

Can Insulin Resistance and Pre-Diabetes Be Reversed?

Yes. Physical activity and weight loss help the body respond better to insulin. By losing weight and being more physically active, people with insulin resistance or pre-diabetes may avoid developing type 2 diabetes.

The Diabetes Prevention Program (DPP) and other large studies have shown that people with pre-diabetes can often prevent or delay diabetes if they lose a modest amount of weight by cutting fat and calorie intake and increasing physical activity—for example, walking thirty minutes a day five days a week. Losing just 5 to 7 percent of body weight prevents or delays diabetes by nearly 60 percent. In the DPP, people aged sixty or older who made lifestyle changes lowered their chances of developing diabetes by 70 percent. Many participants in the lifestyle intervention group returned to normal blood glucose levels and lowered their risk for developing heart disease and other problems associated with diabetes. The DPP also showed that the diabetes drug metformin reduced the risk of developing diabetes by 31 percent.

People with insulin resistance or pre-diabetes can help their body use insulin normally by being physically active, making wise food choices, and reaching and maintaining a healthy weight. Physical activity helps muscle cells use blood glucose for energy by making the cells more sensitive to insulin.

Body Mass Index (BMI)

BMI is a measurement of body weight relative to height. Adults aged twenty or older can use the BMI table below to find out whether they are normal weight, overweight, obese, or extremely obese. To use the table, follow these steps:

- Find the person's height in the left-hand column.

- Move across the row to the number closest to that person's weight.

41

- Check the number at the top of that column.

The number at the top of the column is the person's BMI. The words above the BMI number indicate whether the person is normal weight, overweight, obese, or extremely obese. People who are overweight, obese, or extremely obese should consider talking with a doctor about ways to lose weight to reduce the risk of diabetes.

The BMI table has certain limitations. It may overestimate body fat in athletes and others who have a muscular build and underestimate body fat in older adults and others who have lost muscle. BMI for children and teens must be determined based on age and sex in addition to height and weight. Information about BMI in children and teens, including a BMI calculator, is available from the Centers for Disease Control and Prevention (CDC).

Can Medicines Help Reverse Insulin Resistance or Pre-Diabetes?

Clinical trials have shown that people at high risk for developing diabetes can be given treatments that delay or prevent onset of diabetes. The first therapy should always be an intensive lifestyle modification program because weight loss and physical activity are much more effective than any medication at reducing diabetes risk.

Several drugs have been shown to reduce diabetes risk to varying degrees. No drug is approved by the U.S. Food and Drug Administration to treat insulin resistance or pre-diabetes or to prevent type 2 diabetes. The American Diabetes Association recommends that metformin is the only drug that should be considered for use in diabetes prevention. Other drugs that have delayed diabetes have side effects or haven't shown long-lasting benefit. Metformin use was recommended only for very high risk individuals who have both forms of pre-diabetes (IGT and IFG), have a BMI of at least 35, and are younger than age sixty. In the DPP, metformin was shown to be most effective in younger, heavier patients.

Hope Through Research

Researchers continue to follow DPP participants to learn about the long-term effects of the study. Other research sponsored by the National Institutes of Health builds on the findings from the DPP, including research focusing on lowering diabetes risk in children. Once considered an adult disease, type 2 diabetes is becoming more common in children, and researchers are seeking ways to reverse this trend.

Table 5.1. Body Mass Index

	Normal						Overweight					Obese										Extreme Obesity														
BMI	19	20	21	22	23	24	25	26	27	28	29	30	31	32	33	34	35	36	37	38	39	40	41	42	43	44	45	46	47	48	49	50	51	52	53	54
Height (inches)												Body Weight (pounds)																								
58	91	96	100	105	110	115	119	124	129	134	138	143	148	153	158	162	167	172	177	181	186	191	196	201	205	210	215	220	224	229	234	239	244	248	253	258
59	94	99	104	109	114	119	124	128	133	138	143	148	153	158	163	168	173	178	183	188	193	198	203	208	212	217	222	227	232	237	242	247	252	257	262	267
60	97	102	107	112	118	123	128	133	138	143	148	153	158	163	168	174	179	184	189	194	199	204	209	215	220	225	230	235	240	245	250	255	261	266	271	276
61	100	106	111	116	122	127	132	137	143	148	153	158	164	169	174	180	185	190	195	201	206	211	217	222	227	232	238	243	248	254	259	264	269	275	280	285
62	104	109	115	120	126	131	136	142	147	153	158	164	169	175	180	186	191	196	202	207	213	218	224	229	235	240	246	251	256	262	267	273	278	284	289	295
63	107	113	118	124	130	135	141	146	152	158	163	169	175	180	186	191	197	203	208	214	220	225	231	237	242	248	254	259	265	270	278	282	287	293	299	304
64	110	116	122	128	134	140	145	151	157	163	169	174	180	186	192	197	204	209	215	221	227	232	238	244	250	256	262	267	273	279	285	291	296	302	308	314
65	114	120	126	132	138	144	150	156	162	168	174	180	186	192	198	204	210	216	222	228	234	240	246	252	258	264	270	276	282	288	294	300	306	312	318	324
66	118	124	130	136	142	148	155	161	167	173	179	186	192	198	204	210	216	223	229	235	241	247	253	260	266	272	278	284	291	297	303	309	315	322	328	334
67	121	127	134	140	146	153	159	166	172	178	185	191	198	204	211	217	223	230	236	242	249	255	261	268	274	280	287	293	299	306	312	319	325	331	338	344
68	125	131	138	144	151	158	164	171	177	184	190	197	203	210	216	223	230	236	243	249	256	262	269	276	282	289	295	302	308	315	322	328	335	341	348	354
69	128	135	142	149	155	162	169	176	182	189	196	203	209	216	223	230	236	243	250	257	263	270	277	284	291	297	304	311	318	324	331	338	345	351	358	365
70	132	139	146	153	160	167	174	181	188	195	202	209	216	222	229	236	243	250	257	264	271	278	285	292	299	306	313	320	327	334	341	348	355	362	369	376
71	136	143	150	157	165	172	179	186	193	200	208	215	222	229	236	243	250	257	265	272	279	286	293	301	308	315	322	329	338	343	351	358	365	372	379	386
72	140	147	154	162	169	177	184	191	199	206	213	221	228	235	242	250	258	265	272	279	287	294	302	309	316	324	331	338	346	353	361	368	375	383	390	397
73	144	151	159	166	174	182	189	197	204	212	219	227	235	242	250	257	265	272	280	288	295	302	310	318	325	333	340	348	355	363	371	378	386	393	401	408
74	148	155	163	171	179	186	194	202	210	218	225	233	241	249	256	264	272	280	287	295	303	311	319	326	334	342	350	358	365	373	381	389	396	404	412	420
75	152	160	168	176	184	192	200	208	216	224	232	240	248	256	264	272	279	287	295	303	311	319	327	335	343	351	359	367	375	383	391	399	407	415	423	431
76	156	164	172	180	189	197	205	213	221	230	238	246	254	263	271	279	287	295	304	312	320	328	336	344	353	361	369	377	385	394	402	410	418	426	435	443

Source: Adapted from *Clinical Guidelines on the Identification, Evaluation, and Treatment of Overweight and Obesity in Adults: The Evidence Report,* National Institutes of Health, 1998.

The National Institute of Diabetes and Digestive and Kidney Diseases (NIDDK) sponsors the HEALTHY study, which is part of a broad research initiative called STOPP T2D (Studies to Treat or Prevent Pediatric Type 2 Diabetes). The study seeks to improve the treatment and prevention of type 2 diabetes in youth, exploring the roles of nutrition, physical activity, and behavior change in lowering risk for type 2 diabetes in children. The participating forty-two middle schools are randomly assigned to a program group implementing changes or a comparison group. Students in the program group have healthier choices from the cafeteria and vending machines; longer, more intense periods of physical activity; and activities and awareness campaigns that promote long-term healthy behaviors.

The NIDDK also sponsors the TODAY (Treatment Options for Type 2 Diabetes in Adolescents and Youth) study, which focuses on treatment of type 2 diabetes in children and teens at thirteen sites. The TODAY study will evaluate the effects of three treatment approaches on control of blood glucose levels, insulin production, insulin resistance, and other outcomes. Each approach involves medication, but one of the three treatment groups will also receive an intensive lifestyle intervention to help the participants lose weight and increase physical fitness.

Participants in clinical trials can play a more active role in their own healthcare, gain access to new research treatments before they are widely available, and help others by contributing to medical research.

Sources

Grundy SM, et al. Diagnosis and management of the metabolic syndrome: an American Heart Association/National Heart, Lung, and Blood Institute scientific statement. *Circulation*. 2005;112:2735–52.

Chapter 6

Type 2 Diabetes

Type 2 diabetes is a chronic (lifelong) disease marked by high levels of sugar (glucose) in the blood. Type 2 diabetes is the most common form of diabetes.

Causes

Diabetes is caused by a problem in the way your body makes or uses insulin. Insulin is needed to move blood sugar (glucose) into cells, where it is stored and later used for energy.

When you have type 2 diabetes, the body does not respond correctly to insulin. This is called insulin resistance. Insulin resistance means that fat, liver, and muscle cells do not respond normally to insulin. As a result blood sugar does not get into cells to be stored for energy.

When sugar cannot enter cells, abnormally high levels of sugar build up in the blood. This is called hyperglycemia. High levels of blood sugar often trigger the pancreas to produce more and more insulin, but it is not enough to keep up with the body's demand.

People who are overweight are more likely to have insulin resistance, because fat interferes with the body's ability to use insulin.

Type 2 diabetes usually occurs gradually. Most people with the disease are overweight at the time of diagnosis. However, type 2 diabetes can also develop in those who are thin, especially the elderly.

Family history and genetics play a large role in type 2 diabetes. Low activity level, poor diet, and excess body weight (especially around the waist) significantly increase your risk for type 2 diabetes.

Other risk factors include:

- age greater than forty-five years;
- high-density lipoprotein (HDL) cholesterol of less than 35 mg/dL or triglyceride level of greater than 250 mg/dL;
- high blood pressure;
- history of gestational diabetes;
- polycystic ovarian syndrome;
- previously identified impaired glucose tolerance by your doctor;
- race/ethnicity (African Americans, Hispanic Americans, and Native Americans all have high rates of diabetes).

Symptoms

Often, people with type 2 diabetes have no symptoms at all. If you do have symptoms, they may include:

- blurred vision;
- erectile dysfunction;
- fatigue;
- frequent or slow-healing infections;
- increased appetite;
- increased thirst;
- increased urination.

Exams and Tests

Type 2 diabetes is diagnosed with the following blood tests:

- **Fasting blood glucose level:** Diabetes is diagnosed if higher than 126 mg/dL on two occasions.
- **Hemoglobin A1c test:** This test has been used in the past to help patients monitor how well they are controlling their blood glucose levels. In 2010, the American Diabetes Association recommended that the test be used as another option for diagnosing diabetes and identifying pre-diabetes. Levels indicate:

- Normal: Less than 5.7 percent;

- Pre-diabetes: Between 5.7 and 6.4 percent;

- Diabetes: 6.5 percent or higher.

- **Oral glucose tolerance test:** Diabetes is diagnosed if glucose level is higher than 200 mg/dL after two hours.

- **Random (non-fasting) blood glucose level:** Diabetes is suspected if higher than 200 mg/dL and accompanied by the classic symptoms of increased thirst, urination, and fatigue (this test must be confirmed with a fasting blood glucose test).

You should see your healthcare provider every three months. At these visits, you can expect your healthcare provider to:

- check your blood pressure;

- check the skin and bones on your feet and legs;

- check the sensation in your feet;

- examine the back part of the eye with a special lighted instrument called an ophthalmoscope.

The following tests will help you and your doctor monitor your diabetes and prevent complications:

- Have your blood pressure checked at least every year (blood pressure goals should be 130/80 mm/Hg or lower).

- Have your glycosylated hemoglobin (HbA1c) checked every six months if your diabetes is well controlled; otherwise every three months.

- Have your cholesterol and triglyceride levels checked yearly (aim for low-density lipoprotein [LDL] levels below 70–100 mg/dL).

- Get yearly tests to make sure your kidneys are working well (microalbuminuria and serum creatinine).

- Visit your ophthalmologist at least once a year, or more often if you have signs of diabetic retinopathy.

- See the dentist every six months for a thorough dental cleaning and exam. Make sure your dentist and hygienist know that you have diabetes.

Treatment

The immediate goal of treatment is to lower high blood glucose levels. The long-term goals of treatment are to prevent diabetes-related complications.

The primary treatment for type 2 diabetes is exercise and diet.

Learn These Skills

You should learn basic diabetes management skills. They will help prevent complications and the need for medical care. These skills include:

- how to test and record your blood glucose;

- what to eat and when;

- how to take medications, if needed;

- how to recognize and treat low and high blood sugar;

- how to handle sick days;

- where to buy diabetes supplies and how to store them.

It may take several months to learn the basic skills. Always continue to educate yourself about the disease and its complications. Learn how to control and live with diabetes. Over time, stay current on new research and treatments.

Self-Testing

Self-testing refers to being able to check your blood sugar at home yourself. It is also called self-monitoring of blood glucose (SMBG). Regular self-testing of your blood sugar tells you and your healthcare provider how well your diet, exercise, and diabetes medications are working.

A device called a glucometer can provide an exact blood sugar reading. There are different types of devices. Usually, you prick your finger with a small needle called a lancet. This gives you a tiny drop of blood. You place the blood on a test strip and put the strip into the device. Results are available in thirty to forty-five seconds.

A healthcare provider or diabetes educator will help set up an at-home testing schedule for you. Your doctor will help you set your blood sugar goals:

- Most people with type 2 diabetes only need to check their blood sugar once or twice a day.

- If your blood sugar levels are under control, you may only need to check them a few times a week.

- Tests may be done when you wake up, before meals, and at bedtime.

- More frequent testing may be needed when you are sick or under stress.

The results of the test can be used to adjust meals, activity, or medications to keep your blood sugar levels in an appropriate range. Testing can identify high and low blood sugar levels before serious problems develop.

Keep a record for yourself and your healthcare provider. This will be a big help if you are having trouble managing your diabetes.

Diet and Weight Control

People with type 2 diabetes should eat at about the same times each day and try to be consistent with the types of food they choose. This helps to prevent blood sugar from becoming extremely high or low. Meal planning includes choosing healthy foods, eating the right amount of food, and eating meals at the right time. You should work closely with your doctor, nurse, and registered dietitian to learn how much fat, protein, and carbohydrates you need in your diet. Your meal plans should fit your daily lifestyle and habits, and should try to include foods that you like.

Managing your weight and eating a well-balanced diet are important. Some people with type 2 diabetes can stop taking medications after losing weight (although they still have diabetes).

Bariatric (weight loss) surgery may be considered for very overweight patients who are not well managed with diet and medications.

Regular Physical Activity

Regular exercise is important for everyone, but especially if you have diabetes. Regular aerobic exercise lowers your blood sugar level without medication and helps burn excess calories and fat so you can manage your weight.

Exercise can help your overall health by improving blood flow and blood pressure. It decreases insulin resistance even without weight loss. Exercise also increases the body's energy level, lowers tension, and improves your ability to handle stress.

Consider the following when starting an exercise routine:

- Always check with your healthcare provider before starting an exercise program.

- Ask your healthcare provider whether you have the right footwear.

- Choose an enjoyable physical activity that is appropriate for your current fitness level.

- Exercise every day, and at the same time of day, if possible.

- Monitor blood glucose levels at home before and after exercise.

- Carry food that contains a fast-acting carbohydrate in case blood glucose levels get too low during or after exercise.

- Wear a diabetes identification bracelet and carry a cell phone in case of emergency.

- Drink extra fluids that do not contain sugar before, during, and after exercise.

- You may need to modify your diet or medication if you exercise longer or more intensely, to keep blood glucose levels in the correct range.

Medications to Treat Diabetes

If diet and exercise do not help maintain normal or near-normal blood glucose levels, your doctor may prescribe medication. Since these drugs help lower your blood sugar levels in different ways, your doctor may have you take more than one. These drugs may also be given along with insulin, if needed.

Some of the most common types of medication are listed below. They are taken by mouth or injection:

- Alpha-glucosidase inhibitors (such as acarbose) decrease the absorption of carbohydrates from the digestive tract to lower after-meal glucose levels.

- Biguanides (metformin) tell the liver to produce less glucose and help muscle and fat cells and the liver absorb more glucose from the bloodstream. This lowers blood sugar levels.

- Injectable medications (including exenatide, mitiglinide, pramlintide, sitagliptin, and saxagliptin) can lower blood sugar.

- Meglitinides (including repaglinide and nateglinide) trigger the pancreas to make more insulin in response to the level of glucose in the blood.

- Sulfonylureas (like glimepiride, glyburide, and tolazamide) trigger the pancreas to make more insulin. They are taken by mouth.

- Thiazolidinediones (such as rosiglitazone and pioglitazone) help muscle and fat cells and the liver absorb more blood sugar when insulin is present. Rosiglitazone may increase the risk of heart problems. Talk to your doctor.

If you continue to have poor blood glucose control despite lifestyle changes and taking medicines by mouth, your doctor will prescribe insulin. Insulin may also be prescribed if you have had a bad reaction to other medicines. Insulin must be injected under the skin using a syringe or insulin pen device. It cannot be taken by mouth.

Insulin preparations differ in how fast they start to work and how long they work. Your healthcare provider will determine the appropriate type of insulin to use and will tell you what time of day to use it.

More than one type may be mixed together in an injection to achieve the best blood glucose control. Usually injections are needed one to four times a day. Your doctor or diabetes educator will show you how to give yourself an injection.

Some people with type 2 diabetes find they no longer need medication if they lose weight and increase activity. When they reach their ideal weight, their own insulin and a careful diet can control their blood glucose levels.

It is not known whether hypoglycemia medications taken by mouth are safe for use in pregnancy. Women who have type 2 diabetes and take these medications may be switched to insulin during pregnancy and while breastfeeding.

Medications to Prevent Complications

Since those with diabetes have a much higher chance of developing heart disease, kidney disease, and other medical problems, they may need to take certain medicines to treat these problems or prevent them from happening.

An angiotensin-converting enzyme (ACE) inhibitor (or angiotensin receptor blocker, or ARB) is often recommended:

- as the first choice medicine for treating high blood pressure in persons with diabetes;

- for those who have signs of early kidney disease.

ACE inhibitors include captopril (Capoten®), enalapril (Vasotec®), quinapril (Accupril®), benazepril (Lotensin®), ramipril (Altace®), perindopril (Aceon®), and lisinopril (Prinivil®, Zestril®).

Statin drugs are usually the first choice to treat an abnormal cholesterol level. Aim for LDL cholesterol level less than 100 mg/dL (less than 70 mg/dL in high-risk patients).

Aspirin to prevent heart disease is most often recommended for persons with diabetes who:

- are forty or older;
- have a history of heart problems;
- have a family history of heart disease;
- have high blood pressure or high cholesterol;
- smoke.

Foot Care

People with diabetes are more likely to have foot problems. Diabetes can damage nerves, which means you may not feel an injury to the foot until a large sore or infection develops. Diabetes can also damage blood vessels.

In addition, diabetes affects the body's immune system. This decreases the body's ability to fight infection. Small infections can quickly get worse and cause the death of skin and other tissues. Amputation may be needed.

To prevent injury to the feet, check and care for your feet every day.

Outlook (Prognosis)

The risk of long-term complications from diabetes can be reduced. If you control your blood glucose and blood pressure, you can reduce your risk of death, stroke, heart failure, and other complications. Reduction of HbA1c by even 1 percent can decrease your risk for complications by 25 percent.

Possible Complications

After many years, diabetes can lead to serious problems with your eyes, kidneys, nerves, heart, blood vessels, and other areas in your body.

If you have diabetes, your risk of a heart attack is the same as someone who has already had a heart attack. Both women and men with diabetes are at risk. You may not even have the typical signs of a heart attack.

In general, complications include:

- cataracts;
- damage to blood vessels that supply the legs and feet (peripheral vascular disease);
- diabetic retinopathy (eye disease);
- foot sores or ulcers, which can result in amputation;
- glaucoma;
- high blood pressure;
- high cholesterol;
- kidney disease and kidney failure (diabetic nephropathy);
- macular edema;
- nerve damage, which causes pain and numbness in the feet, as well as a number of other problems with the stomach and intestines, heart, and other body organs;
- stroke;
- worsening of eyesight or even blindness.

Other complications include:

- erection problems;
- infections of the skin, female genital tract, and urinary tract.

When to Contact a Medical Professional

Call 911 immediately if you have:

- chest pain or pressure;
- fainting or unconsciousness;
- seizure;
- shortness of breath.

These symptoms can quickly get worse and become emergency conditions (such as convulsions or hypoglycemic coma).

Call your doctor also if you have:

- numbness, tingling, pain in your feet or legs;

- problems with your eyesight;

- sores or infections on your feet;

- symptoms of high blood sugar (being very thirsty, having blurry vision, having dry skin, feeling weak or tired, needing to urinate a lot);

- symptoms of low blood sugar (weak or tired, trembling, sweating, feeling irritable, unclear thinking, fast heartbeat, double or blurry vision, feeling uneasy).

Prevention

Diabetes screening is recommended for:

- overweight children who have other risk factors for diabetes, starting at age ten and repeating every two years;

- overweight adults (BMI greater than 25) who have other risk factors;

- adults over forty-five every three years.

You can help prevent type 2 diabetes by keeping a healthy body weight and an active lifestyle.

To prevent complications of diabetes, visit your healthcare provider or diabetes educator at least four times a year. Talk about any problems you are having.

Stay up-to-date with all your vaccinations and get a flu shot every year.

To prevent diabetes-related foot problems, you should:

- Check and care for your feet *every day*, especially if you already have known nerve or blood vessel damage or current foot problems.

- Get a foot exam by your healthcare provider at least twice a year and learn whether you have nerve damage.

- Improve control of your blood sugar.

- Make sure you are wearing the right kind of shoes.

- Stop smoking if you smoke.

Alternative Names

Non-insulin-dependent diabetes; Diabetes—type 2; Adult-onset diabetes

References

American Diabetes Association. Diagnosis and classification of diabetes mellitus. *Diabetes Care*. 2010;33 Suppl 1:S62–S69.

American Diabetes Association. Standards of medical care in diabetes—2010. *Diabetes Care*. 2010;33 Suppl 1:S11–S61.

Eisenbarth GS, Polonsky KS, Buse JB. Type 1 Diabetes Mellitus. In: Kronenberg HM, Melmed S, Polonsky KS, Larsen PR. Kronenberg: *Williams Textbook of Endocrinology. 11th ed.* Philadelphia, Pa: Saunders Elsevier; 2008:chap 31.

U.S. Preventive Services Task Force. Screening for type 2 diabetes mellitus in adults: U.S. Preventive Services Task Force recommendation statement. *Ann Intern Med*. 2008 Jun 3;148(11):846–54.

In the clinic. Type 2 diabetes. *Ann Intern Med*. 2007;146:ITC-1-15.

Buchwald H, Estok R, Fahrbach K, Banel D, Jensen MD, Pories WJ, Bantle JP, Sledge I. Weight and type 2 diabetes after bariatric surgery: systematic review and meta-analysis. *Am J Med*. 2009 Mar;122(3):248–56.e5. Review. PubMed PMID: 19272486.

Chapter 7

Gestational Diabetes

What is gestational diabetes?

Gestational diabetes is diabetes that is found for the first time when a woman is pregnant. Out of every one hundred pregnant women in the United States, three to eight get gestational diabetes. Diabetes means that your blood glucose (also called blood sugar) is too high. Your body uses glucose for energy. But too much glucose in your blood can be harmful. When you are pregnant, too much glucose is not good for your baby.

What causes gestational diabetes?

Changing hormones and weight gain are part of a healthy pregnancy. But both changes make it hard for your body to keep up with its need for a hormone called insulin. When that happens, your body doesn't get the energy it needs from the food you eat.

What is my risk of gestational diabetes?

To learn your risk for gestational diabetes, check each item that applies to you. Talk with your doctor about your risk at your first prenatal visit:

Excerpted from "What I Need to Know about Gestational Diabetes," National Institute of Diabetes and Digestive ad Kidney Diseases, National Institutes of Health, NIH Publication No. 06-5129, April 2006. Revised by David A. Cooke, MD, FACP, February 2011.

- I have a parent, brother, or sister with diabetes.

- I am African American, American Indian, Asian American, Hispanic/Latino, or Pacific Islander.

- I am twenty-five years old or older.

- I am overweight.

- I have had gestational diabetes before, or I have given birth to at least one baby weighing more than nine pounds.

- I have been told that I have "pre-diabetes," a condition in which blood glucose levels are higher than normal, but not yet high enough for a diagnosis of diabetes. Other names for it are "impaired glucose tolerance" and "impaired fasting glucose."

If you checked any of these risk factors, ask your healthcare team about testing for gestational diabetes.

You are at high risk if you are very overweight, have had gestational diabetes before, have a strong family history of diabetes, or have glucose in your urine.

You are at average risk if you checked one or more of the risk factors.

You are at low risk if you did not check any of the risk factors.

When will I be checked for gestational diabetes?

Your doctor will decide when you need to be checked for diabetes depending on your risk factors:

- If you are at high risk, your blood glucose level may be checked at your first prenatal visit. If your test results are normal, you will be checked again sometime between weeks twenty-four and twenty-eight of your pregnancy.

- If you have an average risk for gestational diabetes, you will be tested sometime between weeks twenty-four and twenty-eight of pregnancy.

- If you are at low risk, your doctor may decide that you do not need to be checked.

How is gestational diabetes diagnosed?

Your healthcare team will check your blood glucose level. Depending on your risk and your test results, you may have one or more of the following tests.

Fasting blood glucose or random blood glucose test. Your doctor may check your blood glucose level using a test called a fasting blood glucose test. Before this test, your doctor will ask you to fast, which means having nothing to eat or drink except water for at least eight hours. Or your doctor may check your blood glucose at any time during the day. This is called a random blood glucose test.

These tests can find gestational diabetes in some women, but other tests are needed to be sure diabetes is not missed.

Screening glucose challenge test. For this test, you will drink a sugary beverage and have your blood glucose level checked an hour later. This test can be done at any time of the day. If the results are above normal, you may need further tests.

Oral glucose tolerance test. If you have this test, your healthcare provider will give you special instructions to follow. For at least three days before the test, you should eat normally. Then you will fast for at least eight hours before the test.

The healthcare team will check your blood glucose level before the test. Then you will drink a sugary beverage. The staff will check your blood glucose levels one hour, two hours, and three hours later. If your levels are above normal at least twice during the test, you have gestational diabetes.

Table 7.1. Above-Normal Results for the Oral Glucose Tolerance

Test	Result
Fasting	95 or higher
At 1 hour	180 or higher
At 2 hours	155 or higher
At 3 hours	140 or higher

Note: Some labs use other numbers for this test. These numbers are for a test using a drink with 100 grams of glucose.

How will gestational diabetes affect my baby?

Untreated or uncontrolled gestational diabetes can mean problems for your baby, including the following:

- Being born very large and with extra fat; this can make delivery difficult and more dangerous for your baby

- Low blood glucose right after birth

- Breathing problems

If you have gestational diabetes, your healthcare team may recommend some extra tests to check on your baby, such as the following:

- An ultrasound exam, to see how your baby is growing

- "Kick counts" to check your baby's activity (the time between the baby's movements) or special "stress" tests

Working closely with your healthcare team will help you give birth to a healthy baby.

Both you and your baby are at increased risk for type 2 diabetes for the rest of your lives.

How will gestational diabetes affect me?

Often, women with gestational diabetes have no symptoms. However, gestational diabetes may do the following things:

- Increase your risk of high blood pressure during pregnancy

- increase your risk of a large baby and the need for cesarean section at delivery

The good news is that your gestational diabetes will probably go away after your baby is born. However, you will be more likely to get type 2 diabetes later in your life. You may also get gestational diabetes again if you get pregnant again.

Some women wonder whether breastfeeding is okay after they have had gestational diabetes. Breastfeeding is recommended for most babies, including those whose mothers had gestational diabetes.

Gestational diabetes is serious, even if you have no symptoms. Taking care of yourself helps keep your baby healthy.

How is gestational diabetes treated?

Treating gestational diabetes means taking steps to keep your blood glucose levels in a target range. You will learn how to control your blood glucose using the following methods:

- A meal plan

- Physical activity

- Medication (if needed)

Meal plan. You will talk with a dietitian or a diabetes educator who will design a meal plan to help you choose foods that are healthy for you and your baby. Using a meal plan will help keep your blood glucose in your target range. The plan will provide guidelines on which foods to eat, how much to eat, and when to eat. Choices, amounts, and timing are all important in keeping your blood glucose levels in your target range.

You may be advised to do the following things:

- Limit sweets

- Eat three small meals and one to three snacks every day

- Be careful about when and how much carbohydrate-rich food you eat; your meal plan will tell you when to eat carbohydrates and how much to eat at each meal and snack

- Include fiber in your meals in the form of fruits, vegetables, and whole-grain crackers, cereals, and bread

Physical activity. Physical activity, such as walking and swimming, can help you reach your blood glucose targets. Talk with your healthcare team about the type of activity that is best for you. If you are already active, tell your healthcare team what you do.

Medication. Some women are unable to achieve good blood sugar control despite following a meal plan and increasing physical activity. In these cases, medication may be added to improve control.

Traditionally, insulin has been used, in addition to a meal plan and physical activity, to reach their blood glucose targets. This remains a common treatment choice, and can work well. If necessary, your healthcare team will show you how to give yourself insulin. Insulin is not harmful for your baby. It cannot move from your bloodstream to the baby's.

In recent years, studies have shown that a group of oral medications called sulfonylureas can also be used for gestational diabetes. While their use in gestational diabetes is relatively new, they have been used to treat type 2 diabetes for many years. The most commonly used drugs are glyburide, glipizide, and glimepiride. A number of studies have concluded that they are safe in pregnancy, and they work as well as insulin.

Metformin is another oral medication used for type 2 diabetes, and it is sometimes used to treat gestational diabetes. Some studies have concluded it is safe and effective in gestational diabetes. However, some experts argue against using it in pregnancy, since metformin can travel from the mother's blood to the baby. More research is necessary to confirm the medication is safe for babies.

How will I know whether my blood glucose levels are on target?

Your healthcare team may ask you to use a small device called a blood glucose meter to check your levels on your own. You will learn the following things:

- How to use the meter
- How to prick your finger to obtain a drop of blood
- What your target range is
- When to check your blood glucose

You may be asked to check your blood glucose at the following times:

- When you wake up
- Just before meals
- One or two hours after breakfast
- One or two hours after lunch
- One or two hours after dinner

Table 7.2 shows blood glucose targets for most women with gestational diabetes. Talk with your healthcare team about whether these targets are right for you.

Each time you check your blood glucose, write down the results in a record book. Take the book with you when you visit your healthcare team. If your results are often out of range, your healthcare team will suggest ways you can reach your targets.

Table 7.2. Blood Glucose Targets for Most Women with Gestational Diabetes

On awakening	not above 95
One hour after a meal	not above 140
Two hours after a meal	not above 120

Will I need to do other tests on my own?

Your healthcare team may teach you how to test for ketones in your morning urine or in your blood. High levels of ketones are a sign that your body is using your body fat for energy instead of the food you eat. Using fat for energy is not recommended during pregnancy. Ketones may be harmful for your baby.

If your ketone levels are high, your healthcare providers may suggest that you change the type or amount of food you eat. Or you may need to change your meal times or snack times.

After I have my baby, how can I find out whether my diabetes is gone?

You will probably have a blood glucose test six to twelve weeks after your baby is born to see whether you still have diabetes. For most women, gestational diabetes goes away after pregnancy. You are, however, at risk of having gestational diabetes during future pregnancies or getting type 2 diabetes later.

How can I prevent or delay getting type 2 diabetes later in life?

You can do a lot to prevent or delay type 2 diabetes:

- Reach and maintain a reasonable weight. Even if you stay above your ideal weight, losing 5 to 7 percent of your body weight is enough to make a big difference. For example, if you weigh two hundred pounds, losing ten to fourteen pounds can greatly reduce your chance of getting diabetes.

- Be physically active for thirty minutes most days. Walk, swim, exercise, or go dancing.

- Follow a healthy eating plan. Eat more grains, fruits, and vegetables. Cut down on fat and calories. A dietitian can help you design a meal plan.

Remind your healthcare team to check your blood glucose levels regularly. Women who have had gestational diabetes should continue to be tested for diabetes or pre-diabetes every one to two years. Diagnosing diabetes or pre-diabetes early can help prevent complications such as heart disease later.

Your child's risk for type 2 diabetes may be lower if you breastfeed your baby and if your child maintains a healthy weight.

Chapter 8

Other Types of Diabetes Mellitus

A number of other types of diabetes exist. A person may exhibit characteristics of more than one type. For example, in latent autoimmune diabetes in adults (LADA), also called type 1.5 diabetes or double diabetes, people show signs of both type 1 and type 2 diabetes.

Other types of diabetes include those caused by the following:

- Genetic defects of the beta cell—the part of the pancreas that makes insulin—such as maturity-onset diabetes of the young (MODY) or neonatal diabetes mellitus (NDM)

- Genetic defects in insulin action, resulting in the body's inability to control blood glucose levels, as seen in leprechaunism and the Rabson-Mendenhall syndrome

- Diseases of the pancreas or conditions that damage the pancreas, such as pancreatitis and cystic fibrosis

- Excess amounts of certain hormones resulting from some medical conditions—such as cortisol in Cushing syndrome—that work against the action of insulin

- Medications that reduce insulin action, such as glucocorticoids, or chemicals that destroy beta cells

- Infections, such as congenital rubella and cytomegalovirus

Excerpted from "Diabetes Overview," National Institute of Diabetes and Digestive and Kidney Diseases, National Institutes of Health, NIH Publication No. 09-3873, November 2008.

- Rare immune-mediated disorders, such as stiff-man syndrome, an autoimmune disease of the central nervous system

- Genetic syndromes associated with diabetes, such as Down syndrome and Prader-Willi syndrome

Latent Autoimmune Diabetes in Adults (LADA)

People who have LADA show signs of both type 1 and type 2 diabetes. Diagnosis usually occurs after age thirty. Researchers estimate that as many as 10 percent of people diagnosed with type 2 diabetes have LADA. Some experts believe that LADA is a slowly developing kind of type 1 diabetes because patients have antibodies against the insulin-producing beta cells of the pancreas.

Most people with LADA still produce their own insulin when first diagnosed, like those with type 2 diabetes. In the early stages of the disease, people with LADA do not require insulin injections. Instead, they control their blood glucose levels with meal planning, physical activity, and oral diabetes medications. However, several years after diagnosis, people with LADA must take insulin to control blood glucose levels. As LADA progresses, the beta cells of the pancreas may no longer make insulin because the body's immune system has attacked and destroyed them, as in type 1 diabetes.

Diabetes Caused by Genetic Defects of the Beta Cell

Genetic defects of the beta cell cause several forms of diabetes. For example, monogenic forms of diabetes result from mutations, or changes, in a single gene. In most cases of monogenic diabetes, the gene mutation is inherited. In the remaining cases, the gene mutation develops spontaneously. Most mutations in monogenic diabetes reduce the body's ability to produce insulin. Genetic testing can diagnose most forms of monogenic diabetes.

NDM and MODY are the two main forms of monogenic diabetes. NDM is a form of diabetes that occurs in the first six months of life. Infants with NDM do not produce enough insulin, leading to an increase in blood glucose. NDM can be mistaken for the much more common type 1 diabetes, but type 1 diabetes usually occurs after the first six months of life.

MODY usually first occurs during adolescence or early adulthood. However, MODY sometimes remains undiagnosed until later in life. A number of different gene mutations have been shown to cause MODY, all of which limit the pancreas's ability to produce insulin. This process leads to the high blood glucose levels characteristic of diabetes.

Diabetes Caused by Genetic Defects in Insulin Action

A number of types of diabetes result from genetic defects in insulin action. Changes to the insulin receptor may cause mild hyperglycemia—high blood glucose—or severe diabetes. Symptoms may include acanthosis nigricans, a skin condition characterized by darkened skin patches, and, in women, enlarged and cystic ovaries plus virilization and the development of masculine characteristics such as excess facial hair. Two syndromes in children, leprechaunism and the Rabson-Mendenhall syndrome, cause extreme insulin resistance.

Diabetes Caused by Diseases of the Pancreas

Injuries to the pancreas from trauma or disease can cause diabetes. This category includes pancreatitis, infection, and cancer of the pancreas. Cystic fibrosis and hemochromatosis can also damage the pancreas enough to cause diabetes.

Diabetes Caused by Endocrinopathies

Excess amounts of certain hormones that work against the action of insulin can cause diabetes. These hormones and their related conditions include growth hormone in acromegaly, cortisol in Cushing syndrome, glucagon in glucagonoma, and epinephrine in pheochromocytoma.

Diabetes Caused by Medications or Chemicals

A number of medications and chemicals can interfere with insulin secretion, leading to diabetes in people with insulin resistance. These medications and chemicals include pentamidine, nicotinic acid, glucocorticoids, thyroid hormone, phenytoin (Dilantin®), and Vacor®, a rat poison.

Diabetes Caused by Infections

Several infections are associated with the occurrence of diabetes, including congenital rubella, coxsackievirus B, cytomegalovirus, adenovirus, and mumps.

Rare Immune-Mediated Types of Diabetes

Some immune-mediated disorders are associated with diabetes. About one-third of people with stiff-man syndrome develop diabetes.

In other autoimmune diseases, such as systemic lupus erythematosus, patients may have anti-insulin receptor antibodies that cause diabetes by interfering with the binding of insulin to body tissues.

Other Genetic Syndromes Sometimes Associated with Diabetes

Many genetic syndromes are associated with diabetes. These conditions include Down syndrome, Klinefelter syndrome, Huntington chorea, porphyria, Prader-Willi syndrome, and diabetes insipidus.

Chapter 9

Diabetes Insipidus

What Is Diabetes Insipidus?

Diabetes insipidus, sometimes called water diabetes, is a rare endocrine (hormonal) condition. The symptoms of diabetes insipidus are an excessive thirst, passing large amounts of dilute urine and a general feeling of weakness.

Although similar in name to diabetes mellitus (sugar diabetes), diabetes insipidus is a completely unrelated condition.

What Causes Diabetes Insipidus?

Diabetes insipidus can be caused either by a defect in the hypothalamus or the pituitary gland in the brain (central diabetes insipidus) or a defect in the kidney (nephrogenic diabetes insipidus).

These defects cause problems with a hormone called anti-diuretic hormone (ADH, also known as vasopressin). ADH is secreted by the hypothalamus and pituitary gland and affects the functioning of the kidney, where it is responsible for reabsorption of water. For various reasons, this doesn't happen in diabetes insipidus and the body doesn't retain water but instead passes large volumes of very dilute urine. Someone with diabetes insipidus may pass up to 18 liters (38 pints) of urine a day compared with a healthy person's 1.5 liters (3 pints).

Central Diabetes Insipidus

Central diabetes insipidus is caused by not having enough ADH (anti-diuretic hormone).

When there isn't enough ADH to tell the kidneys to conserve water, large amounts of dilute urine are passed; the person has a pronounced thirst, will become dehydrated, and in advanced cases will develop low blood pressure.

What Causes Central Diabetes Insipidus?

Central diabetes insipidus is generally caused by damage to the hypothalamus and/or pituitary gland, both of which are located in the brain. This damage may be a result of:

- brain surgery;
- autoimmune destruction of the hypothalamus;
- brain tumor;
- injury to the head;
- infections such as encephalitis (inflammation of the brain) or meningitis (inflammation of the membrane surrounding the brain); or
- rare causes such as genetic disorders causing inherited disease.

People with this condition drink large amounts of fluid because of the extreme thirst that occurs in response to the water loss.

Nephrogenic Diabetes Insipidus

Nephrogenic diabetes insipidus is not caused by a lack of ADH but by the kidneys failing to respond to the message that ADH is telling them—which is to reabsorb water.

What Causes Nephrogenic Diabetes Insipidus?

Nephrogenic diabetes insipidus can be a result of chronic (long-lasting) kidney disease. It can also be due to a rare inherited disorder called congenital nephrogenic diabetes insipidus. This disorder more commonly affects men, but women can carry the gene and pass it to their children. Rarely, pregnant women can develop diabetes insipidus during their pregnancy—this is known as gestational diabetes insipidus.

Other causes include:

- low blood-potassium levels;
- high blood-calcium levels;
- sickle cell anemia; and
- medicines such as lithium (used to treat bipolar mood disorders) and tetracycline (an antibiotic).

As with central diabetes insipidus, excessive amounts of watery (dilute) urine are passed and excessive thirst causes a high intake of fluids. If, however, inadequate fluids are consumed the excessive amounts of dilute urine passed may cause dehydration.

In approximately 30 percent of cases of diabetes insipidus, no cause is found.

How Is Diabetes Insipidus Treated?

In very mild cases no treatment for diabetes insipidus may be necessary. However, in most cases of central diabetes insipidus a synthetic form of the missing ADH hormone (desmopressin) is given by tablet, injection, or by nasal spray. If treated appropriately, people with central diabetes insipidus can restore their urine output to normal and some even find that their condition improves spontaneously over time.

In cases of nephrogenic diabetes insipidus, medications are used to reduce the volume of urine passed, while the levels of salts (such as sodium) in the blood must be monitored closely. Dietary changes may be advised.

What You Should Do If You Have Diabetes Insipidus

It is important for people with diabetes insipidus to work with their doctors to accurately diagnose the severity of the condition and the underlying cause, and to decide on the form of treatment.

People with diabetes insipidus should wear some kind of medical identification, such as a MedicAlert bracelet.

Part Two

Identifying and Managing Diabetes

Chapter 10

Diabetes: Assessing Your Risk

Types of Diabetes

The three main kinds of diabetes are type 1, type 2, and gestational diabetes.

Type 1 Diabetes

Type 1 diabetes, formerly called juvenile diabetes or insulin-dependent diabetes, is usually first diagnosed in children, teenagers, or young adults. In this form of diabetes, the beta cells of the pancreas no longer make insulin because the body's immune system has attacked and destroyed them. Treatment for type 1 diabetes includes taking insulin shots or using an insulin pump, making wise food choices, exercising regularly, controlling blood pressure and cholesterol, and taking aspirin daily—for some.

Type 2 Diabetes

Type 2 diabetes, formerly called adult-onset or non-insulin-dependent diabetes, is the most common form of diabetes. People can develop type 2 diabetes at any age, even during childhood. This form of diabetes usually begins with insulin resistance, a condition in which

Excerpted from "Am I at Risk for Type 2 Diabetes?" National Institute of Diabetes and Digestive and Kidney Diseases, National Institutes of Health, NIH Publication No. 09-4805, November 2008.

fat, muscle, and liver cells do not use insulin properly. At first, the pancreas keeps up with the added demand by producing more insulin. In time, however, it loses the ability to secrete enough insulin in response to meals. People who are overweight and inactive are more likely to develop type 2 diabetes. Treatment includes taking diabetes medicines, making wise food choices, exercising regularly, controlling blood pressure and cholesterol, and taking aspirin daily—for some.

Gestational Diabetes

Some women develop gestational diabetes late in pregnancy. Although this form of diabetes usually goes away after the baby is born, a woman who has had gestational diabetes is more likely to develop type 2 diabetes later in life. Gestational diabetes is caused by the hormones of pregnancy or a shortage of insulin.

What Are the Signs and Symptoms of Type 2 Diabetes?

Nearly six million people in the United States have type 2 diabetes and do not know it. Many have no signs or symptoms. Symptoms can also be so mild that you might not even notice them. Some people have symptoms but do not suspect diabetes. Symptoms include the following:

* Increased thirst
* Increased hunger
* Fatigue
* Increased urination, especially at night
* Weight loss
* Blurred vision
* Sores that do not heal

Many people do not find out they have the disease until they have diabetes complications, such as blurry vision or heart trouble. If you find out early that you have diabetes, then you can get treatment to prevent damage to your body.

Should I Be Tested for Diabetes?

Anyone forty-five years old or older should consider getting tested for diabetes. If you are forty-five or older and overweight getting tested is strongly recommended. If you are younger than forty-five, overweight, and have one or more of the risk factors, you should consider getting tested. Ask your doctor for a fasting blood glucose test or an oral glucose tolerance test. Your doctor will tell you if you have normal blood glucose, pre-diabetes, or diabetes.

What Does Having Pre-Diabetes Mean?

Pre-diabetes means your blood glucose is higher than normal but lower than the diabetes range. In 2007, at least fifty-seven million American adults had pre-diabetes. Having pre-diabetes also means you are at risk for getting type 2 diabetes and heart disease. However, you can reduce the risk of getting diabetes and even return to normal blood glucose levels with modest weight loss through healthy eating and moderate physical activity. If you are told you have pre-diabetes, have your blood glucose checked again in one to two years.

Besides Being Older and Overweight, What Other Factors Increase My Risk for Type 2 Diabetes?

To find out your risk for type 2 diabetes, check each item that applies to you:

- I have a parent, brother, or sister with diabetes.

- My family background is Alaska Native, American Indian, African American, Hispanic/Latino, Asian American, or Pacific Islander.

- I have had gestational diabetes, or I gave birth to at least one baby weighing more than nine pounds.

- My blood pressure is 140/90 mm Hg or above, or I have been told that I have high blood pressure.

- My cholesterol levels are not normal. My high-density lipoprotein (HDL) cholesterol—"good" cholesterol—is below 35 mg/dL, or my triglyceride level is above 250 mg/dL.

- I am fairly inactive. I exercise fewer than three times a week.

- I have polycystic ovary syndrome, also called PCOS (women only).

- On previous testing, I had impaired fasting glucose (IFG) or impaired glucose tolerance (IGT).

- I have other clinical conditions associated with insulin resistance, such as a condition called acanthosis nigricans, characterized by a dark, velvety rash around my neck or armpits.

- I have a history of cardiovascular disease.

The more items you checked, the higher your risk.

How Can I Reduce My Risk?

You can do a lot to lower your chances of getting diabetes. Exercising regularly, reducing fat and calorie intake, and losing a little weight can help you reduce your risk of developing type 2 diabetes. Lowering blood pressure and cholesterol levels also helps you stay healthy.

If you are overweight, then take these steps:

- Reach and maintain a reasonable body weight.

- Make wise food choices most of the time.

- Be physically active every day.

If you are fairly inactive, then take this step:

- Be physically active every day.

If your blood pressure is too high, then take these steps:

- Reach and maintain a reasonable body weight.

- Make wise food choices most of the time.

- Reduce your intake of sodium and alcohol.

- Be physically active every day.

- Talk with your doctor about whether you need medicine to control your blood pressure.

If your cholesterol or triglyceride levels are too high, then take these steps:

- Make wise food choices most of the time.

- Be physically active every day.

- Talk with your doctor about whether you need medicine to control your cholesterol levels.

Making Changes to Lower My Risk

Making big changes in your life is hard, especially if you are faced with more than one change. Your doctor, a dietitian, or a counselor can help you make a plan. Consider making changes to lower your risk of diabetes.

Chapter 11

Metabolic Syndrome Increases Diabetes Risk

The metabolic syndrome, also known as metabolic syndrome X, was first described in 1988. It was recognized as a common clustering of clinical symptoms strongly associated with cardiovascular disease. Over the past two decades, there has been considerable research and study of the metabolic syndrome, and some of its elements are now better understood. Nevertheless, many unknowns remain, and experts continue to debate whether the metabolic syndrome is a distinct disease or a combination of several different disorders.

Defining the Metabolic Syndrome

Several definitions of the metabolic syndrome have been issued since it was first described. However, they were considered unsatisfactory because they required complex testing to make the diagnosis. The 2005 American Heart Association/National Heart, Blood, and Lung Institute definition is simpler and based on common tests, and it is now the most widely used standard. Under this definition, a person is said to have the metabolic syndrome if at least three of five elements are present:

- Waist circumference greater than forty inches in men or thirty-five inches in women; a smaller standard, thirty-five inches in men or thirty-one inches in women, is recommended for Asian Americans

"The Metabolic Syndrome," by David A. Cooke, M.D., ©2010. This article originally appeared in *When Your Doctor Says Diabetes*, edited by David A. Cooke, M.D. (Omnigraphics, 2010).

- Fasting triglycerides greater than 150 mg/dl (milligrams per deciliter); or on medication for elevated triglycerides

- High-density lipoprotein (HDL) cholesterol less than 40 mg/dl in men or 50 mg/dl in women; or on medication for low HDL cholesterol

- Systolic blood pressure greater than 130 mmHg (millimeters of mercury) or diastolic blood pressure greater than 85 mmHg; or on medication for elevated blood pressure

- Fasting glucose greater than 100 mg/dl; or on medication for elevated glucose

In the United States, it is estimated that about 25 percent of people aged twenty-five to fifty-nine meet this definition of the metabolic syndrome, and more than 40 percent of people older than sixty have the condition.

The fact that these particular elements are so frequently seen together has led many researchers to suspect they are all manifestations of a single underlying disease. However, this point remains very controversial, and research to date has not provided a clear answer.

Causes of the Metabolic Syndrome

Obesity is believed to play a critical role in the metabolic syndrome. Rates of obesity have been rapidly increasing in the United States in recent decades, and high rates of the metabolic syndrome are directly linked to obesity. While obesity is not required for a diagnosis of the metabolic syndrome, nearly all people with the metabolic syndrome are obese.

Excess fat is believed to be the root cause of the metabolic syndrome. Most people think of fat as inert tissue. In fact, fat tissue is very hormonally active and constitutes a major endocrine organ in the human body.

Fat can be stored in a number of locations in the body, including the trunk, hips, legs, and surrounding the abdominal organs. Its location in a given person is determined by genetic, hormonal, and gender-specific factors. Research suggests the location of a person's fat has more than cosmetic significance.

Not all fat seems to be the same. Fat deposits around the abdominal organs, known as visceral fat, behave somewhat differently than other fat. Abdominal obesity typically reflects increased amounts of visceral fat, which is why waist circumference is considered in the definition of metabolic syndrome

Visceral fat is located next to the abdominal organs, so hormones from visceral fat release into the blood and drain directly into the liver. The liver has a central role in metabolism, which amplifies the effects of the fat hormones. These interactions trigger a complex cascade of metabolic changes that lead to elevated levels of blood fats, low levels of HDL cholesterol, resistance to the effects of insulin, and increases in blood pressure.

These hormonal effects also appear to interact with the immune system. The metabolic syndrome promotes inflammation, which appears critical to the development of atherosclerosis. Markers of inflammation are frequently elevated in the blood of people with the metabolic syndrome, and high levels are known to predict cardiovascular disease. Additionally, active inflammation promotes blood clotting, which is often the inciting event in a heart attack or stroke.

Excess visceral fat appears to be necessary for the metabolic syndrome to develop, but it may not be enough by itself. It is believed that a number of genetic variations affect the risk for the metabolic syndrome and that the condition is at least partially hereditary. Not all obese individuals develop the metabolic syndrome, and some people show symptoms of the metabolic syndrome with much less obesity than others.

There are definite racial differences in the frequency of the metabolic syndrome, which cannot simply be explained by differences in rates of obesity. The metabolic syndrome is more common in white men than African American men, and people of Mexican, Native American, and Pacific Islander descent seem to have higher risk than whites. Many people of Asian descent develop the abnormalities of the metabolic syndrome with only mild obesity, which is why a smaller waist circumference is used in the clinical definition. Studies have also shown increased risk for the metabolic syndrome within individual families.

It has been speculated that the genes that predispose a person to the metabolic syndrome may reflect adaptations that were useful over most of human history. Some of these metabolic changes allow for more efficient metabolism when food is scarce and may reduce the risk of starvation. However, under conditions where food is plentiful, their effects are more harmful.

Dietary factors are also important. The metabolic syndrome is much more common among people who follow Western-style diets and is more common in cities than in rural areas.

Finally, lack of exercise also appears to be a major contributing factor. Poor physical fitness and little leisure-time physical activity are strongly correlated with the metabolic syndrome.

The Significance of the Metabolic Syndrome

The metabolic syndrome is critical in that it strongly predicts cardiovascular disease. People with the metabolic syndrome were 1.5 to 2.7 times more likely to have heart attacks or strokes in several large population studies. The risk of developing diabetes is approximately three times the average. Other studies have found the overall risk of death for people with the metabolic syndrome to be 37 to 60 percent higher than for people without it. Given how many people have the metabolic syndrome, this may translate into millions of deaths and billions of dollars in medical costs each year.

The metabolic syndrome is also strongly associated with fatty liver disease, polycystic ovary syndrome, gout, and sleep apnea. There should be a higher suspicion for these disorders if the metabolic syndrome is present.

Despite these associations and a workable definition, there is still disagreement over whether the metabolic syndrome is actually a disease versus a collection of different conditions. It was originally believed insulin resistance was the root cause of the metabolic syndrome, but it appears the metabolic syndrome can exist in its absence. Some experts argue that the metabolic syndrome is a single disorder with several different effects. Others argue it is not really a condition but simply the presence of several individual cardiac risk factors.

The data so far have not been conclusive. Some studies have found that people with the metabolic syndrome have a higher risk of cardiovascular disease than would be expected from their individual diseases. However, other studies have concluded that the cardiovascular risks seen with the metabolic syndrome are no higher than the risks of the individual diseases present. Indeed, several studies have found that making a diagnosis of the metabolic syndrome predicts risk no better than other assessment methods. Experts continue to disagree over whether the metabolic syndrome is more than the sum of its parts.

Treatment of the Metabolic Syndrome

Whether or not the metabolic syndrome has a special effect on risk, it is clear that people with the condition are in danger of developing cardiovascular disease. There is broad agreement that modifiable risk factors should be treated.

Weight loss is probably the most important and effective measure for treating the metabolic syndrome. Losing 7 to 10 percent of initial body weight over six to twelve months sharply improves the abnormalities of the metabolic syndrome. One study found a 41 percent reduction in the incidence of the metabolic syndrome, and another found a 58 percent reduction in the development of diabetes, with weight loss and lifestyle changes. Studies of patients who have undergone weight loss surgery have found dramatic reductions in the rate of the metabolic syndrome.

Increasing exercise is closely tied to weight loss and improvement in the metabolic syndrome. Increased exercise causes hormonal signaling that offsets many of the metabolic syndrome changes and improves insulin resistance. Most experts recommend physical activity of thirty to sixty minutes daily.

Dietary change is also important in achieving weight loss and treating the metabolic syndrome. It is controversial whether any particular diet is superior for treating the metabolic syndrome, but reducing caloric intake is clearly necessary. Many experts recommend a low-fat diet, with no more than 25 to 35 percent of daily calories from fat and no more than 7 percent from saturated fats. Increased intake of fruits, vegetables, and whole grains is also commonly recommended.

Treatment of hypertension is important. Blood pressure should be reduced to no more than 140/90 mmHg, and the American Diabetes Association recommends less than 130/80 mmHg for people with diabetes or kidney disease. If this cannot be achieved through weight loss, diet, and exercise, medication should be used to help reach these targets.

Improving cholesterol levels is a major goal. The recommendations for diabetics are low-density lipoprotein (LDL) cholesterol less than 100 mg/dl, triglycerides less than 150 mg/dl, and HDL cholesterol greater than 40 mg/dl in men and 50 mg/dl in women. Some authorities recommend the same cholesterol targets for people with the metabolic syndrome, even if they do not have diabetes. Statin medications for high cholesterol are known to reduce the risk of and have beneficial effects on heart disease. Fibrate medications, niacin, and fish oil may also be beneficial, but evidence supporting these is much weaker.

Tight blood sugar control for diabetics with the metabolic syndrome is strongly recommended. As with blood pressure and cholesterol, it is preferable to achieve this through lifestyle changes, but medication should be used if necessary.

It has been suggested that certain medications for diabetes, such as metformin, rosiglitazone, and pioglitazone, may be particularly useful in treating the metabolic syndrome. These medications reduce insulin resistance, and rosiglitazone and pioglitazone appear to reduce visceral fat deposits. However, their benefit over other medications for treating the metabolic syndrome has not been proven. In trials of these medications in people who have the metabolic syndrome without diabetes, the benefits have not been large enough to recommend routine use.

Addressing other cardiovascular risk factors is also important. Smoking cessation is critical, as smoking sharply increases cardiovascular risk when combined with the metabolic syndrome. Low-dose daily aspirin therapy may be recommended for some people given that it reduces risk of heart attack and stroke in high-risk individuals.

If the metabolic syndrome is truly a distinct disorder, it is possible a medication could be developed to treat the core abnormality. In theory, this could treat several individual diseases at the same time. However, researchers have not yet found a single root cause for the disorder.

Conclusion

The metabolic syndrome is very common in the United States, and rates are increasing. It carries a high risk for developing diabetes, heart attack, and stroke. The sheer number of people affected by the condition means many people suffer disability or death from its complications, and the costs of treating the disease are enormous.

Researchers continue to look for additional interventions to address the underlying causes of the disease. It is possible a drug for treating the metabolic syndrome as a whole will eventually be developed.

Until that time, weight loss, dietary change, and increased exercise are clearly effective treatments for the metabolic syndrome and can lead to a cure if they are maintained. Addressing modifiable risk factors such as high blood pressure, high cholesterol, elevated blood sugars, and smoking reduces the risk of bad outcomes.

Chapter 12

Tests Used to Diagnose Diabetes

Chapter Contents

Section 12.1

Blood Glucose Test

"Glucose Test—Blood," © 2010 A.D.A.M., Inc. Reprinted with permission.

A blood glucose test measures the amount of sugar (glucose) in a sample of your blood.

How the Test Is Performed

Blood is typically drawn from a vein, usually from the inside of the elbow or the back of the hand. The site is cleaned with germ-killing medicine (antiseptic). The healthcare provider wraps an elastic band around the upper arm to apply pressure to the area and make the vein swell with blood.

Next, the healthcare provider gently inserts a needle into the vein. The blood collects into an airtight vial or tube attached to the needle. The elastic band is removed from your arm.

Once the blood has been collected, the needle is removed, and the puncture site is covered to stop any bleeding.

In infants or young children, a sharp tool called a lancet may be used to puncture the skin and make it bleed. The blood collects into a small glass tube called a pipette, or onto a slide or test strip. A bandage may be placed over the area if there is any bleeding.

How to Prepare for the Test

The test may be done while you are fasting or at random.

If you are having a fasting glucose blood test, you should *not* eat or drink for six hours before the test.

A random glucose test can be done at any time of the day, but results depend on what you drink or eat before the test, as well as your activity.

How the Test Will Feel

When the needle is inserted to draw blood, some people feel moderate pain, while others feel only a prick or stinging sensation. Afterward, there may be some throbbing.

Why the Test Is Performed

Your doctor may order this test if you have signs of diabetes. It is also used to monitor patients who have the disease.

The carbohydrates you eat eventually end up as glucose in the blood. Glucose is a major source of energy for most cells of the body, including those in the brain.

Normal Results

Levels vary according to the laboratory, but in general up to 100 milligrams per deciliter (mg/dL) are considered normal.

Persons with levels between 100 and 126 mg/dL may have impaired fasting glucose or pre-diabetes. These levels are considered to be risk factors for type 2 diabetes and its complications.

Diabetes is typically diagnosed when fasting blood glucose levels are 126 mg/dL or higher.

Normal value ranges may vary slightly among different laboratories. Talk to your doctor about the meaning of your specific test results.

What Abnormal Results Mean

Greater than normal levels (hyperglycemia) may indicate:

- acromegaly (very rare);
- Cushing syndrome (rare);
- diabetes mellitus;
- impaired fasting glucose (also called "pre-diabetes");
- hyperthyroidism;
- pancreatic cancer;
- pancreatitis;
- pheochromocytoma (very rare);
- too little insulin;
- too much food.

Lower than normal levels (hypoglycemia) may indicate:

- hypopituitarism;
- hypothyroidism;
- insulinoma (very rare);

- too little food;
- too much insulin.

This test also may be performed for:
- acute adrenal crisis;
- Cushing syndrome caused by adrenal tumor;
- Cushing syndrome—exogenous;
- delirium;
- dementia;
- dementia due to metabolic causes;
- diabetic hyperglycemic hyperosmolar coma;
- diabetic ketoacidosis;
- diabetic nephropathy/sclerosis;
- ectopic Cushing syndrome;
- epilepsy;
- generalized tonic-clonic seizure;
- glucagonoma;
- islet of Langerhans tumor;
- multiple endocrine neoplasia (MEN) I;
- pituitary Cushing (Cushing disease);
- syphilis;
- syphilis—primary;
- syphilis—secondary;
- syphilis—tertiary;
- type 1 diabetes;
- type 2 diabetes;
- transient ischemic attack (TIA).

Risks

Veins and arteries vary in size from one patient to another and from one side of the body to the other. Obtaining a blood sample from some people may be more difficult than from others.

Other risks associated with having blood drawn are slight but may include:

- excessive bleeding;
- fainting or feeling light-headed;
- hematoma (blood accumulating under the skin);
- infection (a slight risk any time the skin is broken).

Considerations

Many forms of severe stress (for example, trauma, stroke, heart attack, and surgery) can temporarily increase blood glucose levels.

Drugs that can increase glucose measurements include the following:

- Atypical antipsychotics, especially olanzapine
- Corticosteroids
- Diazoxide
- Intravenous dextrose
- Diuretics
- Epinephrine
- Estrogens
- Glucagon
- Isoniazid
- Lithium
- Phenothiazines
- Phenytoin
- Salicylates
- Triamterene
- Tricyclic antidepressants

Drugs that can decrease glucose measurements include the following:

- Acetaminophen
- Alcohol
- Anabolic steroids

- Clofibrate

- Disopyramide

- Gemfibrozil

- Monoamine oxidase inhibitors (MAOIs)

- Pentamidine

- Sulfonylurea medications (such as glipizide, glyburide, and glimepiride)

Alternative Names

Random blood sugar; blood sugar level; fasting blood sugar

References

American Diabetes Association. Standards of medical care in diabetes—2009. *Diabetes Care*. 2009;32:S13–S61.

Inzucchi SE, Sherwin RS. Type 2 diabetes mellitus. In: Goldman L, Ausiello D, eds. *Cecil Medicine. 23rd ed*. Philadelphia, Pa: Saunders Elsevier; 2007:chap 248.

Section 12.2

Glucose Tolerance Test

The glucose tolerance test is a laboratory method to check how the body breaks down (metabolizes) blood sugar.

How the Test Is Performed

The most common glucose tolerance test is the oral glucose tolerance test (OGTT). You cannot eat or drink anything after midnight before the test. For the test, you will be asked to drink a liquid containing a certain amount of glucose. Your blood will be taken before you do this, and again every thirty to sixty minutes after you drink the solution. The test takes up to three hours.

The intravenous glucose tolerance test (IGTT) is rarely used. In this test, glucose is injected into your vein for three minutes. Blood insulin levels are measured before the injection, and again at one and three minutes after the injection.

How to Prepare for the Test

Make sure you eat normally for several days before the test.

Do not eat or drink anything for twelve hours before the test. You cannot eat during the test.

Ask your healthcare provider if you are using medications that can interfere with the test results.

How the Test Will Feel

Some people feel nauseated or sweaty after drinking the glucose for the test.

When the needle is inserted to draw blood, some people feel moderate pain. Others feel only a prick or stinging sensation. Afterward, there may be some throbbing.

Why the Test Is Performed

Glucose is the sugar the body uses for energy. Patients with untreated diabetes have high blood glucose levels. Glucose tolerance tests are one of the tools used to diagnose diabetes.

Above-normal blood glucose levels can be used to diagnose type 2 diabetes or high blood glucose during pregnancy (gestational diabetes). Insulin levels may also be measured. (Insulin is the hormone produced by the pancreas that moves glucose from the bloodstream into cells.)

The oral glucose tolerance test is used to screen pregnant women for gestational diabetes between twenty-four and twenty-eight weeks of pregnancy. It may also be used in cases where the disease is suspected, despite a normal fasting blood glucose level.

Normal Results

Normal blood values for a 75-gram oral glucose tolerance test used to check for type 2 diabetes:

- Fasting: 60–100 mg/dL
- One hour: less than 200 mg/dL
- Two hours: less than 140 mg/dL.

Between 140 and 200 mg/dL is considered impaired glucose tolerance (sometimes called "pre-diabetes"). This group is at increased risk for developing diabetes. Greater than 200 mg/dL is a sign of diabetes mellitus.

Normal blood values for a 50-gram oral glucose tolerance test used to screen for gestational diabetes:

- One hour: equal to or less than 140 mg/dL

Normal blood values for a 100-gram oral glucose tolerance test used to screen for gestational diabetes:

- Fasting: less than 95 mg/dL
- One hour: less than 180 mg/dL
- Two hours: less than 155 mg/dL
- Three hours: less than 140 mg/dL

Note: mg/dL = milligrams per deciliter

Normal value ranges may vary slightly among different laboratories. Talk to your doctor about the meaning of your specific test results.

What Abnormal Results Mean

Greater than normal levels of glucose may mean you have diabetes or gestational diabetes.

However, high glucose levels may be related to another medical problem (for example, Cushing syndrome).

Risks

Veins and arteries vary in size from one patient to another and from one side of the body to the other. Obtaining a blood sample from some people may be more difficult than from others.

Other risks associated with having blood drawn are slight but may include:

- excessive bleeding;

- fainting or feeling light-headed;

- hematoma (blood accumulating under the skin);

- infection (a slight risk any time the skin is broken).

Considerations

Factors that may affect the test results:

- acute stress (for example, from surgery or an infection);

- vigorous exercise.

Several drugs may cause glucose intolerance, including:

- beta-blockers (for example, propranolol);

- certain psychiatric medications;

- corticosteroids (for example, prednisone);

- oral contraceptives (birth control pills);

- thiazide diuretics (for example, hydrochlorothiazide).

Before having the test, let your healthcare provider know if you are taking any of these medications.

Alternative Names

Oral glucose tolerance test

References

American Diabetes Association. Standards of medical care in diabetes—2009. *Diabetes Care*. 2009;32:S13–S61.

Section 12.3

Urine Glucose Test

"Glucose Test—Urine," © 2010 A.D.A.M., Inc. Reprinted with permission.

The glucose urine test measures the amount of sugar (glucose) in a urine sample. The presence of glucose in the urine is called glycosuria or glucosuria.

How the Test Is Performed

A urine sample is needed.

Usually, the healthcare provider checks for glucose in the urine sample using a dipstick made with a color-sensitive pad. The pad contains chemicals that react with glucose. The color that the dipstick changes tells the provider how much glucose is in your urine.

How to Prepare for the Test

Your healthcare provider may tell you to stop taking drugs that may affect the results of the test.

Drugs that may increase urine glucose measurements include:

• aminosalicylic acid;

• cephalosporins;

• chloral hydrate;

• chloramphenicol;

• dextrothyroxine;

• diazoxide;

• diuretics (loop and thiazides);

- estrogens;
- ifosfamide;
- isoniazid;
- levodopa;
- lithium;
- nafcillin;
- nalidixic acid;
- nicotinic acid (large doses).

Other drugs also can cause false negative or false positive results, depending on the type of test strip used. Talk to your doctor.

How the Test Will Feel

The test involves only normal urination, and there is no discomfort.

Why the Test Is Performed

This test is most commonly used to screen for diabetes.

Normal Results

Glucose is not usually found in urine. If it is, further testing is needed.

What Abnormal Results Mean

Greater than normal levels of glucose may be a sign of:

- diabetes mellitus;
- glucose release from the kidneys into the urine (renal glycosuria);
- pregnancy.

Note: Results may vary slightly among different laboratories. Talk to your doctor about the meaning of your specific test results.

Risks

There are no risks.

Alternative Names

Urine sugar test; urine glucose test; glucosuria test

References

Bazari H. Approach to the patient with renal disease. In: Goldman L, Ausiello D, eds. *Cecil Medicine. 23rd ed*. Philadelphia, Pa: Saunders Elsevier; 2007:chap 115.

Chapter 13

The Diabetes Treatment Team

Healthcare providers should be your primary source for individualized information and advice about your diabetes. They can help you develop a treatment plan to manage the disease and prevent or, at least, minimize associated health complications.

"A joint effort—almost camaraderie—between you and your healthcare provider is often required to successfully manage type 2 diabetes," said Daniel W. Jones, M.D. and past president of the American Heart Association.

When working with your healthcare providers, it's important that you do your part. This includes:

- researching your family history of diabetes and associated risks and providing that information;

- adhering to the treatment plan they recommend including making lifestyle changes and taking medications;

- monitoring your critical health numbers;

- being open and honest about how well you are adhering to the treatment plan;

- seeing your healthcare provider as often as recommended.

"Your Diabetes Healthcare Team," reprinted with permission from www.heart.org. © 2010 American Heart Association, Inc.

In some cases, managing diabetes requires a multidisciplinary approach with medical professionals who have expertise in specific fields. Your healthcare team may include the following.

Your Family Doctor (General Practitioner)

If you have diabetes, you should see your family doctor more than once a year. Your doctor's staff may include nurse practitioners and physician assistants, as well. Supported by staff, your doctor will:

- provide you with valuable information about diabetes and how to treat it;

- focus on your specific diabetes problems and your overall health;

- talk to you about lifestyle changes you can make to lessen the effects of the disease and prevent complications;

- refer you to other professionals with specialized knowledge that can help treat diabetes and its effects, as needed.

When meeting with your family doctor, you might want to get answers to the following questions:

- What is my blood sugar level and what should my target number be?

- What is my blood pressure and what should my target number be?

- What is my blood cholesterol and what should my target number be?

- Am I overweight or obese? How much weight should I lose?

- What are my risk factors for cardiovascular disease, such as heart disease or stroke? What are the warning signs?

- What types of foods should I eat? What should I avoid?

- What are the best types of physical activities for me? How active do I need to be?

- Are there medications I should take to help me manage my diabetes?

Diabetes Educators

These healthcare professionals specialize in providing care and education to people with diabetes. They can be nurses, dietitians, pharmacists, doctors, exercise physiologists, podiatrists, and social workers, among others. Many are also certified diabetes educators (CDEs), meaning they have met additional care criteria.

Diabetes educators provide patients comprehensive care by:

- counseling them on how to incorporate healthy eating and regular physical activity into their life;

- helping them understand how their medications work

- teaching them how to monitor their blood glucose to avoid the risk of complications;

- assisting them in solving problems associated with diabetes, including making emotional adjustments;

- creating a customized self-management plan based on the patients' specific needs, age, school or work schedule, daily activities, family demands, eating habits, and health problems.

When meeting with your diabetes educator, you might want to get answers to the following questions:

- What do my blood sugar results mean, and when should I call my doctor?

- What type of physical activity/exercise is right for me?

- What do I need to know about healthy eating and meal planning?

- What should be my "sick day" plan?

- What should I do if I start to get sick at work?

- How do my diabetes medications affect other prescription or over-the-counter drugs?

- What should I do if I can't remember something we talked about?

Dietitians

Dietitians can help you understand dietary dos and don'ts, a must for managing your diabetes. Being consistent about what you eat, when you eat, and how much you eat is crucial, but without the help of a nutritional expert, it can be frustrating and confusing trying to figure it all out. Dietitians undergo rigorous academic training and extensive practical experience. Plus, they keep their food and nutrition knowledge up to date by completing ongoing professional education programs.

When meeting with your dietitian, you might want to get answers to the following questions:

- How does food affect my blood glucose?

- Can I eat foods with sugar in them?

- How can I eat and keep my blood glucose levels at a healthy level?

- Why should I eat about the same amount at the same times each day?

- How much of each type of food should I eat each day?

- What should I eat when I feel sick?

- What foods can I eat a lot of?

- Can I drink alcohol?

Pharmacists

Your pharmacist can be a valuable resource for education and information about the medications you take for diabetes and other conditions. Pharmacists are trained in the science and clinical use of both prescription and over-the-counter medications.

Consider these helpful tips for building a successful relationship with your pharmacist:

- Even though you may have several doctors, fill all your prescriptions at the same pharmacy. Then all your medication records will be in one place, and your pharmacist can alert you to any potential drug interactions of medications prescribed by different doctors.

- Check with your pharmacists before taking over-the-counter drugs and herbal supplements since they can interact with your prescription medications and cause side effects.

- Read the label. If you're unsure whether the medication is what your doctor prescribed or if the dosage seems incorrect, ask your pharmacist.

- To prevent any adverse reactions, both your doctor and pharmacist should know all the allergies you have to medications, foods, or anything else.

To get the most from your medication, ask your pharmacist the following questions:

- When is the best time to take this medication? Should it be taken before or after I eat?

- How will this drug interact with my current medications?

  Are there any foods I should avoid?

- What are the side effects?

- What is the best way to store this medication?

- What should I do if I miss a dosage?

- Is there a generic version of this medication?

Endocrinologists (Hormone Doctors)

Endocrinologists treat patients who have disorders of the endocrine gland, such as diabetes, as well as other problems like thyroid diseases and hormonal disorders. In many cases, your endocrinologist may become your primary doctor when it comes to managing your diabetes. If this becomes true for you, be prepared to talk about your lifestyle in detail and ask questions about your condition.

Podiatrists (Foot Doctors)

A podiatrist is certified and trained to prevent, diagnose, and treat conditions associated with the foot and ankle. The American Diabetes Association recommends that all people with diabetes receive an annual foot exam to examine and assess their feet. Why? Because over time, 20 to 40 percent of people with diabetes develop neuropathy—nerve damage in their feet and lower legs. This loss of feeling may prevent patients from feeling heat, cold, or pain; in fact, they can even get cut or otherwise injured on their feet and legs and not realize it. Untreated cuts can lead to infections, ulcerations, and in severe cases, amputation.

As a preventive measure, your family doctor may send you to a podiatrist to help with early recognition and management of feet and leg issues. Your visits may be more frequent if you have other foot-risk conditions.

Your podiatrist will:

- check your pulses and the circulation in your feet;

- look for cuts, bruises, or infections;

- check the sensation in your feet;
- educate you about:
  - your risks;
  - how to manage your feet;
  - the importance of daily foot monitoring;
  - proper foot and nail care;
  - proper footwear.

Ophthalmologists/Optometrists (Eye Doctors)

Ophthalmologists and optometrists are doctors who specialize in treating the eyes, which can be affected by diabetes. "Retinopathy" is a general term used for all disorders of the retina caused by diabetes, and it's very common in people with type 1 and type 2 diabetes.

Upon diagnosis of type 2 diabetes, patients are strongly advised to have a comprehensive eye exam right away by an ophthalmologist or optometrist who knows about diabetes and how to manage retinopathy. After that, yearly exams are recommended unless retinopathy is progressing.

Cardiologists (Heart Doctors)

Cardiologists are doctors who are specially certified to treat problems of the cardiovascular system, which includes the heart and arteries. Cardiologists also treat related conditions such as high blood pressure, high cholesterol, chest pain, heart failure, heart attacks, stroke, congenital heart defects, and arrhythmia. Cardiologists may recommend a variety of tests to diagnose a patient's condition.

Role of Family and Friends

In addition to your healthcare team, your friends and family can be vital to managing your diabetes, helping with your emotional well-being, and supporting you in case of an emergency.

With diabetes, there are often important choices and items to remember about your healthcare. Having a friend or family member around to help you make those decisions can be helpful. Choose one member of your family to come with you to your healthcare visits and help you with your diabetes management.

Your healthcare providers are bound by law to keep your medical information confidential. However, your family members may wish to speak with them to get answers to questions and find support to deal with their feelings. If you are not opposed to this, you can provide your healthcare providers with a list of people with whom they have your permission to discuss your medical condition.

Chapter 14

Diabetes Control: Why It's Important

People who have diabetes may hear or read a lot about controlling, or managing, the condition. But what is diabetes control and why is it so important?

What Is Diabetes Control?

When you hear your doctors or healthcare providers talk about "diabetes control," they're usually referring to how close your blood sugar, or glucose, is kept to the desired range. Having too much or too little sugar in your blood can lead you to feel sick now and can cause health problems later.

Managing diabetes is like a three-way balancing act: The medications you take (insulin or pills), the food you eat, and the amount of exercise you get all need to be in sync.

Diabetes can get out of control if someone:

- doesn't take diabetes medicines as directed;

- doesn't follow the meal plan (like eating too much or not enough food without adjusting diabetes medicines);

"Diabetes Control: Why It's Important," July 2009, reprinted with permission from www.kidshealth.org. Copyright © 2009 The Nemours Foundation. This information was provided by KidsHealth, one of the largest resources online for medically reviewed health information written for parents, kids, and teens. For more articles like this one, visit www.KidsHealth.org, or www.TeensHealth.org.

- doesn't get regular exercise or exercises more or less than usual without making changes to his or her diabetes plan;

- has an illness or too much stress;

- doesn't check blood sugar levels enough.

What Can Happen If Diabetes Is Not Under Control?

Out-of-control blood sugar levels can lead to short-term problems like hypoglycemia, hyperglycemia, or diabetic ketoacidosis. In the long run, not controlling diabetes can also damage the vessels that supply blood to important organs, like the heart, kidneys, eyes, and nerves. This means that heart disease and stroke, kidney disease, vision problems, and nerve problems can happen to people with diabetes.

These problems don't usually show up in kids or teens who have had the disease for only a few years, but they can happen to adults with diabetes. Kids and teens with diabetes who don't control their blood sugar levels can be late going into puberty and might not end up as tall as they would have otherwise.

The good news is that keeping blood sugar levels under control can help keep you healthy and prevent health problems from happening later.

How Do People Know When Diabetes Is Under Control?

If you have diabetes, your doctor or diabetes healthcare team will tell you what your blood sugar levels should be (usually called a target range). If you have diabetes, you're trying to keep your blood sugar level as close to the target range as possible. As you get older, your target range may change.

The only way to know if your blood sugar level is close to your target range is to measure your blood sugar level several times a day with a glucose meter. Your diabetes healthcare team will help you determine when and how often you should be checking your blood sugar level. Checking it regularly and keeping a record of the test results is very important—this helps you and your diabetes healthcare team make adjustments to your diabetes management plan as needed.

The glucose meter tells you what your blood sugar level is at the moment you test. But another type of blood sugar test, the glycosylated hemoglobin (pronounced: gly-koh-sih-lay-tid he-muh-glo-bin and also known as the hemoglobin A1c or HbA1c) test, will help you and your doctor know how your blood sugar control was over the two to three months before the test was done. In general, the lower your HbA1C level, the better you're doing at controlling your diabetes.

Getting Control

Keeping blood sugar levels close to normal will be challenging at times. However, you can help keep your blood sugar levels in a healthy range with these steps:

- Take your insulin or pills when you're supposed to.
- Follow your meal plan.
- Get regular exercise.
- Check your blood sugar levels often and make changes with the help of your diabetes healthcare team.
- Visit your doctor and diabetes healthcare team regularly.
- Learn as much as possible about diabetes.

Chapter 15

Glucose Monitoring

Chapter Contents

Section 15.1

What Is Blood Glucose Monitoring?

"Blood Glucose Monitoring," © 2010 A.D.A.M., Inc.
Reprinted with permission.

Blood glucose monitoring refers to the ongoing measurement of blood sugar (glucose). Monitoring can be done at any time using a portable device called a glucometer.

How the Test Is Performed

The traditional glucose meter comes with test strips, small needles called lancets, and a logbook for recording your numbers. There are many different kinds of these meters, but they all work essentially the same way.

A complete testing kit can be purchased from a pharmacy without a prescription. Your doctor or nurse can help you choose the equipment that's right for you, help you set it up, and teach you how to use it.

You will prick your finger with the lancet and place a drop of blood on a special strip. This strip uses a chemical substance to determine the amount of glucose in the blood. (Newer monitors can use blood from other areas of the body besides the fingers, reducing discomfort.) The meter displays your blood sugar results as a number on a digital display.

How to Prepare for the Test

Have all test items within reach before starting—timing is important. Clean the needle prick area with soap and water or an alcohol swab. Completely dry the skin before pricking.

How the Test Will Feel

There is a sharp prick.

Why the Test Is Performed

This test reveals your blood sugar level.

If you have diabetes, you can use it to carefully monitor your blood sugar levels at home. Regularly checking your blood sugar level is one of the most important steps you can take in managing the disease. It provides your doctor with important information regarding the control of your blood sugar.

When you keep track of your blood sugar you will:

- start to see patterns that will help you plan meals, activities, and what time of day to take your medications;

- learn how certain foods affect your blood sugar levels;

- see how exercise can improve your numbers.

Testing allows you to respond quickly to high blood sugar (hyperglycemia) or low blood sugar (hypoglycemia). This might include diet adjustments, exercise, and insulin (as instructed by your healthcare provider).

Your doctor may order a blood sugar test to screen for diabetes.

Normal Results

- Before meals: 70–130 milligrams per deciliter (mg/dL)

- After meals: Less than 180 mg/dL

Values can vary depending on physical activity, meals, and insulin administration. Normal value ranges may vary slightly among different laboratories. Talk to your doctor about the meaning of your specific test results.

What Abnormal Results Mean

Low levels indicate hypoglycemia. Have something to eat. You may need to change the next insulin dose, and possibly future insulin doses as well.

If levels are too high, this indicates hyperglycemia. You may need additional insulin.

Risks

There is a slight chance of infection at the puncture site. A small amount of bleeding may occur after the puncture.

Considerations

The correct procedure must be followed or the results will not be accurate.

Alternative Names

Home glucose monitoring; self-monitoring of blood glucose

References

American Diabetes Association. Standards of medical care in diabetes—2010. *Diabetes Care*. 2010 Jan;33 Suppl 1:S11–61.

Section 15.2

Glucose Meters

"Glucose Testing Devices,"
U.S. Food and Drug Administration, March 18, 2010.

What does this test do?

This is a home-use test kit to measure blood sugar (glucose) in your blood.

What is glucose?

Glucose is blood sugar that your body uses as a source of energy. Unless you have diabetes, you body regulates the amount of glucose in your blood. People with diabetes have poorly controlled blood glucose.

What type of test is this?

This is a quantitative test—you find out the amount of glucose present in your sample.

Why should you do this test?

You should do this test if you have diabetes and you need to monitor your blood sugar (glucose) levels. You can use the results to help you determine your daily adjustments in treatment, know if you have dangerously high or low levels of glucose, and understand how your diet and exercise change your glucose levels.

The Diabetes Control and Complications Trial (1993) showed that good glucose control using home monitors led to fewer complications.

How often should you test your glucose?

Follow your doctor's recommendations about how often you test your glucose. You may need to test yourself several times each day to determine adjustments in your treatment.

What should your glucose levels be?

Your fasting blood glucose level (after not eating for eight to ten hours) should be lower than 126 mg/dL. Your blood glucose level immediately after eating should be lower than 200 mg/dL.

How accurate is this test?

The accuracy of this test depends on many factors including the following:

- The quality of your meter.
- The quality of your test strips.
- How well you do the test.
- Your hematocrit (the amount of red blood cells in the blood). If you have a high hematocrit, you may test low for blood glucose. Or, if you have a low hematocrit, you may test high for glucose. If you know your hematocrit is low or high, discuss with your healthcare provider how it may affect your glucose testing.
- Interfering substances (some substances, such as vitamin C and uric acid, may interfere with your glucose testing). Check the package insert for your meter and test strips to find out what substances may affect the testing accuracy.
- Altitude, temperature, and humidity (high altitude, low and high temperatures, and humidity can cause unpredictable effects on glucose results). Check the meter and test strip package inserts for more information. Store and handle the meter and strips according to instructions.

How do you do this test?

Before you self-monitor your blood glucose, you must read and understand the instructions for your meter. In general, you prick your finger with a lancet to get a drop of blood. Place the blood on a disposable "test strip" that is coated with chemicals that react with glucose. Then place the test strip in your meter. Some meters measure the amount of electricity that passes through the test strip. Others measure how much light reflects from it. In the United States, meters report results in milligrams of glucose per deciliter of blood or mg/dl.

You can get information about your meter and test strips from several different sources including the toll-free number in the user manual or the manufacturer's website. If you have an urgent problem, always contact your healthcare provider or a local emergency room for advice.

How do you choose a glucose meter?

You can purchase more than twenty-five different types of meters. They differ in several ways including the following:

- Amount of blood needed for each test
- How easy it is to use
- Pain associated with using the product
- Accuracy
- Testing speed
- Overall size
- Ability to store test results in memory
- Cost of the meter
- Cost of the test strips used
- Doctor's recommendation
- Technical support provided by the manufacturer
- Special features such as automatic timing, error codes, large display screen, or spoken instructions or results

Talk to your healthcare practitioner about glucose meters and how to use them.

How do you compare your home test glucose values with the laboratory values?

Most home blood glucose meters in the United States measure glucose in whole blood. Most lab tests, in contrast, measure glucose in plasma. Plasma is blood without the cells. A lab test of your blood glucose will be about 10 to 15 percent higher than the value given by your meter. Look at the instructions for your meter to find out if it gives its results as "whole blood" or "plasma equivalent." Many meters now sold give values that are "plasma equivalent," which means they can be compared more directly to lab test values.

Should you use generic or "third party" test strips?

You may choose test strips that are made by a different company than the one that made the meter. Sometimes, generic test strips are cheaper. If you choose generic test strips:

- make sure the generic strips will work with your meter. Check the label of the test strips to make sure they will work with the make and model of your meter. Just because the generic test strip looks like it will work does not mean that it will work.

- watch for inconsistent results. If you get poor results, try strips made or recommended by the maker of your meter until you again get consistent results.

How can you check your meter's performance?

There are three ways to make sure your meter works properly:

1. Use liquid control solution:

    - every time you open a new container of test strips;

    - occasionally as you use the container of test strips;

    - whenever you get unusual results.

    You test a drop of these solutions just like you test a drop of your blood. The value you get should match that written on the liquid control solution bottle.

2. Use electronic checks. Every time you turn on your meter, it does an electronic check. If it detects a problem it will give you an error code. Look in your owner's manual to see what the error codes mean and how to fix the problem.

3. Compare your meter with a laboratory meter. Take your meter with you to your next appointment with your healthcare provider. Ask your provider to watch your technique to make sure you are using the meter correctly. Ask your healthcare provider have your blood tested with a routine laboratory method. If

the values you obtain on your glucose meter match the laboratory values, then your meter is working well and you are using good technique.

What should you do if your meter malfunctions?

If your meter malfunctions, you should tell your healthcare professional and the company that made your meter and strips.

Can you test blood glucose from sites other than your fingers?

Some new meters allow you to test blood from the base of your thumb, upper arm, forearm, thigh, or calf. If your glucose changes rapidly, these other sites may not give you accurate results. You should probably use your fingers to get your blood for testing if any of the following applies:

- You have just taken insulin.
- You think your blood sugar is low.
- You are not aware of symptoms when you become hypoglycemic.
- The site results do not agree with the way you feel.
- You have just eaten.
- You have just exercised.
- You are ill.
- You are under stress.

Section 15.3

Goals for Blood Glucose Control

People who have diabetes should be testing their blood glucose regularly at home. Regular blood glucose testing helps you determine how well your diabetes management program of meal planning, exercising, and medication (if necessary) is doing to keep your blood glucose as close to normal as possible. The results of the nationwide Diabetes Control and Complications Trial (DCCT) show that the closer you keep your blood glucose to normal, the more likely you are to prevent diabetes complications such as eye disease, nerve damage, and other problems. For some people, other medical conditions, age, or other issues may cause your physician to establish somewhat higher blood glucose targets for you.

Table 15.1 outlines the usual blood glucose ranges for a person who does and does not have diabetes. Use this as a guide to work with your physician and your healthcare team to determine what your target goals should be, and to develop a program of regular blood glucose monitoring to manage your condition.

Table 15.1. Blood Glucose Goals

Time of Check	Goal plasma blood glucose ranges for people without diabetes	Goal plasma blood glucose ranges for people with diabetes
Before breakfast (fasting)	< 110	90–130
Before lunch, supper, and snack	< 110	90–130
Two hours after meals	< 140	< 180
Bedtime	< 120	110–150
A1C (also called glycosylated hemoglobin A1c, HbA1c or glycohemoglobin A1c)	< 6 percent	< 7 percent

Section 15.4

When to Test Blood Glucose and How to Avoid Inaccuracies

When to Test Blood Glucose

Ask your healthcare team when it is best to check your blood glucose and how often you should test. You may want to check at different times of the day to get an idea of how well your treatment program is working for you. The best times to check are before breakfast, before lunch, before dinner, and before bedtime snack. Sometimes it is helpful to check blood glucose two to four hours after a meal to see the effect of food on your glucose levels.

There are times when you will want to check your blood glucose more often than usual. You may think of other times as well:

- During periods of stress, illness, or surgery.

- When you are pregnant.

- When low blood glucose is suspected.

- When blood glucose levels are erratic.

- When there are changes made in your treatment program, such as a change in medication doses, meal plan, or activity.

- When taking new medications, like steroids.

Little Things That Can Have a Big Impact on Your Blood Glucose Reading

Things That Can Affect Your Blood Glucose Reading

- A dirty meter.

- Outdated test strips.

- If test strips are not compatible with the meter you're using, results may be inaccurate or no result will be obtained. If the wrong strip is used, it may not even fit into the slot or it may fit, but the meter won't turn on.

- Substances left on your hands. For example, if there is a sugary substance on the finger used for lancing, even if it's a small amount that can't be seen, a high blood glucose reading can result.

- Temperature changes (heat/humidity/cold air).

- Not a big enough blood sample on the test strip.

- Wet fingers. Fluid mixes with blood and can cause an inaccurate reading.

How to Avoid an Inaccurate Blood Glucose Reading

- Before using the meter for the first time and then again every few weeks, check your meter using the control solution. Control solution is only good for three months once opened. Label the control solution bottle with the date you open it. Check the date and shake control solution before using. The value the control solution gives should be in the target range printed on the strips container.

- Make sure strips are not expired. Check the date on the strip container.

- Make sure code on strip container matches the code on the meter.

- Wash hands in warm water and dry them off after.

- Massage hands before checking.

- Select site on one side of the center of a fingertip. Rotate sites for each check.

- Apply gentle pressure to lanced finger to help the drop of blood form on the surface.

- Completely fill the strip target area with blood.

Section 15.5

Continuous Glucose Monitoring

Excerpted from "Continuous Glucose Monitoring," National Institute
of Diabetes and Digestive and Kidney Diseases, National Institutes of
Health, NIH Publication No. 09-4551, October 2008.

What Is Glucose Monitoring?

Glucose monitoring helps people with diabetes manage the disease
and avoid its associated problems. A person can use the results of glucose monitoring to make decisions about food, physical activity, and
medications. The most common way to check glucose levels involves
pricking a fingertip with an automatic lancing device to obtain a blood
sample and then using a glucose meter to measure the blood sample's
glucose level.

Many types of glucose meters are available, and all are accurate
and reliable if used properly. Some meters use a blood sample from a
less sensitive area than the fingertip, such as the upper arm, forearm,
or thigh.

What Is Continuous Glucose Monitoring?

Continuous glucose monitoring (CGM) systems use a tiny sensor
inserted under the skin to check glucose levels in tissue fluid. The sensor stays in place for several days to a week and then must be replaced.
A transmitter sends information about glucose levels via radio waves
from the sensor to a pager-like wireless monitor. The user must check
blood samples with a glucose meter to program the devices. Because
currently approved CGM devices are not as accurate and reliable as
standard blood glucose meters, users should confirm glucose levels
with a meter before making a change in treatment.

CGM systems are more expensive than conventional glucose monitoring, but they may enable better glucose control. CGM devices produced by Abbott, DexCom, and Medtronic have been approved by the
U.S. Food and Drug Administration (FDA) and are available by prescription. These devices provide real-time measurements of glucose

levels, with glucose levels displayed at five-minute or one-minute intervals. Users can set alarms to alert them when glucose levels are too low or too high. Special software is available to download data from the devices to a computer for tracking and analysis of patterns and trends, and the systems can display trend graphs on the monitor screen.

What Are the Prospects for an Artificial Pancreas?

To overcome the limitations of current insulin therapy, researchers have long sought to link glucose monitoring and insulin delivery by developing an artificial pancreas. An artificial pancreas is a system that will mimic, as closely as possible, the way a healthy pancreas detects changes in blood glucose levels and responds automatically to secrete appropriate amounts of insulin. Although not a cure, an artificial pancreas has the potential to significantly improve diabetes care and management and to reduce the burden of monitoring and managing blood glucose.

An artificial pancreas based on mechanical devices requires at least three components:

- A CGM system

- An insulin delivery system

- A computer program that "closes the loop" by adjusting insulin delivery based on changes in glucose levels

With recent technological advances, the first steps have been taken toward closing the loop. The first pairing of a CGM system with an insulin pump—the MiniMed Paradigm REAL-Time System—is not an artificial pancreas, but it does represent the first step in joining glucose monitoring and insulin delivery systems using the most advanced technology available.

Points to Remember

- Glucose monitoring helps people with diabetes manage the disease and avoid its associated problems.

- The most common way to check glucose levels involves pricking a fingertip to obtain a blood sample and using a glucose meter to measure the glucose level in the sample.

- Continuous glucose monitoring (CGM) systems use a tiny sensor inserted under the skin to check glucose levels in tissue fluid. A transmitter sends glucose measurements to a wireless monitor.

- An artificial pancreas based on mechanical devices will consist of a CGM system, an insulin delivery system, and a computer program to adjust insulin delivery based on changes in glucose levels.

Hope through Research

The National Institute of Diabetes and Digestive and Kidney Diseases (NIDDK) and the National Institutes of Health (NIH) have encouraged and supported research that has helped researchers explore and develop improved glucose sensing technologies. NIDDK support was instrumental in the development of two CGM devices. One device is on the market and the other is under review by the FDA. Research supported by the NIDDK and NIH is contributing to the development of an artificial pancreas that will combine continuous glucose sensing with insulin delivery in a "closed-loop" system.

Chapter 16

Routine Medical Examinations and Recommended Vaccinations

Chapter Contents

Section 16.1

Recommended Diabetes Tests and Checkups

"Diabetes: Tests and Checkups,"
© 2010 A.D.A.M., Inc. Reprinted with permission.

You can live an active lifestyle when you take control of your diabetes care. Still, you must have regular health checkups and tests. These visits will give you a chance to:

- ask your doctor or nurse questions;
- learn more about diabetes.

See Your Doctor

See your diabetes doctor every three to six months. During this exam, your doctor should check your:

- blood pressure;
- weight;
- feet.

See your dentist every six months.

Eye Exams

An eye doctor should check your eyes at least once a year. If you have eye problems because of diabetes, you will probably see your eye doctor more often.

Foot Exams

Your doctor should check the pulses in your feet and your reflexes at least once a year. The doctor should also look for calluses, infections, and sores.

The doctor should check every year for loss of feeling or sensation, using a special instrument.

If you have had foot ulcers before, see your doctor every three to six months. It is always a good idea to ask your doctor to check your feet.

Hemoglobin A1C (HbA1C)

An HbA1C lab test shows the average amount of sugar in your blood over three months. It shows how well you are controlling your diabetes.

The normal level is less than 6 percent. Most people with diabetes should have an HbA1C of less than 7 percent. Higher numbers mean that your diabetes control is not as good.

Cholesterol

A cholesterol test measures cholesterol and triglycerides in your blood. You should have the test on an empty stomach after not eating overnight.

Adults with type 2 diabetes should have this test every year. People with high cholesterol may have this test more often.

Kidney Tests

Once a year, you should have a urine test. It looks for a protein called "albumin." Because the test looks for small amounts of albumin, it is sometimes called a test for microalbuminuria. You will have more of this protein in your blood if you have early kidney damage due to diabetes. But the level of this protein in urine can also be higher for other reasons.

Your doctor will also check your kidney function with a blood test every year.

References

American Diabetes Association. Standards of medical care in diabetes—2010. *Diabetes Care*. 2010 Jan;33 Suppl 1:S11–61.

Inzucchi SE and Sherwin RS. Type 2 diabetes mellitus. In: Goldman L and Ausiello D, eds. *Cecil Medicine. 23rd ed.* Saunders; 2007:chap 248.

In the clinic. Type 2 diabetes. *Ann Intern Med*. 2010 Mar 2;152(5): ITC1–16.

Section 16.2

A1C Testing

Excerpted from "If You Have Diabetes . . . Know Your Blood Sugar Numbers," National Diabetes Education Program, National Institutes of Health, NIH Publication No. 98-4350, July 2005. Revised by David A. Cooke, MD, FACP, February 2010.

What is the A1C test?

The A1C test is a simple lab test that reflects your average blood glucose level over the last three months. A small blood sample to check your A1C can be taken at any time of the day, and is not affected by eating before the test.

Why should I have an A1C test?

The A1C test is the best test for you and your healthcare team to know how well your treatment plan is working over time. The test shows if your blood glucose levels have been close to normal or too high. The higher the amount of glucose in your blood, the higher your A1C result will be. A high A1C result will increase your chances for serious health problems.

In 2010, the American Diabetes Association recommended the A1c test as an option for making a diagnosis of diabetes. Previously, it was recommended only for monitoring blood sugar control in people with known diabetes. Some doctors now test A1c routinely to screen for diabetes.

What is a good A1C goal?

You and your healthcare team should discuss the A1C goal that is right for you. For most people with diabetes, the A1C goal is less than 7. An A1C higher than 7 means that you have a greater chance of eye disease, kidney disease, or nerve damage. Lowering your A1C—by any amount—can improve your chances of staying healthy. If your number is 7 or more, or above your goal, ask your healthcare team about changing your treatment plan to bring your A1C number down.

Traditionally, it was believed that lower A1c numbers were better. Clearly, diabetics with an A1c less than 7 have fewer complications than those with higher levels. However, recent studies have suggested that using medications to achieve very low A1c numbers (less than 6) may increase risk of death. Very low A1c levels may also be less safe in people with serious heart disease or advanced diabetic complications. Most experts currently aim for an A1c between 6.5 and 7, but a higher target may be appropriate for certain patients.

Table 16.1. What Your A1C Numbers Mean

Level of Control	A1C Number
Normal	5.6 or less
Goal	less than 7
Take action	7 or more

If I am pregnant, what is my A1C goal?

Keeping your A1C less than 6 if you are pregnant will help ensure a healthy baby. If possible, women should plan ahead and work to get their A1C below 6 before getting pregnant. However, hypoglycemia (low blood sugar) is harmful to the mother and baby, and a higher A1c may be targeted if hypoglycemia occurs frequently.

How often do I need an A1C test?

Ask for an A1C test at least twice a year. Get the test more often if your blood glucose stays too high or if your treatment plan changes.

What about home testing for A1C?

You and your healthcare team should decide if home testing is a good idea for you. If so, be sure to do the test the correct way and discuss the results with your doctor.

Section 16.3

Ketone Testing

What are ketones?

Ketones are produced when the body burns fat for energy or fuel. They are also produced when you lose weight or if there is not enough insulin to help your body use sugar for energy. Without enough insulin, glucose builds up in the blood. Since the body is unable to use glucose for energy, it breaks down fat instead. When this occurs, ketones form in the blood and spill into the urine. These ketones can make you very sick.

How can I test for ketones?

You can test to see if your body is making any ketones by doing a simple urine test. There are several products available for ketone testing and they can be purchased, without a prescription, at your pharmacy. The test result can be negative, or show small, moderate, or large quantities of ketones.

When should I test for ketones?

- Anytime your blood glucose is over 250 mg/dl for two tests in a row.

- When you are ill. Often illness, infections, or injuries will cause sudden high blood glucose and this is an especially important time to check for ketones.

- When you are planning to exercise and the blood glucose is over 250 mg/dl.

- If you are pregnant, you should test for ketones each morning before breakfast and any time the blood glucose is over 250 mg/dl.

If ketones are positive, what does this mean?

There are situations when you might have ketones without the blood glucose being too high. Positive ketones are not a problem when blood glucose levels are within range and you are trying to lose weight.

It is a problem if blood glucose levels are high and left untreated. Untreated high blood glucose with positive ketones can lead to a life-threatening condition called diabetic ketoacidosis (DKA).

What should I do if the ketone test is positive?

Call your diabetes educator or physician, as you may need additional insulin. Drink plenty of water and fluids containing no calories to "wash out" the ketones. Continue testing your blood glucose every three to four hours, testing for ketones if the blood glucose is over 250 mg/dl. Do not exercise if your blood glucose is over 250 mg/dl and ketones are present.

Section 16.4

Microalbumin and Microalbumin/Creatinine Ratio Testing

"Microalbumin and Microalbumin/Creatinine Ratio Testing," http://www
.labtestsonline.org/understanding/analytes/microalbumin/multiprint.html#
© 2010 American Association for Clinical Chemistry. Reprinted with permission. For additional information about clinical lab testing, visit the Lab
Tests Online website at www.labtestsonline.org.

Also known as: Urine microalbumin; Albumin-to-Creatinine ratio; ACR
Formal name: Microalbumin and Microalbumin/Creatinine Ratio
Related tests: Albumin; Creatinine; Glucose; A1C

At a Glance

Why Get Tested?

To get screened for a possible kidney disorder or for early damage to the kidneys in those with diabetes.

When to Get Tested?

Annually after a diagnosis of diabetes or hypertension,

Sample Required?

A random, timed, overnight, or twenty-four-hour urine sample.

Test Preparation Needed?

None.

The Test Sample

What Is Being Tested?

The microalbumin test is an early indicator of kidney failure. It measures the tiny amounts of albumin that the body begins to release into the urine several years before significant kidney damage becomes apparent. Albumin is a protein that is produced in the liver. It is present in high concentrations in the blood, but when the kidneys are functioning properly, virtually no albumin is allowed to leak through into the urine. If a person's kidneys become damaged or diseased, however, they begin to lose their ability to filter proteins out of the urine. This is frequently seen in chronic diseases, such as diabetes and hypertension, with increasing amounts of protein in the urine reflecting increasing kidney failure.

Since the albumin molecule is small, it is one of the first proteins to be detected in the urine with kidney damage. Patients who have consistently detectible amounts of albumin in their urine (microalbuminuria) have an increased risk of developing progressive kidney failure and cardiovascular disease in the future. Microalbumin measurements can be obtained using urine collected over a twenty-four-hour period, for a specified amount of time (e.g., four hours or overnight), or randomly (spot).

Creatinine, a byproduct of muscle metabolism, is normally excreted into the urine on a consistent basis. Its level in the urine is relatively stable. Since the concentration (or dilution) of urine varies throughout the day, this property of creatinine allows its measurement to be used as a corrective factor in random/spot urine samples. When a creatinine measurement is performed along with a random microalbumin, the result is the microalbumin/creatinine ratio (also called the albumin/creatinine ratio [ACR]), which the American Diabetes Association states is the preferred test for screening for microalbuminuria.

How Is the Sample Collected for Testing?

You will be asked to collect either a random sample of urine while you are at the doctor's office or laboratory, a timed urine sample (such as four hours or overnight), or you may be requested to collect a complete twenty-four-hour urine sample. Your doctor or the laboratory will give you a container and instructions for properly collecting a timed or twenty-four-hour urine sample.

Is Any Test Preparation Needed to Ensure the Quality of the Sample?

No test preparation is needed.

The Test

How Is It Used?

The random microalbumin test or microalbumin/creatinine ratio is frequently ordered as a screening test on patients with chronic conditions, such as diabetes and hypertension, that put them at an increased risk of developing kidney failure. Studies have shown that identifying the very early stages of kidney disease (microalbuminuria) helps patients and doctors adjust treatment. With better control of diabetes and hypertension by maintaining tight glycemic control and reducing blood pressure, the progression of diabetic kidney disease can be slowed or prevented.

A timed microalbumin test (four-hour or overnight) may be ordered as an alternative screening tool. If significant amounts of microalbumin are detected with these screening tests, they may be confirmed with a twenty-four-hour microalbumin test.

When Is It Ordered?

The National Kidney Foundation recommends that everyone with diabetes between twelve and seventy years of age have a urine test for microalbuminuria at least once a year. According to the American Diabetes Association, everyone with type 1 diabetes should get tested annually, starting five years after onset, and all those with type 2 diabetes should start at the time of diagnosis. If microalbuminuria is detected, it should be confirmed by retesting and, if positive on two of three determinations over a three- to six-month period, it is considered to be present and appropriate treatment should be given.

Patients with hypertension may be tested at regular intervals, with the frequency determined by their doctor.

What Does the Test Result Mean?

Moderately increased microalbumin levels in urine indicate that a person is in one of the very early phases of developing kidney disease. Very high levels are an indication that kidney disease is present in a more severe form. Normal levels are an indication that kidney function is normal.

Is There Anything Else I Should Know?

Studies have shown that elevated levels of urinary albumin in people with diabetes or hypertension are associated with increased risk of developing cardiovascular disease (CVD), even if those levels are within the normal reference range. More recently, research has been focused on trying to determine if increased levels of albumin in the urine are also indicative of CVD risk in those who do not have diabetes or high blood pressure.

Common Questions

What Is the Difference between Albumin, Prealbumin, and Microalbumin Tests?

The prealbumin test measures a protein that reflects your nutritional status, particularly before and after surgery, or if you are hospitalized or taking nutritional supplements. Albumin testing is more often used to test for liver or kidney disease or to learn if your body is not absorbing enough amino acids. Albumin can also be used to monitor nutritional status. However, prealbumin changes more quickly, making it more useful for detecting changes in short-term nutritional status than albumin. The microalbumin test measures very small levels of albumin in your urine and may indicate whether you are at risk for developing kidney disease.

Is Microalbumin Just Smaller Molecules of Albumin?

Microalbumin tests for a small amount of albumin, not smaller molecules.

What Is the Test Finding in My Urine?

If you are diabetic, each year your doctor will test a sample of your urine to see if your kidneys are leaking albumin, even in small amounts. It is good news if your kidneys are not leaking even small amounts of albumin.

Are There Other Reasons for Having Increased Microalbumin Levels in Urine?

Yes, microalbuminuria is not specific for diabetes. It may also be associated with hypertension (high blood pressure), some lipid abnormalities, and several immune disorders. Elevated results may also be caused by vigorous exercise, blood in the urine, urinary tract infection, dehydration, and some drugs.

Section 16.5

Glomerular Filtration Rate Testing

Glomerular filtration rate (GFR) is a test used to check how well the kidneys are working. Specifically, it estimates how much blood passes through the tiny filters in the kidneys, called glomeruli, each minute.

How the Test Is Performed

Blood is drawn from a vein, usually from the inside of the elbow or the back of the hand. The site is cleaned with germ-killing medicine (antiseptic). The healthcare provider wraps an elastic band around the upper arm to apply pressure to the area and make the vein swell with blood.

Next, the healthcare provider gently inserts a needle into the vein. The blood collects into an airtight vial or tube attached to the needle. The elastic band is removed from your arm.

Once the blood has been collected, the needle is removed, and the puncture site is covered to stop any bleeding.

In infants or young children, a sharp tool called a lancet may be used to puncture the skin and make it bleed. The blood collects into a small glass tube called a pipette, or onto a slide or test strip. A bandage may be placed over the area if there is any bleeding.

The blood sample is sent to a lab, where the creatinine level is tested. The lab specialist combines your creatinine level with several other factors to estimate your glomerular filtration rate (GFR). Different formulas are used for adults and children. The formula will include some or all of the following:

- Age
- Creatinine measurement
- Gender
- Height
- Race
- Weight

How to Prepare for the Test

Certain drugs can interfere with test results. Tell your doctor about all medicines you are taking, including over-the-counter ones.

How the Test Will Feel

When the needle is inserted to draw blood, some people feel moderate pain, while others feel only a prick or stinging sensation. Afterward, there might be some throbbing.

Why the Test Is Performed

The GFR test measures how well your kidneys are filtering a waste called creatinine, which is produced by the muscles. When the kidneys aren't working as well as they should, creatinine builds up in the blood.

Your doctor may order this test if there are signs that your kidneys are not working properly. It may also be done to see how far kidney disease has progressed.

The test is recommended for people with chronic kidney disease and those at risk for it due to:

- diabetes;
- family history of kidney disease;
- frequent urinary tract infections;
- heart disease;

- high blood pressure;

- urinary blockage.

Normal Results

According to the National Kidney Foundation, normal results range from 90–120 mL/min. Older people will have lower normal GFR levels, because GFR decreases with age.

Normal value ranges can vary slightly among different laboratories. Talk to your doctor about what your specific test results mean.

What Abnormal Results Mean

Levels below 60 mL/min for three or more months are a sign of chronic kidney disease. Those with GFR results below 15 mL/min are a sign of kidney failure.

Risks

Veins and arteries vary in size from one patient to another and from one side of the body to the other. Obtaining a blood sample from some people may be more difficult than from others.

Other risks associated with having blood drawn are slight, but can include:

- excessive bleeding;

- fainting or feeling light-headed;

- hematoma (blood accumulating under the skin);

- infection (a slight risk any time the skin is broken).

Considerations

The creatinine clearance test, which involves a twenty-four-hour urine collection, can also provide an estimate of kidney function. However, this method is not always accurate.

GFR can increase during pregnancy.

Alternative Names

GFR; estimated GFR; eGFR

References

K/DOQI clinical practice guidelines for chronic kidney disease: evaluation, classification, and stratification. Kidney Disease Outcome Quality Initiative. *Am J Kidney Dis*. 2002;39(2 Suppl 1):S1–246.

Johnson CA, Levey AS, Coresh J, Levin A, Lau J, Eknoyan G. Clinical practice guidelines for chronic kidney disease in adults: Part II. Glomerular filtration rate, proteinuria, and other markers. *Am Fam Physician*. 2004;70:1091–97.

Snyder S, Pendergraph B. Detection and evaluation of chronic kidney disease. *Am Fam Physician*. 2005;72:1723–32, 1733–34.

Section 16.6

Recommended Vaccinations for Diabetes

"Take Charge of Your Diabetes: Vaccinations," Centers for Disease Control and Prevention, March 12, 2010.

If you have diabetes, take extra care to keep up-to-date on your vaccinations (also called immunizations). Vaccines can prevent illnesses that can be very serious for people with diabetes. This section talks about some vaccines you need to know about.

Influenza Vaccine

Influenza (often called the flu) is not just a bad cold. It's a serious illness that can lead to pneumonia and even death. The flu spreads when influenza viruses pass from one person to the nose or throat of others. Signs of the flu may include sudden high fever, chills, body aches, sore throat, runny nose, dry cough, and headache.

The flu is a serious illness that can put you in the hospital. A yearly flu shot can help prevent this.

People with diabetes who come down with the flu may become very sick and may even have to go to a hospital. If you get the flu, you'll need to take special care of yourself.

You can help keep yourself from getting the flu by getting a flu shot every year. Everyone with diabetes—even pregnant women—should get a yearly flu shot. The best time to get one is between October and mid-November, before the flu season begins. This vaccine is fully covered under Medicare Part B.

Pneumococcal Vaccine

Pneumococcal disease is a major source of illness and death. It can cause serious infections of the lungs (pneumonia), the blood (bacteremia), and the covering of the brain (meningitis). Pneumococcal polysaccharide vaccine (often called PPV) can help prevent this disease.

PPV can be given at the same time as the flu vaccine—or at any time of the year. Most people have to take PPV only once in their life. Ask your healthcare provider whether you might need a second vaccination. This vaccine is fully covered under Medicare Part B.

Tetanus/Diphtheria (Td) Toxoid

Tetanus (or lockjaw) and diphtheria are serious diseases. Tetanus is caused by a germ that enters the body through a cut or wound. Diphtheria spreads when germs pass from one person to the nose or throat of others.

You can help prevent tetanus and diphtheria with a combined shot called Td toxoid. Most people get Td toxoid as part of their routine childhood vaccinations, but all adults need a Td booster shot every ten years. Other vaccines may be given at the same time as Td toxoid.

Other Vaccines

You may need vaccines to protect you against other illnesses. Ask your healthcare provider if you need any of these:

- Measles/Mumps/Rubella vaccine
- Hepatitis A and B vaccines
- Varicella (chicken pox) vaccine
- Polio vaccine
- Vaccines for travel to other countries

How to Get More Information

Call the immunization program in your state health department to find out where you can get vaccinations in your area. Keep your vaccination records up-to-date so you and your healthcare provider will know what vaccines you may need.

Part Three

Medications and Diabetes Care

Chapter 17

Diabetes Medicines: What You Need to Know

What Do Diabetes Medicines Do?

Over time, high levels of blood glucose, also called blood sugar, can cause health problems. These problems include heart disease, heart attacks, strokes, kidney disease, nerve damage, digestive problems, eye disease, and tooth and gum problems. You can help prevent health problems by keeping your blood glucose levels on target.

Everyone with diabetes needs to choose foods wisely and be physically active. If you can't reach your target blood glucose levels with wise food choices and physical activity, you may need diabetes medicines. The kind of medicine you take depends on your type of diabetes, your schedule, and your other health conditions.

Diabetes medicines help keep your blood glucose in your target range. The target range is suggested by diabetes experts and your doctor or diabetes educator.

What Targets Are Recommended for Blood Glucose Levels?

The National Diabetes Education Program uses blood glucose targets set by the American Diabetes Association (ADA) for most people

Excerpted from "What I Need to Know about Diabetes Medicines," National Institute of Diabetes and Digestive and Kidney Diseases, National Institutes of Health, NIH Publication No. 08-4222, March 2008.

with diabetes. To learn your daily blood glucose numbers, you'll check your blood glucose levels on your own using a blood glucose meter.

Target blood glucose levels for most people with diabetes are as follows:

- Before meals: 70 to 130 mg/dL

- One to two hours after the start of a meal: Less than 180 mg/dL

Also, you should ask your doctor for a blood test called the A1C at least twice a year. The A1C will give you your average blood glucose for the past three months. The target A1C result for people with diabetes is less than 7 percent.

Your personal A1C goal might be higher or lower than 7 percent. Keeping your A1C as close to normal as possible—below 6 percent without having frequent low blood glucose—can help prevent long-term diabetes problems. Doctors might recommend other goals for very young children, older people, people with other health problems, or those who often have low blood glucose.

Talk with your doctor or diabetes educator about whether the target blood glucose levels and A1C result listed here are best for you. Both ways of checking your blood glucose levels are important.

If your blood glucose levels are not on target, you might need a change in how you take care of your diabetes. The results of your A1C test and your daily blood glucose checks can help you and your doctor make decisions about the following things:

- What you eat

- When you eat

- How much you eat

- What kind of exercise you do

- How much exercise you do

- The type of diabetes medicines you take

- The amount of diabetes medicines you take

What Happens to Blood Glucose Levels in People with Diabetes?

Blood glucose levels go up and down throughout the day and night in people with diabetes. High blood glucose levels over time can result in heart disease and other health problems. Low blood glucose levels can make you feel shaky or pass out. But you can learn how to make sure your blood glucose levels stay on target—not too high and not too low.

What Makes Blood Glucose Levels Go Too High?

Your blood glucose levels can go too high if the following are true:

- You eat more than usual
- You're not physically active
- You're not taking enough diabetes medicine
- You're sick or under stress
- You exercise when your blood glucose level is already high

Some diabetes medicines can also lower your blood glucose too much. Ask your doctor whether your diabetes medicines can cause low blood glucose.

Medicines for My Diabetes

Medicines for Type 1 Diabetes

Type 1 diabetes, once called juvenile diabetes or insulin-dependent diabetes, is usually first found in children, teenagers, or young adults. If you have type 1 diabetes, you must take insulin because your body no longer makes it. You also might need to take other types of diabetes medicines that work with insulin.

Medicines for Type 2 Diabetes

Type 2 diabetes, once called adult-onset diabetes or non-insulin-dependent diabetes, is the most common form of diabetes. It can start when the body doesn't use insulin as it should, a condition called insulin resistance. If the body can't keep up with the need for insulin, you may need diabetes medicines. Many choices are available. Your doctor might prescribe two or more medicines. The ADA recommends that most people start with metformin, a kind of diabetes pill.

Medicines for Gestational Diabetes

Gestational diabetes is diabetes that occurs for the first time during pregnancy. The hormones of pregnancy or a shortage of insulin can cause gestational diabetes. Most women with gestational diabetes control it with meal planning and physical activity. But some women need insulin to reach their target blood glucose levels.

Medicines for Other Types of Diabetes

If you have one of the rare forms of diabetes, such as diabetes caused by other medicines or monogenic diabetes, talk with your doctor about what kind of diabetes medicine would be best for you.

Types of Diabetes Medicines

Diabetes medicines come in several forms.

Insulin

If your body no longer makes enough insulin, you'll need to take it. Insulin is used for all types of diabetes. Your doctor can help you decide which way of taking insulin is best for you.

Taking injections. You'll give yourself shots using a needle and syringe. The syringe is a hollow tube with a plunger. You will put your dose of insulin into the tube. Some people use an insulin pen, which looks like a pen but has a needle for its point.

Using an insulin pump. An insulin pump is a small machine about the size of a cell phone, worn outside of your body on a belt or in a pocket or pouch. The pump connects to a small plastic tube and a very small needle. The needle is inserted under the skin and stays in for several days. Insulin is pumped from the machine through the tube into your body.

Using an insulin jet injector. The jet injector, which looks like a large pen, sends a fine spray of insulin through the skin with high-pressure air instead of a needle.

What Does Insulin Do?

Insulin helps keep blood glucose levels on target by moving glucose from the blood into your body's cells. Your cells then use glucose for energy. In people who don't have diabetes, the body makes the right amount of insulin on its own. But when you have diabetes, you and your doctor must decide how much insulin you need throughout the day and night.

What Are the Possible Side Effects of Insulin?

Possible side effects include the following:

- Low blood glucose
- Weight gain

How and When Should I Take My Insulin?

Your plan for taking insulin will depend on your daily routine and your type of insulin. Some people with diabetes who use insulin need to take it two, three, or four times a day to reach their blood glucose targets. Others can take a single shot. Your doctor or diabetes educator will help you learn how and when to give yourself insulin.

Types of Insulin

Each type of insulin works at a different speed. For example, rapid-acting insulin starts to work right after you take it. Long-acting insulin works for many hours. Most people need two or more types of insulin to reach their blood glucose targets.

Diabetes Pills

Along with meal planning and physical activity, diabetes pills help people with type 2 diabetes or gestational diabetes keep their blood glucose levels on target . Several kinds of pills are available. Each works in a different way. Many people take two or three kinds of pills. Some people take combination pills. Combination pills contain two kinds of diabetes medicine in one tablet. Some people take pills and insulin.

Your doctor may ask you to try one kind of pill. If it doesn't help you reach your blood glucose targets, your doctor may ask you to do one or more of the following:

- Take more of the same pill
- Add another kind of pill
- Change to another type of pill
- Start taking insulin
- Start taking another injected medicine

If your doctor suggests that you take insulin or another injected medicine, it doesn't mean your diabetes is getting worse. Instead, it means you need insulin or another type of medicine to reach your blood glucose targets. Everyone is different. What works best for you depends on your usual daily routine, eating habits, and activities, and your other health conditions.

Injections Other Than Insulin

In addition to insulin, two other types of injected medicines are now available. Both work with insulin—either the body's own or injected— to help keep your blood glucose from going too high after you eat. Neither is a substitute for insulin.

What Do I Need to Know about Side Effects of Medicines?

A side effect is an unwanted problem caused by a medicine. For example, some diabetes medicines can cause nausea or an upset stomach when you first start taking them. Before you start a new medicine, ask your doctor about possible side effects and how you can avoid them. If the side effects of your medicine bother you, tell your doctor.

Chapter 18

Oral Diabetes Medications

Alpha-Glucosidase Inhibitors

Table 18.1. Types of Alpha-Glucosidase Inhibitors

Brand Name	Generic Name
Glyset®	miglitol
Precose®	acarbose

What Does This Type of Pill Do?

This type of pill helps keep your blood glucose from going too high after you eat, a common problem in people with diabetes. It works by slowing down the digestion of foods high in carbohydrates, such as rice, potatoes, bread, milk, and fruit.

Who Should Not Take Glyset or Precose?

Talk with your doctor about whether to take this type of pill if any of the following are true:

- You have bowel disease or other intestinal conditions

- You have advanced kidney or liver disease

- You are pregnant, planning to get pregnant, or breastfeeding

---

Excerpted from "What I Need to Know about Diabetes Medicines," National Institute of Diabetes and Digestive and Kidney Diseases, National Institutes of Health, NIH Publication No. 08-4222, March 2008.

What Are the Possible Side Effects?

This type of pill doesn't cause low blood glucose by itself. But your risk of having low blood glucose goes up if you also take either of the following:

- Diabetes pills that cause low blood glucose

- Insulin

Your doctor may ask you to take a lower dose of your other diabetes medicines while you take this type of pill.

Taking Glyset or Precose may cause stomach pain, gas, bloating, or diarrhea. These symptoms usually go away after you have taken these pills for a while.

If You Take Glyset or Precose: What You Need to Know about Low Blood Glucose

If you take Glyset or Precose, only glucose tablets or glucose gel will bring your blood glucose level back to normal quickly. Other quick-fix foods and drinks won't raise your blood glucose as quickly because Glyset and Precose slow the digestion of other quick-fix foods and drinks.

Biguanide

Table 18.2. Types of Biguanides

Brand Name	Generic Name
Glucophage®	metformin
Glucophage XR®	metformin—long-acting
Riomet®	metformin—liquid

What Does This Type of Medicine Do?

This type of medicine, which comes in pill or liquid form, lowers the amount of glucose made by your liver. Then your blood glucose levels don't go too high. This type of medicine also helps treat insulin resistance. With insulin resistance, your body doesn't use insulin the way it should. When your insulin works properly, your blood glucose levels stay on target and your cells get the energy they need. This type of medicine improves your cholesterol levels. It also may help you lose weight.

Who Should Not Take Glucophage, Glucophage XR, or Riomet?

Talk with your doctor about whether to take this type of medicine if any of the following are true:

- You have advanced kidney or liver disease

- You drink excessive amounts of alcoholic beverages

- You are pregnant, planning to get pregnant, or breastfeeding

What Are the Possible Side Effects?

This type of pill doesn't cause low blood glucose by itself. But your risk of having low blood glucose goes up if you also take either of the following:

- Diabetes pills that cause low blood glucose

- Insulin

Your doctor may ask you to take a lower dose of your other diabetes medicines while you take this type of pill.

You may have nausea, diarrhea, or an upset stomach when you first start taking this type of medicine. These side effects are likely to go away after a while.

Rarely, a serious condition called lactic acidosis occurs as a side effect of taking this medicine. Call your doctor right away if any of the following occur:

- You become weak and tired

- You become dizzy

- You feel very cold

- You have trouble breathing

- You have unusual muscle pain and stomach problems

- You have a sudden change in the speed or steadiness of your heartbeat

Sometimes you'll need to stop taking this type of medicine for a short time so you can avoid developing lactic acidosis. If you have severe vomiting, diarrhea, or a fever, or if you can't keep fluids down, call your doctor right away. You should also talk with your doctor well

149

ahead of time about stopping this type of medicine if either of the following are true:

- You'll be having special x-rays that require an injection of dye
- You'll be having surgery

Your doctor will tell you when it's safe to start taking your medicine again.

D-Phenylalanine Derivative

Table 18.3. Types of D-Phenylalanine Derivatives

Brand Name	Generic Name
Starlix®	nateglinide

What Does This Type of Pill Do?

This type of pill helps your body make more insulin for a short period of time right after meals. The insulin helps keep your blood glucose from going too high after you eat, a common problem in people with diabetes.

Who Should Not Take Starlix?

Talk with your doctor about whether to take this type of pill if either of the following are true:

- You are pregnant, planning to get pregnant, or breastfeeding
- You have liver disease

What Are the Possible Side Effects?

Possible side effects are as follows:

- Low blood glucose, also called hypoglycemia
- Weight gain
- Dizziness

Dipeptidyl Peptidase-4 (DPP-4) Inhibitors

Table 18.4. Types of Dipeptidyl Peptidase-4 (DDP-4) Inhibitors

Brand Name	Generic Name
Januvia®	sitagliptin phosphate

What Does This Type of Pill Do?

This type of pill lowers your blood glucose by helping your body make more insulin when it's needed, especially right after meals. It also helps keep your liver from putting stored glucose into your blood.

Who Should Not Take Januvia?

Talk with your doctor about whether to take this type of pill if any of the following are true:

- You are pregnant, planning to get pregnant, or breastfeeding
- You have kidney disease
- You have type 1 diabetes and you have a condition called diabetic ketoacidosis

What Are the Possible Side Effects?

This type of pill doesn't cause low blood glucose by itself. But your risk of having low blood glucose goes up if you also take either of the following:

- Diabetes pills that cause low blood glucose
- Insulin

Your doctor may ask you to take a lower dose of your other diabetes medicines while you take this type of pill.

Possible side effects are as follows:

- A cold
- Runny nose
- Sore throat
- Headache

If you take Januvia and have kidney problems, your healthcare provider might order blood tests to see how well your kidneys are working.

Meglitinides

Table 18.5. Types of Meglitinides

Brand Name	Generic Name
Prandin®	repaglinide

What Does This Type of Pill Do?

This type of pill helps your body make more insulin for a short period of time right after meals. The insulin helps keep your blood glucose from going too high after you eat, a common problem in people with diabetes.

Who Should Not Take Prandin?

Talk with your doctor about whether to take this type of pill if either of the following are true:

- You are pregnant, planning to get pregnant, or breastfeeding
- You have liver disease

What Are the Possible Side Effects?

Prandin can cause the following:

- Low blood glucose, also called hypoglycemia
- Weight gain
- Upset stomach
- Back pain or a headache

Sulfonylureas

Table 18.6. Types of Sulfonylureas

Brand Name	Generic Name
Amaryl®	glimepiride
DiaBeta®	glyburide
Diabinese®	chlorpropamide
Glucotrol®	glipizide
Glucotrol XL®	glipizide (long-acting)
Glynase®	glyburide
Micronase®	glyburide

Available only in generic form:

tolazamide

tolbutamide

What Does This Type of Pill Do?

This type of pill helps your body make more insulin. The insulin helps lower your blood glucose.

Who Should Not Take Sulfonylureas?

Talk with your doctor about whether to take this type of pill if either of the following are true:

- You are allergic to sulfa drugs
- You are pregnant, planning to get pregnant, or breastfeeding

What Are the Possible Side Effects?

Possible side effects include the following:

- Low blood glucose, also called hypoglycemia
- Upset stomach
- Skin rash
- Weight gain

Thiazolidinediones

Table 18.7. Types of Thiazolidinediones

Brand Name	Generic Name
Actos®	pioglitazone
Avandia®	rosiglitazone

What Does This Type of Pill Do?

This type of pill helps treat insulin resistance. With insulin resistance, your body doesn't use insulin the way it should. Thiazolidinediones help your insulin work properly. Then your blood glucose levels stay on target and your cells get the energy they need.

Who Should Not Take Actos or Avandia?

If you have heart failure, you should not take this type of pill. This type of pill can cause congestive heart failure or make it worse.

Studies have shown that Avandia is associated with an increased risk for heart attacks and chest pain or discomfort from blocked blood vessels.

This type of pill can cause congestive heart failure. Congestive heart failure is a condition in which your heart no longer pumps properly. Then your body keeps too much fluid in your legs, ankles, and lungs.

If you already have congestive heart failure, this type of pill can make it worse.

Call your doctor right away if you have signs of heart failure. Warning signs include the following:

- Having swelling in your legs or ankles

- Gaining a lot of weight in a short time

- Having trouble breathing

- Having a cough

- Being very tired

You should also talk with your doctor about whether to take this type of pill if either of the following are true:

- You are pregnant, planning to get pregnant, or breastfeeding

- You have liver disease

What Are the Possible Side Effects?

Congestive heart failure is the most serious side effect.

This type of pill doesn't cause low blood glucose by itself. But your risk of having low blood glucose goes up if you also take either of the following:

- Diabetes pills that cause low blood glucose

- Insulin

Your doctor may ask you to take a lower dose of your other diabetes medicines while you take this type of pill.

Possible side effects, in addition to the side effects related to heart failure, are as follows:

- Anemia, a condition that can make you feel very tired

- An increased risk of getting pregnant even if you're taking birth control pills

Women who take Actos, Avandia, or combination diabetes pills containing pioglitazone or rosiglitazone may have an increased risk of bone fractures.

If you take Actos or Avandia, your healthcare provider should make sure your liver is working properly. Call your doctor right away if you have any signs of liver disease: nausea, vomiting, stomach pain, tiredness, dark-colored urine, or loss of appetite.

Combination Diabetes Pills

Combination pills contain two different types of diabetes medications. Several combination pills are available. They are shown in Table 18.8.

Table 18.8. Types of Combination Diabetes Pills

Brand Name	Generic Name
Actoplus Met®	pioglitazone + metformin
Avandamet®	rosiglitazone + metformin
Avandaryl®	rosiglitazone + glimepiride
Duetact®	pioglitazone + glimepiride
Glucovance®	glyburide + metformin
Janumet®	sitagliptin + metformin
Metaglip®	glipizide + metformin

What Does Actoplus Met Do?

Actoplus Met is a combination of two types of pills. One pill lowers the amount of glucose made by your liver. Both types help your insulin work the way it should.

What Does Avandamet Do?

Avandamet is a combination of two types of pills. One pill lowers the amount of glucose made by your liver. Both types help your insulin work the way it should.

What Does Avandaryl Do?

Avandaryl is a combination of two types of pills. One pill helps your insulin work the way it should. The other pill helps your body make more insulin.

What Does Duetact Do?

Duetact is a combination of two types of pills. One pill helps your insulin work the way it should. The other pill helps your body make more insulin.

What Does Glucovance Do?

Glucovance is a combination of two types of pills. One pill helps your body make more insulin. The other pill lowers the amount of glucose made by your liver and helps your insulin work the way it should.

What Does Janumet Do?

Janumet is a combination of two types of pills. One pill helps your body make more insulin when it's needed, especially right after meals. It also helps keep your liver from putting stored glucose into your blood. The other pill lowers the amount of glucose made by your liver and helps your insulin work the way it should.

What does Metaglip do?

Metaglip is a combination of two types of pills. One pill helps your body make more insulin. The other pill lowers the amount of glucose made by your liver and helps your insulin work the way it should.

Chapter 19

Injectable Non-Insulin Diabetes Medications

Amylin Mimetic

Table 19.1. Types of Amylin Mimetics

Brand Name	Generic Name
Symlin®	pramlintide acetate

What Does This Medicine Do?

Symlin helps keep your blood glucose from going too high after you eat, a common problem in people with diabetes. It works by helping food move more slowly through your stomach. Symlin helps keep your liver from putting stored glucose into your blood. It also may prevent hunger, helping you eat less and maybe lose weight.

Symlin is for people who already take insulin. However, you should always use a separate syringe to inject Symlin. Symlin is not used in place of insulin, but taking Symlin may change the amount of insulin you take.

Who Should Not Take Symlin?

Talk with your doctor about whether you should take this type of medicine if any of the following are true:

Excerpted from "What I Need to Know about Diabetes Medicines," National Institute of Diabetes and Digestive and Kidney Diseases, National Institutes of Health, NIH Publication No. 08-4222, March 2008.

157

- You can't tell when you are having low blood glucose, a condition called hypoglycemia unawareness

- You have recently had severe low blood glucose

- You have stomach problems caused by diabetes-related nerve damage

- You are pregnant, planning to get pregnant, or breastfeeding

Symlin has not been studied for use in children.

There may be times when you should not take your usual dose of Symlin. If you're having surgery or you're sick and can't eat, you should not take your Symlin. Ask your doctor about other times to not take it.

What Are the Possible Side Effects?

Symlin can cause the following:

- Nausea and vomiting—most often when you first start taking Symlin

- Swelling, redness, or itching of the skin where Symlin is injected

- Headache

- Decreased appetite

- Stomach pain and indigestion

- Tiredness

- Dizziness

This type of medicine doesn't cause low blood glucose by itself, but your risk of having low blood glucose is higher because Symlin is always taken along with insulin.

Incretin Mimetic

Table 19.2. Types of Incretin Mimetics

Brand Name	Generic Name
Byetta®	exenatide

What Does This Medicine Do?

Byetta helps your body make more insulin when it's needed. It helps keep your blood glucose from going too high after you eat, a common problem in people with diabetes. It works by helping food move more slowly through your stomach. Byetta helps keep your liver from putting stored glucose into your blood. It also may prevent hunger, helping you eat less and maybe lose weight.

Byetta is not used in place of insulin.

Who Should Not Take Byetta?

Talk with your doctor about whether you should take this type of medicine if any of the following are true:

- You have severe stomach or digestive problems
- You have any symptoms of kidney disease or are on dialysis
- You are pregnant, planning to get pregnant, or breastfeeding
- You have type 1 diabetes

Byetta has not been studied for use in children.

What Are the Possible Side Effects?

Byetta can cause the following:

- Nausea and vomiting—most often when you first start taking Byetta
- Headache
- Diarrhea
- Dizziness

Byetta also can cause an acid stomach or make you feel nervous.

If You Take Byetta: What You Need to Know about Problems with Your Kidneys

Talk with your doctor right away if you notice any of the following:

- Changes in the color of your urine, how often you urinate, or the amount you urinate
- Swelling of your hands or feet
- Tiredness
- Changes in your appetite or digestion
- A dull ache in your mid to lower back

This type of medicine doesn't cause low blood glucose by itself, but your risk of having low blood glucose goes up if you also take either of the following:

- Diabetes pills that cause low blood glucose
- Insulin

Your doctor may ask you to take a lower dose of your other diabetes medicines while you take this type of medicine.

Chapter 20

Insulin Basics

The ultimate goal of insulin therapy is to mimic normal insulin levels. Unfortunately, current insulin replacement therapy can only approximate normal insulin levels. Insulin therapy for diabetes ranges from one injection a day to multiple injections and using an insulin pump (continuous subcutaneous insulin infusion—CSII). The more frequent the insulin injections, the better the approximation of natural or normal insulin levels. Discuss with your medical provider the insulin regimen that is best for you.

Normal or Non-Diabetic Blood Sugar Levels and Insulin Release from the Pancreas

Natural insulin (i.e., insulin released from your pancreas) keeps your blood sugar in a very narrow range. Overnight and between meals, the normal, non-diabetic blood sugar ranges between 60–100mg/dl and 140 mg/dl or less after meals and snacks.

To keep the blood sugar controlled overnight, during fasting, and between meals, your body releases a low, background level of insulin. When you eat, there is a large burst of insulin. This surge of insulin is needed to dispose of all the carbohydrate or sugar that is getting absorbed from your meal. All of this happens automatically!

More about Natural Insulin Release

Insulin is continuously released from the pancreas into the bloodstream. Although the insulin is quickly destroyed (five to six minutes) the effect on cells may last one to one and a half hours. When your body needs more insulin, the blood levels quickly rise, and the converse— when you need less, the blood levels rapidly fall. The situation is different when you have diabetes and are getting insulin replacement therapy. Once you have injected a dose of insulin, it is going to get absorbed into your bloodstream whether you need it or not.

At mealtime, a little insulin is released even as you are first smelling or chewing the food. This gets your body ready to receive the sugar load from the meal. Then as you eat and the food is digested, the sugar levels rise, which causes a surge of insulin. The insulin levels rapidly climb and peak in about forty-five minutes to one hour before falling back to the background or basal levels. The situation is different when you have diabetes and are getting insulin replacement therapy. You have to calculate how much carbohydrate you are going to eat and how much insulin you will need. And you have to try to mimic natural overnight fasting (or between meals) and mealtime insulin release with injected insulin.

Principles of Insulin Replacement

When you have diabetes and don't have enough of your own insulin, or cannot take other medications to control your blood sugar, you will need to start insulin therapy.

The insulin therapy tries to mimic natural or non-diabetic insulin secretion. There are two components of insulin therapy.

Background or Basal Insulin Replacement

- Controls glucose overnight and between meals by keeping fat in fat tissue and curbing glucose production from the liver.

- Provides a low, continuous level of insulin.

- Can be a long-acting insulin, which you inject once or twice daily such as the insulin analogs, insulin glargine, insulin detemir, and NPH.

- Or can be a rapid-acting insulin continuously infused under the skin, if you are using an insulin pump.

- Represents about 50 percent or half of the body's daily insulin requirements.

Bolus Insulin Replacement

There are two kinds of bolus replacement:

- **Mealtime bolus:** To cover the carbohydrate in the meal or snack.

- **High blood sugar correction bolus:** Provides extra insulin to return the blood sugar back to the target level when your blood sugar is too high.

Bolus insulin is usually provided by rapid-acting insulin analogs, such as insulin aspart, insulin Lispro, and insulin glulisine or regular insulin.

This represents about 10 to 20 percent of the daily insulin requirement at each meal, or about 50 percent of the body's daily insulin needs.

Some people with diabetes need just background/basal insulin replacement, others will need just bolus insulin replacement, and still others will need both basal and bolus insulin schedules. Talk with your provider about the insulin regimen that is most suitable for you.

Chapter 21

Types of Insulin

Human insulin and insulin analogs are available for insulin replacement therapy. Insulins also are classified by the timing of their action in your body—specifically, how quickly they start to act, when they have a maximal effect, and how long they act.

Insulin analogs have been developed because human insulins have limitations when injected under the skin. In high concentrations, such as in a vial or cartridge, human (and also animal insulin) clumps together. This clumping causes slow and unpredictable absorption from the subcutaneous tissue and a dose-dependent duration of action (i.e. the larger the dose, the longer the effect or duration). In contrast, insulin analogs have a more predictable duration of action. The rapid-acting insulin analogs work more quickly, and the long-acting insulin analogs last longer and have a more even, "peakless" effect.

Background

Insulin has been available since 1925. It was initially extracted from beef and pork pancreases. In the early 1980s, technology became available to produce human insulin synthetically. Synthetic human insulin has replaced beef and pork insulin in the United States. And now, insulin analogs are replacing human insulin.

Characteristics of Insulin

Insulins are categorized by differences in:

- Onset (how quickly they act).

- Peak (how long it takes to achieve maximum impact).

- Duration (how long they last before they wear off).

- Concentration (Insulins sold in the United States have a concentration of 100 units per ml or U100. In other countries, additional concentrations are available. Note: If you purchase insulin abroad, be sure it is U100.)

- Route of delivery (whether they are injected under the skin or given intravenously).

Insulin is usually injected into the fatty tissue just under the skin. This is also called subcutaneous tissue.

Table 21.1. shows how the different types of insulins act.

Types of Insulin

There are three main groups of insulins: fast-acting, intermediate-acting, and long-acting insulin.

Fast-Acting Insulin

Fast-acting insulin:

- is absorbed quickly from your fat tissue (subcutaneous) into the bloodstream;

- is used to control the blood sugar during meals and snacks and to correct high blood sugars;

- includes rapid-acting insulin analogs and regular human insulin.

Rapid-acting insulin analogs. Rapid-acting insulin analogs (insulin aspart, insulin lispro, insulin glulisine) have an onset of action of five to fifteen minutes, peak effect in one to two hours, and duration of action that lasts four to six hours. With all doses, large and small, the onset of action and the time to peak effect is similar, The duration of insulin action is, however, affected by the dose—so a few units may last four hours or less, while twenty-five or thirty units may last five to six hours. As a general rule, assume that these insulins have duration of action of four hours.

Regular human insulin. Regular human insulin has an onset of action of one half hour to one hour, peak effect in two to four hours, and duration of action of six to eight hours. The larger the dose the faster the onset of action, but the longer the time to peak effect and the longer the duration of the effect.

Intermediate-Acting Insulin

Intermediate-acting insulin:

- is absorbed more slowly, and lasts longer;
- is used to control the blood sugar overnight, while fasting, and between meals;
- includes NPH human insulin and pre-mixed insulin.

NPH human insulin. NPH human insulin has an onset of insulin effect of one to two hours, a peak effect of four to six hours, and duration of action of more than twelve hours. Very small doses will have an earlier peak effect and shorter duration of action, while higher doses will have a longer time to peak effect and prolonged duration.

Pre-mixed insulin. Pre-mixed insulin is NPH pre-mixed with either regular human insulin or a rapid- acting insulin analog. The insulin action profile is a combination of the short- and intermediate-acting insulins.

Long-Acting Insulin

Long-acting insulin:

- is absorbed slowly, has a minimal peak effect, and a stable plateau effect that lasts most of the day;
- is used to control the blood sugar overnight, while fasting, and between meals;
- includes long-acting insulin analogs.

Long-acting insulin analogs. Long-acting insulin analogs (insulin glargine, insulin detemir) have an onset of insulin effect in one and a half to two hours. The insulin effect plateaus over the next few hours and is followed by a relatively flat duration of action that lasts twelve to twenty-four hours for insulin detemir and twenty-four hours for insulin glargine.

Compare insulin actions in Table 21.1.

Table 21.1. Table of Insulin Action

Type of Insulin	Onset	Peak	Duration	Appearance
Fast-acting				
Regular	½–1 hr.	2–4 hr.	6–8 hr.	clear
Lispro/ Aspart/ Glulisine	<15 min.	1–2 hr.	4–6 hr.	clear
Intermediate-acting				
NPH	1–2 hr.	6–10 hr.	12+ hr.	cloudy
Long-acting				
Detemir	1 hr.	Flat, Max effect in 5 hrs.	12–24 hr.	clear
Glargine	1½ hr.	Flat, Max effect in 5 hrs.	24 hr.	clear

Chapter 22

Administering Insulin Correctly

Chapter Contents

Section 22.1

Determining the Correct Dosage

Your provider will prescribe an insulin dose regimen for you; however, you still need to calculate some of your insulin doses. Your insulin dose regimen provides formulas that allow you to calculate how much bolus insulin to take at meals and snacks, or to correct high blood sugars.

First, some basic things to know about insulin.

Approximately 40 to 50 percent of the total daily insulin dose is to replace insulin overnight, when you are fasting, and between meals. This is called background or basal insulin replacement. The basal or background insulin dose usually is constant from day to day.

The other 50 to 60 percent of the total daily insulin dose is for carbohydrate coverage (food) and high blood sugar correction. This is called the bolus insulin replacement.

Bolus: Carbohydrate Coverage

The bolus dose for food coverage is prescribed as an insulin to carbohydrate ratio. The insulin to carbohydrate ratio represents how many grams of carbohydrate are covered or disposed of by one unit of insulin.

Generally, one unit of rapid-acting insulin will dispose of 12–15 grams of carbohydrate. This range can vary from 4–30 grams or more of carbohydrate depending on an individual's sensitivity to insulin. Insulin sensitivity can vary according to the time of day, from person to person, and is affected by physical activity and stress.

Bolus: High Blood Sugar Correction (Also Known as Insulin Sensitivity Factor)

The bolus dose for high blood sugar correction is defined as how much one unit of rapid-acting insulin will drop the blood sugar.

Generally, to correct a high blood sugar, one unit of insulin is needed to drop the blood glucose by 50 mg/dl. This drop in blood sugar can range from 15–100 mg/dl or more, depending on individual insulin sensitivities, and other circumstances.

Examples

Read some examples and therapeutic principles on how to calculate the carbohydrate coverage dose, high blood sugar correction dose, and the total mealtime insulin dose.

Example #1: Carbohydrate Coverage at a Meal

First, you have to calculate the carbohydrate coverage insulin dose using this formula: CHO insulin dose = Total grams of carbohydrate (CHO) in the meal ÷ grams of CHO disposed by 1 unit of insulin (the grams of CHO disposed of by 1 unit of insulin is the bottom number or denominator of the Insulin:CHO ratio).

For Example #1, assume:

- you are going to eat 60 grams of carbohydrate for lunch;

- your insulin: CHO ratio is 1:10.

To get the CHO insulin dose, plug the numbers into the formula: CHO insulin dose = Total grams of CHO in the meal (60 g) ÷ grams of CHO disposed by 1 unit of insulin (10) = 6 units.

You will need 6 units of rapid-acting insulin to cover the carbohydrate.

Example #2: High Blood Sugar Correction Dose

Next, you have to calculate the high blood sugar correction dose.

High blood sugar correction dose = (Actual blood sugar – target blood sugar) ÷ correction factor.

For Example #2, assume:

- 1 unit will drop your blood sugar 50 points (mg/dl) and the high blood sugar correction factor is 50;

- pre-meal blood sugar target is 120 mg/dl;

- your actual blood sugar before lunch is 220 mg/dl.

Now, calculate the difference between your actual blood sugar and target blood sugar: 220 – 120 mg/dl = 100 mg/dl.

To get the high blood sugar correction insulin dose, plug the numbers into this formula: Correction dose = Difference between actual and target blood glucose (100mg/dl) ÷ correction factor (50) = 2 units of rapid-acting insulin.

So, you will need an additional 2 units of rapid acting insulin to "correct" the blood sugar down to a target of 120 mg/dl.

Example #3: Total Mealtime Dose

Finally, to get the total mealtime insulin dose, add the CHO insulin dose together with the high blood sugar correction insulin dose: CHO Insulin Dose + High Blood Sugar Correction Dose = Total Meal Insulin Dose.

For Example #3, assume:

- the carbohydrate coverage dose is 6 units of rapid-acting insulin;

- the high blood sugar correction dose is 2 units of rapid-acting insulin.

Now, add the two doses together to calculate your total meal dose. Carbohydrate coverage dose (6 units) + high sugar correction dose (2 units) = 8 units total meal dose!

The total lunch insulin dose is 8 units of rapid-acting insulin.

Example #4: Formulas Commonly Used to Create Insulin Dose Recommendations

This example illustrates a method for calculating your background/basal and bolus doses and estimated daily insulin dose when you need full insulin replacement. Bear in mind, this may be too much insulin if you are newly diagnosed or still making a lot of insulin on your own. And it may be too little if you are very resistant to the action of insulin. Talk to your provider about the best insulin dose for you as this is a general formula and may not meet your individual needs.

The initial calculation of the basal/background and bolus doses requires estimating your total daily insulin dose.

Total Daily Insulin Requirement

The general calculation for the body's daily insulin requirement is: Total Daily Insulin Requirement(in units of insulin) = Weight in Pounds ÷ 4.

Alternatively, if you measure your body weight in kilograms: Total Daily Insulin Requirement (in units of insulin) = 0.55 x Total Weight in Kilograms.

Example 1

If you are measuring your body weight in pounds: Assume you weigh 160 lbs.

In this example: TOTAL DAILY INSULIN DOSE = 160 lb ÷ 4 = 40 units of insulin/day.

Example 2

If you are measuring your body weight in kilograms: Assume your weight is 70Kg.

In this example: TOTAL DAILY INSULIN DOSE = 0.55 x 70 Kg = 38.5 units of insulin/day.

If your body is very resistant to insulin, you may require a higher dose. If your body is sensitive to insulin, you may require a lower insulin dose.

Basal/Background and Bolus Insulin Doses

Next, you need to establish the basal/background dose, carbohydrate coverage dose (insulin to carbohydrate ratio), and high blood sugar correction dose (correction factor).

Basal/Background Insulin Dose

Basal/background Insulin Dose = 40–50% of Total Daily Insulin Dose
Example:

- Assume you weigh 160 pounds.

- Your total daily insulin dose (TDI) = 160 lbs ÷ 4 = 40 units.

In this example: Basal/background insulin dose = 50% of TDI (40 units) = 20 units of either long-acting insulin,(such as glargine or detemir) or rapid-acting insulin if you are using an insulin pump (continuous subcutaneous insulin infusion device).

The Carbohydrate Coverage Ratio

500 ÷ Total Daily Insulin Dose = 1 unit insulin covers so many grams of carbohydrate

This can be calculated using the Rule of "500."
Example:

- Assume your total daily insulin dose (TDI) = 160 lbs ÷ 4 = 40 units

In this example: Carbohydrate coverage ratio = 500 ÷ TDI (40 units) = 1 unit insulin/ 12 g CHO.

This example assumes that you have a constant response to insulin throughout the day. In reality, individual insulin sensitivity varies. Someone who is resistant in the morning, but sensitive at midday, will need to adjust the insulin-to-carbohydrate ratio at different mealtimes. In such a case, the background insulin dose would still be approximately 20 units; however, the insulin-to-carbohydrate ratio might be breakfast 1:8 grams, lunch 1:15 grams, and dinner 1:12 grams.

The High Blood Sugar Correction Factor

Correction Factor = 1,800 ÷Total Daily Insulin Dose = 1 unit of insulin will reduce the blood sugar so many mg/dl
This can be calculated using the Rule of "1800."
Example:

- Assume your total daily insulin dose(TDI) = 160 lbs ÷ 4 = 40 units.

In this example: Correction Factor = 1,800 ÷ TDI(40 units) = 1 unit insulin will drop reduce the blood sugar level by 45 mg/dl.

While the calculation is 1 unit will drop the blood sugar 45 mg/dl, to make it easier most people will round up or round down the number so the suggested correction factor may be 1 unit of rapid-acting insulin will drop the blood sugar 40–50 mg/dl.

Please keep in mind, the estimated insulin regimen is an initial "best guess" and the dose may need to be modified to keep your blood sugar on target.

Also, there are many variations of insulin therapy. You will need to work out your specific insulin requirements and dose regimen with your medical provider and diabetes team.

Section 22.2

How to Give an Insulin Injection

"How to Give an Insulin Injection," August 2010, reprinted with permission from www.kidshealth.org. Copyright © 2010 The Nemours Foundation. This information was provided by KidsHealth, one of the largest resources online for medically reviewed health information written for parents, kids, and teens. For more articles like this one, visit www.KidsHealth.org, or www .TeensHealth.org.

1. Get the supplies you'll need:

    - Insulin bottle
    - Syringe
    - Alcohol swabs
    - Container for the used syringe

2. Wash your hands.

3. Check the insulin bottle to make sure it hasn't expired.

4. Remove the lid from the insulin bottle.

5. Wipe the rubber top of the bottle with an alcohol swab.

6. Remove the cap from the syringe.

7. Pull air into the syringe by pulling back on the plunger until its black tip is even with the line showing the dose you'll need.

8. Push the needle through the rubber top of the bottle.

9. Push the plunger so that the air goes from the syringe into the bottle.

10. Turn the insulin bottle and syringe upside down. To pull insulin into the syringe, slowly pull back on the plunger until the top of its black tip is even with the line showing your dose.

11. The most common places to inject insulin are the abdomen (belly), the back of the upper arms, the upper buttocks, and the outer thighs. Choose a place to make the injection, and wipe the skin with an alcohol swab.

12. Gently pinch the skin. Hold the syringe at a ninety-degree angle to the skin, and push the needle all the way in.

13. Let go of the pinched skin, and slowly push the plunger to inject all of the insulin. Wait about five seconds before pulling out the needle. Don't just put the used syringe in the trash. Instead, put it in a plastic or metal container with a tight lid. When the container is full, be sure the lid is closed and put it in the trash.

Chapter 23

External Insulin Pumps

In a healthy person, the pancreas constantly monitors blood sugar, and adjusts its insulin production to maintain a normal blood sugar range. In diabetes, this carefully regulated system has broken down, and insulin from external sources is often needed.

All type 1 diabetics, and some type 2 diabetics, take insulin to control their sugars. However, this often requires multiple daily injections, and doesn't allow for fine control. Insulin pumps have been developed to mimic natural pancreatic function.

The Insulin Pump Device

There are several different models of insulin pumps available. While details differ from pump to pump, all have the same basic elements:

- An insulin solution reservoir

- A pump able to give precise doses of insulin solution

- A tiny, battery-powered computer to control the pump

The devices are about the size of a pager or a small cell phone, and are usually worn on clothing or a belt near the waist. They have a small display screen and multiple control buttons for monitoring and programming the pump.

"Insulin Pumps," by David A. Cooke, M.D., FACP, © 2011 Omnigraphics, Inc.

Insulin flows out of the pump through thin tubing to a plastic needle implanted beneath the skin. The patient can place and remove the plastic needles at home, so the infusion site can be changed every few days.

What Are the Advantages of an Insulin Pump?

Insulin pumps deliver a continuous flow of insulin into the body, which allows for more precise control. Insulin flow can be turned up after a meal and turned down when going to bed. It can be turned down before exercise and turned up before dessert.

Properly timed and dosed injections can mimic normal insulin release patterns. However, there are some diabetics for whom this does not work well. Diabetics with varying work schedules or who travel frequently may be unable to match their injections to their needs.

Some diabetics are able to achieve far better blood sugar control with insulin pumps than with injections. The ability to change insulin levels hour-to-hour may result in fewer episodes of hypoglycemia and less spiking of sugar levels after meals. This can greatly reduce diabetic complications and allow for a more flexible lifestyle.

What Are the Disadvantages of an Insulin Pump?

Pumps are not "set it and forget it" devices. While complex schedules can be programmed into the pumps, frequent glucose monitoring and adjustments are needed. For example, the pump user needs to manually trigger extra doses of insulin at mealtime (boluses), and estimate the required insulin dose. Failing to trigger mealtime boluses or miscalculating insulin requirements will cause wide swings in blood sugars.

Pump users need to be educated about their diabetes and highly motivated. It is necessary to check blood sugars four to eight times a day or more to guide pump adjustments. They are not usually good options for diabetics with limited understanding of their disease, or those who are not technically inclined. Pumps may also not work well for diabetics with poor vision or ability to use their fingers, due to the need to view a small display and operate small buttons.

Insulin pumps are subject to various mechanical complications. The infusion tubing can disconnect from the device, pull out of the skin, or become kinked, all of which can seriously impact glucose control. Pumps can also fail or break, and cannot be exposed to water or strong magnetic fields.

Insulin pumps are very expensive. An insulin pump may cost $10,000 to $20,000 or more, and not all insurers are willing to pay for them. There are high costs associated with the insulin, tubing, needles, and testing supplies needed for using the pump.

As a practical matter, pumps are unaffordable for those without health insurance, or for those with plans that have high co-pays for diabetic supplies. Insurers almost invariably also require documentation that the patient has tried and failed to control their diabetes with insulin injections before they will pay for a pump.

"Closed Loop" Insulin Pumps

The ideal insulin pump would continuously monitor glucose levels and adjust insulin output on its own. No such pump currently exists. However, advances in technology have brought us closer to this goal.

Continuous glucose monitoring systems have recently become available that automatically and frequently measure glucose levels. A small glucose sensor is implanted beneath the skin and lasts several days at a time. These systems can provide nearly "real time" updates in blood sugars.

Pumps paired with a continuous glucose monitoring system are often called "closed loop" systems. The glucose sensor sends information wirelessly to the pump, and sugar readings are displayed on the device's control screen. This makes it easier to adjust the pump settings and quickly judge results.

While promising, this technology still has significant limitations. The continuous sensors do not actually measure glucose levels in the blood, but rather levels in fluid beneath the skin. This tends to be similar to blood glucose levels, but may be inaccurate when blood sugars are rising or falling rapidly. The continuous sensors also require calibration several times per day with conventional blood glucose meters, so they don't eliminate the need for finger stick readings.

Current systems also still require the user to adjust the insulin flow in response to the glucose readings. Engineers have not yet been able to design a pump capable of properly adjusting insulin doses without human input.

Not surprisingly, using a continuous glucose monitoring system also increases the cost of insulin pump therapy. It is possible that these devices improve quality of life and diabetic complications enough to make them cost-effective. However, this has not been proven, and not all insurers will pay for these systems until they have been convincingly shown to improve outcomes.

Future Directions for Insulin Pumps

Insulin pump technology has been evolving rapidly, and it is likely that future devices will be far superior to anything currently available. Further improvements in continuous glucose monitoring systems may reduce lag and increase durability, which will improve their utility in "closed loop" systems. Insulin pumps that can be permanently implanted within the body are also under development, and might be better solutions than the current external pumps. It is also possible that computer software will be developed that will allow the pump to fully self-adjust its insulin output, allowing for an "artificial pancreas." Active research is underway in all of these areas.

Should I Get an Insulin Pump?

If you are using insulin injections to control your blood sugars with good results, there is no reason to switch to a pump. However, if you have frequent and dangerous swings in your sugars, or have a very irregular schedule, a pump might be a better solution for you.

At this point, nearly all insulin pump users are type 1 diabetics. Type 2 diabetics generally need much larger insulin doses than type 1 patients, and this can be impractical with a pump. However, certain type 2 diabetics may be pump candidates.

Your physician can probably tell you whether you should consider a pump. If he or she thinks you might benefit, you will most likely be referred to an "insulin pump clinic" for evaluation. Physicians at these clinics have special training in the use of insulin pump systems. They can perform an individual assessment and decide whether you are likely to succeed with a pump. They can also determine which pump system will be best suited to your needs.

Chapter 24

Emerging and Alternative Insulin Delivery Systems

Chapter Contents

181

Section 24.1

Insulin Inhalers

A new form of inhaled insulin appears to help people with diabetes who must use insulin, with fewer potential risks than an earlier form of inhaled insulin that is no longer on the market.

The new drug, Afrezza®, which is awaiting approval from the U.S. Food and Drug Administration (FDA), works faster, keeps blood sugar levels at a closer to normal level, and has less risk of causing low blood sugar levels (hypoglycemia) than currently available injectable insulins, researchers say. It also appears to have less risk of causing lung problems than its inhaled predecessor, Exubera®.

"Afrezza is an ultra-rapid-acting insulin, and clinical studies have shown us that it has the potential to change diabetes therapy, because in the body, Afrezza looks like the insulin that's normally in a person's body," said Andrea Leone-Bay, vice president of pharmaceutical development for MannKind Corp., manufacturer of Afrezza.

"Afrezza differs a lot from Exubera," she said, both in the way it's made and in the way it works.

Afrezza uses a novel technology called Technosphere, according to Leone-Bay. It's inhaled as a dry powder that dissolves in the lungs. The particles then pass through the lungs into the bloodstream and begin acting almost immediately. Afrezza's action peaks about twelve to fifteen minutes after inhalation, instead of the forty-five to sixty minutes it takes for Exubera to peak, she said.

That fast action helps to keep after-meal blood sugar levels lower, which is a goal for people with diabetes. And Afrezza is less likely to cause hypoglycemia, a common problem that occurs when insulin levels are higher than required for a meal.

The idea of an inhaled insulin appeals to diabetics who must use insulin every time they eat. Currently, the only way to get that insulin is through injection or an insulin pump that must be inserted in a new site under the skin every few days.

In 2006, the first inhaled insulin, Exubera, received FDA approval. However, the drug was pulled from the market in October 2007 by its manufacturer, Pfizer, because of disappointing sales. From the beginning, concerns surfaced about the effects the drug might have on the lungs. One study found a reduction in lung function for some, but of more concern was an increased risk of lung cancer associated with its use. This finding came after Exubera had been pulled from the market, and the sample size wasn't large enough to draw a definitive link between the drug and the increased risk of lung cancer.

Leone-Bay said that cancer studies have been conducted on Afrezza in rats. The rats got a much higher inhalation dose than humans would take, and the researchers didn't find an increase in lung cancer. She said these types of studies weren't done on Exubera.

"They have done the required safety studies and come out clean, but it's only been tested for six months, so long-term isn't known," said Sanjoy Dutta, director of the insulin initiative at the Juvenile Diabetes Research Foundation.

Dutta confirmed that Afrezza is fast acting and less likely to cause low blood sugar. "Just as quickly as it has an onset of action, it also has a quick off mechanism. It doesn't stay around long enough to cause hypoglycemia," he said.

While Afrezza looks promising, it can't replace all injections for people with diabetes. Because it's fast acting, it can't provide the long action of insulin known as basal insulin. It will only replace mealtime insulin.

Afrezza may have an impact on lung function, but Leone-Bay said once people stopped taking Afrezza, this effect went away. The company is conducting clinical trials to assess Afrezza in people with asthma.

Leone-Bay was to explain the Technosphere technology at the American Chemical Society annual meeting in San Francisco. MannKind hopes the technology used in Afrezza might help deliver drugs that treat pain and osteoporosis, too.

Section 24.2

Insulin Pens

Normally, about half of the day's insulin is released as a relatively steady background or basal delivery. When carbs are eaten, a spike or bolus of insulin release occurs from the pancreas. In attempting to mimic the pancreas with a basal/bolus approach that better matches insulin to need, a convenient and precise way to deliver insulin can be very helpful.

The best way for many to mimic the pancreas is with an insulin pen. Pens have been available for a quarter century, but their use in the United States lags behind the wide popularity they have experienced in Europe. Insulin pens allow discrete injections on a just-in-time basis. There is no need to carry a syringe and bottle of insulin and doses can be conveniently dialed up, making dose errors less likely.

An insulin pen looks like a fountain pen and is usually only slightly thicker in size. It has a disposable needle at one end with a cartridge that holds insulin and a dial that is used to select the insulin dose. Pen cartridges hold 150 or 300 units of insulin. Some pens are disposable and thrown away once the insulin is gone, while others are more environmentally friendly with disposable glass cartridges that are replaced when they become empty.

Different pens can deliver insulin in half unit, one unit, or two unit increments. Half-unit pens, such as the NovoPen Junior, are particularly well suited for children and adults on low doses, and come in bright graphic designs. Two unit pens, such as the AutoPen from Owen Mumford, are ideal for those with Type 2 diabetes or others who use large doses of insulin.

Prefilled cartridges are available for common insulins, such as Apidra®, Humalog®, or NovoLog®, and Lantus® or Levemir®. Although we do not recommend them for most people, 70/30 mixtures which contain fixed ratios of 70 percent longer-acting and 30 percent shorter-acting insulin are available for Novolog and Humalog. This works well for people who have difficulty determining correct doses and take doses twice a day, as well as for those not yet ready to take the fixed number of injections required for a basal/bolus approach. Most people who love the convenience of a pen will use one pen with a rapid insulin to cover carbs and lower high readings as needed several times a day. Then they use a second pen to take one or two doses of a flat long-acting basal insulin in separate injections.

Pen Use

To prepare the pen for use, always prime it first. Purge two to five units of insulin into a sink or the air to ensure that the pen is functioning, not clogged, and has insulin in it. Put a needle on before each injection and take the needle off after using it for an injection to avoid insulin loss or evaporation of insulin through the needle. When the pen is not in use, keep its cap on.

The needle on the pen is pushed into the skin and a button is pressed to give the selected dose. Pen needles are available in different lengths and sizes. The needle may be discarded after each use or at the end of the day.

After you inject, leave the needle under the skin while you count to eight. It takes longer for insulin to enter the skin from a pen than from an injection by a needle. If insulin is dripping out of the needle when you take it out, you probably have not received your full dose. Leave it in longer next time.

In storing a pen, avoid freezing and exposure to heat, just as you would with a bottle of insulin. A pen with insulin should be kept unrefrigerated only as long as the insulin in the pen can be kept unrefrigerated.

Section 24.3

Insulin Pills

Reprinted from "Insulin in a Pill,"
© 2010 Technology Review, Inc. 72712-4Y:N1510AS.

In late 2009, Denmark-based Novo Nordisk quietly started phase 1 clinical trials of a pill that it hopes to market as an alternative to insulin injections. Offering patients with diabetes the chance to avoid painful needles has long been the holy grail of some pharmaceutical companies, especially Novo, a leader in diabetes treatment for much of its eighty-seven-year history. Novo's entry into clinical testing puts the company ahead of the pack of drug makers trying to encapsulate insulin into an easy-to-swallow dose.

The fact that Novo entered phase 1 testing with little fanfare is apropos, however, considering the checkered history of insulin drug development. Insulin is a protein that rapidly degrades in the stomach and upper portion of the small intestine, making it almost impossible to deliver orally. Several drug makers have attempted to deliver insulin via the lungs, most notably Pfizer, which introduced its inhalable insulin drug, Exubera®, in 2006. But the product flopped—patients balked at the clumsy inhaler and doctors questioned whether it might endanger the lungs. Several other drug makers, Novo among them, abandoned their attempts to make inhalable insulin in the wake of Exubera's failure.

Theoretically, delivering insulin through the stomach should be ideal: insulin would travel directly to the liver, its primary site of action, in a way that mimics the action of endogenous insulin. Because insulin injections go into muscle and fat, patients who use them are susceptible to hypoglycemia. Mads Krogsgaard Thomsen, Novo's chief scientific officer, says that's why he believes oral insulin could be safer and more convenient than either the injectable or inhalable forms. But he urges caution for now.

The challenge of making an insulin pill that can survive the digestive system has been magnified by the characteristics of the molecule itself. Human insulin is a large and complex protein. So even if it survives being doused by stomach acid, it's unlikely to be easily absorbed by the epithelial cells of the gut. Thus the portion of oral insulin that actually makes it into the bloodstream is under 1 percent. "You can't use human insulin" in a pill, Thomsen says. "It doesn't work."

So Novo's scientists set out to increase the oral viability of insulin tenfold through protein engineering. They embarked on a painstaking, multiyear process designed to answer some key questions: What are the enzymes that attack the molecule, and where do they attack it? The scientists used the insight they gained to design a pill that can transverse the stomach without being broken down, facilitating the transfer of insulin across cells and into the bloodstream.

The drug, called NN1952, will be tested in 150 volunteers over more than a year. The company will examine how the drug is metabolized in patients with type 1 or type 2 diabetes, and in healthy people.

Some doctors say they'll need to see the data before they can get excited about oral insulin. One issue with past attempts was that the pills were affected by food in unexpected ways, says Howard Wolpert, a senior physician at the Joslin Diabetes Center in Boston. "The data from the tests would look okay, and then you'd give it with meals and find the absorption was affected," says Wolpert, who is not participating in the Novo trials. "Getting the insulin absorption to match the carbohydrate absorption creates a confounding variable."

Novo's phase 1 program will include food interaction studies, Thomsen says. Still, the extent to which oral insulin might be able to replace injections is not yet known: The company will test the drug at various doses, with or without meals, and compare it with both injections and placebos. Thomsen believes oral insulin may prove to be most appealing to type 2 diabetics, who aren't dependent on insulin injections because their pancreases are still able to make the protein. Should those patients need an extra boost, however, they may prefer to get it from something other than a needle. "There's a difference between taking a tablet a day and an injection a day," he says.

Other companies are experimenting with different delivery methods for insulin. Generex Biotechnology of Worcester, Massachusetts, is in late-stage testing of an insulin spray that's absorbed through the back of the throat. And MannKind of Valencia, California, is awaiting a verdict from the U.S. Food and Drug Administration on its insulin inhaler.

Sanjoy Dutta, director of the insulin initiative at the Juvenile Diabetes Research Foundation, says the onus will be on all of these companies to prove that the insulin drugs they deliver mark an improvement over what diabetics are injecting today. "We are tremendously interested in insulins that are safer, more efficacious, faster-acting, and compatible with other medications," Dutta says. "If they come orally, that would be icing on the cake."

Chapter 25

Tight Diabetes Control (Intensive Insulin Therapy)

A method of intensive diabetes self-management that involves keeping blood glucose levels as close as possible to normal without causing severe or frequent episodes of hypoglycemia (low blood sugar), in the aim of preventing complications of diabetes. The term "tight control" has been around for decades, as researchers hotly debated whether aggressive blood glucose control could lower the risk of developing diabetic complications, including eye disease, kidney disease, and nerve disease. In recent years, a number of large clinical trials put the debate to rest. Based on the results of these trials, the American Diabetes Association (ADA) began to define tight control in terms of numeric values and urged most people with diabetes to strive for these more stringent goals. Even so, experts say that no single range of blood glucose levels works for everyone, and that these goals must be individualized.

In the Diabetes Control and Complications Trial (DCCT), which ended in 1993, 1,441 people with Type 1 diabetes were randomly assigned to receive either standard diabetes care or intensive insulin therapy. While the standard care group had one or two insulin injections per day, the intensive care group was treated with three or more daily insulin injections or insulin pump therapy, had frequent contact with healthcare providers, and checked their blood glucose level four or more times a day. After an average of 6.5 years of therapy, the standard care group had an average glycosylated hemoglobin (HbA1c) level of about 9 percent, while the intensive care group achieved an HbA1c level of 7 percent. (The HbA1c level indicates a person's average blood glucose level over the previous two to three months and is a good measure of how well blood glucose is being controlled. The average for people who don't have diabetes is less than 6 percent.) More important, researchers found that the intensive care group had significantly lower rates of diabetic eye disease, diabetic kidney disease, and diabetic nerve disease. Years after the completion of the DCCT, the average HbA1c for all participants had leveled to around 8 percent, but those who had practiced tight control during the study continued to have fewer complications.

The results of follow-up studies, published in 2003 and 2005, showed that the DCCT participants who had practiced tight control also lowered their risk of atherosclerosis and heart disease.

An even larger clinical trial, the United Kingdom Prospective Diabetes Study (UKPDS), studied the effects of intensive blood glucose control in over five thousand adults newly diagnosed with Type 2 diabetes. In this study, the standard care group was treated with lifestyle interventions alone (diet and exercise) unless symptoms of severe hyperglycemia (high blood glucose) developed and pharmacologic intervention became necessary. The intensive care group was treated with insulin, metformin, or a sulfonylurea drug such as glyburide (brand names Micronase®, DiaBeta®, Glynase®), or a combination of these. At the end of the study, the standard care group had an average HbA1c of 7.9 percent, while the intensive care group had attained an HbA1c of 7 percent. Although this may not seem like a big difference, the intensive care group had a significantly lower rate of all complications of diabetes. In particular, for each 1 percent reduction in HbA1c level (for example, from 9 percent to 8 percent), there was a 35 percent reduction in the risk of developing microvascular (small-blood-vessel) complications like eye disease, kidney disease, and nerve disease.

Based on this and other powerful evidence, aggressive blood glucose control as practiced in the DCCT and UKPDS has become the goal of self-care for most people with diabetes, and they should expect their doctors to help them achieve tight control.

To reach the target HbA1c of less than 7 percent, the ADA recommends aiming for the following blood glucose levels:

• Average blood glucose levels before meals should be 70–130 mg/dl.

- Blood glucose levels after meals should be less than 180 mg/dl.

If pre-meal blood sugar levels are consistently within the target range but the HbA1c level is still high, the ADA suggests monitoring one or two hours after meals and treating out-of-range numbers appropriately.

Ultimately, blood glucose targets must be tailored to the individual, and tight control is not for everyone. All of the studies demonstrating the value of tight blood glucose control have also shown that it is associated with an increased risk of hypoglycemia. Those who are especially prone to hypoglycemia may need somewhat higher target values. In particular, elderly adults, who can experience stroke or heart attack from episodes of hypoglycemia, and who may have a harder time recognizing symptoms of hypoglycemia, may be advised not to attempt tight control. Some people who already have severe complications (particularly end-stage kidney disease) may also be advised against tight control. Work with a healthcare professional before starting a regimen of tight control.

Tight control has also been associated with weight gain, but such weight gain can be prevented or reversed. The weight gain associated with improved blood glucose control usually comes from absorbing calories that previously were eliminated in urine, overtreating hypoglycemia, and consuming more food after learning to match carbohydrate grams with insulin. Consuming fewer calories and learning to treat hypoglycemia without overtreating it can remedy the situation.

Chapter 26

Avoiding Drug Interactions with Diabetes Medications

People with diabetes often have a number of co-existing health problems. So in addition to insulin or diabetes pills, other drugs are often needed to control these problems—statins for high cholesterol, diuretics or beta-blockers for high blood pressure, antidepressants for depression or neuropathy pain, and a daily aspirin to prevent a heart attack. But some drugs are not supposed to be taken simultaneously, and doctors and pharmacists don't always notice when a person is taking dangerous or risky drug combinations.

What can happen to you if you take several drugs that are not supposed to be taken together? This chapter explains why and how medicines can interact and what a drug interaction may mean for you and your health care.

The Scope of the Problem

Surprisingly, most drug reactions are caused by a small group of commonly prescribed drugs. The nonsteroidal anti-inflammatory drugs (such as ibuprofen), anticoagulants, diuretics, and drugs to treat diabetes are on this list. Adverse drug reactions may add as much as $130 billion a year to the cost of health care in the United States. A significant portion of adverse drug reactions are caused by interacting drugs. This is a huge problem and much research and effort is going into trying to reduce the incidence and risk of these interactions.

It is estimated that people over sixty-five take an average of seven drugs at any one time to treat a variety of illnesses. With this amount of medicine use, the probability that a person will take two prescribed drugs that may interact with one another is very high. In a recent study done in six European countries, investigators reviewed the medicines taken by about 1,600 people and found that 46 percent were taking at least one pair of drugs that could interact. (Studies that include people under age sixty-five have shown somewhat lower percentages of people taking interacting drugs.) Although not all potential drug interactions result in a bad outcome, drug interactions contribute to an increased risk of an adverse event. In fact, up to 7 percent of people who are admitted to hospitals end up there because of an adverse drug reaction.

One might think the risk of drug interactions would be lower in the hospital, where patients are under close medical supervision, but the opposite is true: The problem is even greater for people admitted to a hospital. On average, a person who enters the hospital is treated with ten drugs and has about a 20 percent probability of having a reaction caused by drug interactions.

With all of the drugs on the market today, how many drug interactions are possible? The answer is quite a few. Fortunately, while there are a lot of potential drug interactions, not all of them result in adverse drug reactions. Why this is so is not well understood but may include underreported or unrecognized adverse drug events by the people taking them or their physicians, people simply not taking their medicines consistently, individual differences in tolerance of drug effects, and individual variations in the blood levels of any of the potential interacting drugs.

Why and How Drugs Interact

When you take a drug, most of it must be absorbed into your bloodstream and go to the particular part of the body it needs to affect. After it has produced its effect, the body needs to get it out of the system. Interference with any of these steps, whether drug-induced or from physiological problems, can produce unwanted effects. The most common form of drug interaction occurs when one drug interferes with another drug's elimination from the body.

Drugs are mainly eliminated from the body by two organs, the liver and the kidney. The kidney rids the body of some drugs in the urine.

The liver rids the body of some drugs in the bile via the gallbladder. Both the kidney and the liver sometimes need to metabolize, or chemically change, drugs into forms that are more easily eliminated from the body.

The liver acts as a gatekeeper between the gastrointestinal tract and the rest of the body because it is the first major organ to receive blood (and the drugs absorbed into the blood) from the intestines. In fact, the liver can metabolize some drugs so quickly that after taking one of these drugs by mouth, only a small fraction of the drug is left to travel through the body. But how do your liver and kidneys "know" how to metabolize drugs they've never seen before? Humans didn't suddenly develop ways to eliminate or modify drugs. Rather, through the course of our evolution as a species, our livers now have a large family of enzymes (proteins that modify or metabolize chemicals) to deal with a range of substances. Probably originally developed and retained to deal with foreign chemicals in food or the environment, these enzymes now also serve to break down drugs.

The enzymes come in many different types but the largest family is known as the cytochrome P450's (CYP450). More than a thousand CYP450's have been identified in various species; humans alone have more than fifty distinct genes for CYP450's. These enzymes are very old and have been conserved in the evolutionary sense, meaning that many plants and bacteria have similar enzymes to those now found in humans. Several individual enzymes metabolize the majority of drugs available today. The CYP450 enzymes that are most commonly involved in drug metabolism are CYP3A4, CYP2D6, CYP2C9, CYP2C19, CYP1A2, and CYP2E1. CYP3A4 is the most important enzyme in drug metabolism due to its abundance in the liver and the intestine and its ability to modify many different types of chemicals and drugs. CYP3A4 is involved in the metabolism of more than 60 percent of all drugs that are on the market today.

Inhibition of metabolism. When a drug blocks or inhibits one or more of these CYP450 enzymes, it interferes with the elimination of drugs that are normally metabolized by the blocked enzyme(s). If a drug cannot be metabolized, it is not eliminated as quickly as it should be and can accumulate in the bloodstream, resulting in higher blood levels of the drug. The blocked drug also stays in the bloodstream longer than expected. Both of these situations can lead to trouble.

The once-popular antihistamine terfenadine (Seldane®) was removed from the U.S. market because it caused potentially fatal heart rhythms when given in combination with drugs that block its metabolism. It was found that terfenadine was normally broken down in the body by CYP3A4, but when a CYP3A4-blocking drug such as ketoconazole (an antifungal drug) was given at the same time, the levels of terfenadine were both higher in the bloodstream and higher for a longer time. The high levels caused the heart problem, and because it was difficult to prevent the potentially harmful mixture of drugs, terfenadine was removed from the market in 1998.

Induction of metabolism. Some drugs can increase the levels of a CYP450 enzyme in the body by interacting with the genes for that enzyme. The increased levels of enzyme serve to metabolize drugs faster than normal, which reduces the blood levels of medicines metabolized by that enzyme, making them less effective. This process is called induction, and the drugs that serve to increase the amount of enzymes are called inducers.

Inhibition of excretion. The diabetes drug metformin, on the other hand, is not metabolized by enzymes and is eliminated unchanged in the urine. This means that it is not susceptible to other drugs that inhibit CYP450 enzymes. However, metformin concentrations in the body can be increased by drugs that inhibit its excretion from the kidneys, such as cimetidine (Tagamet®).

Synergism. Drugs can also interact when they have the same intended effect or complementary effects. For instance, this can occur when several drugs are given to prevent blood clots from forming. Although both aspirin and warfarin (Coumadin®) are intended to prevent blood from clotting inappropriately, in combination they can increase the risk of bleeding.

Rosiglitazone (Avandia®) and pioglitazone (Actos®) can produce edema (fluid retention). When these diabetes drugs are given in combination with insulin or metformin, the risk of edema increases. The mechanism behind this interaction is still unknown.

Specific Drug Interactions

Table 26.1 lists common drugs used to treat diabetes as well as other drugs commonly used by people with diabetes that could potentially cause interference. The list is not meant to be comprehensive; there are other drugs used by people who have diabetes that may cause interactions.

You may remember the recent recall of the statin cerivastatin (Baycol®), but perhaps you haven't heard how the drug interaction in that case relates to a diabetes drug. The triglyceride-lowering drug gemfibrozil (Lopid®), an inhibitor of CYP2C8, was connected with an increased incidence of muscle breakdown (rhabdomyolysis) as well as deaths when taken with the cholesterol-lowering drug cerivastatin. The combination causes cerivastatin levels in the blood to increase by up to 600 percent on average because cerivastatin is usually metabolized by CYP2C8 and CYP3A4. Cerivastatin was removed from the market because of the risks.

The same mechanism appears to be occurring with the combination of repaglinide (Prandin®) and gemfibrozil and with rosiglitazone and gemfibrozil. Repaglinide is usually broken down in the body by CYP2C8 and CYP3A4. Gemfibrozil's inhibition of the CYP2C8 enzyme appears to result in increased levels of repaglinide in the blood. The levels are increased so much that on average they essentially convert the dose taken into one 800 percent higher. When repaglinide is given in combination with gemfibrozil and itraconazole (Sporanox®, an antifungal drug and CYP3A4 inhibitor), the increase becomes even more profound (up to 1,940 percent). If your usual dose is a one-milligram tablet of repaglinide, the three-drug interaction would potentially give you the same blood levels of repaglinide as if you had taken nineteen tablets, an overdose rather than the intended dose. Gemfibrozil's CYP2C8-blocking effect also seems to be behind its ability to increase levels of rosiglitazone when the two are taken together.

Why did this take so long to figure out and why was this not understood before repaglinide was put on the market? Although the U.S. Food and Drug Administration (FDA) requires new drugs to undergo studies of potential drug interactions before they can be approved, it's difficult to test a new drug against every known drug, so a method was devised to help target the most likely interactions to study. The method that the FDA and pharmaceutical companies came to rely on is done in vitro (in test tubes) with human enzymes (cloned and expressed in cell culture). The most common human enzymes are used in these studies, and CYP2C8 is not usually one of them. It was not until very recently that this enzyme was found to be blocked by gemfibrozil. It has also not been the practice lately to do interaction studies with more than one drug at a time, even if the blocking of two or more enzymes simultaneously would have potentially significant consequences. The findings from the cerivastatin–gemfibrozil, repaglinide–gemfibrozil, and rosiglitazone–gemfibrozil interactions may spur both the FDA and drug companies to look much closer at how drug interaction studies are done.

Table 26.1. Possible Drug Interactions

Common Diabetes Medicines	Drugs That Can Increase the Concentration of This Diabetes Medicine in the Blood	Drugs That Can Decrease the Concentration of This Diabetes Medicine in the Blood	Other Drugs Affected by This Diabetes Medicine
Insulin			Increased risk of fluid retention and heart failure when taken with pioglitazone or rosiglitazone.
Metformin (Glucophage®, Glucophage XR®; also found in Avandamet®, Glucovance®, Metaglip®)	cimetidine nifedipine		Metformin can decrease blood levels of furosemide.
Nateglinide (Starlix®)	amiodarone cimetidine clarithromycin erythromycin fluconazole fluvastatin grapefruit juice itraconazole ketoconazole lovastatin nefazodone sulfamethoxazole	carbamazepine phenytoin rifampin St. John's wort	Nateglinide may inhibit the metabolism of tolbutamide.
Pioglitazone (Actos®)	amiodarone cimetidine clarithromycin erythromycin gemfibrozil grapefruit juice itraconazole ketoconazole nefazodone trimethoprim	carbamazepine phenytoin rifampin St. John's wort	Pioglitazone can decrease blood concentrations of amlodipine, atorvastatin, diltiazem, felodipine, lovastatin, nifedipine, nisoldipine, nitrendipine, repaglinide, simvastatin, and verapamil. Also, there is an increased risk of fluid retention and heart failure when taken with insulin.

Table 26.1. Possible Drug Interactions, continued

Common Diabetes Medicines	Drugs That Can Increase the Concentration of This Diabetes Medicine in the Blood	Drugs That Can Decrease the Concentration of This Diabetes Medicine in the Blood	Other Drugs Affected by This Diabetes Medicine
Repaglinide (Prandin®)	amiodarone cimetidine clarithromycin erythromycin gemfibrozil grapefruit juice itraconazole ketoconazole nefazodone pioglitazone rosiglitazone trimethoprim	carbamazepine phenytoin rifampin St. John's wort	
Rosiglitazone (Avandia®; also found in Avandamet®)	amiodarone fluconazole fluvastatin gemfibrozil lovastatin sulfamethoxazole trimethoprim	rifampin	Rosiglitazone can decrease blood concentrations of amlodipine, atorvastatin, diltiazem, felodipine, lovastatin, nifedipine, nisoldipine, nitrendipine, repaglinide, simvastatin, and verapamil. Also, there is an increased risk of fluid retention and heart failure when taken with insulin.
Sulfonylureas: glimepiride (Amaryl®), glipizide (Glucotrol®, Glucotrol XL®; also found in Metaglip®), glyburide (DiaBeta®, Glynase®, Micronase®; also found in Glucovance®), tolbutamide (Orinase®)	amiodarone fluconazole fluvastatin lovastatin sulfamethoxazole	rifampin	

Are You at Risk?

With all of these potential interactions, how do you find out if you may be at risk? Start by consulting your physician and your pharmacist. Bring a list of all of the drugs you take (or simply bring the drugs themselves), including prescription drugs, over-the-counter drugs, and any supplements, herbal or otherwise, to a doctor appointment or to your pharmacy. Ask your doctor or pharmacist to look over your list for any potentially dangerous combinations.

Be careful about relying on commercial internet sources for drug information. Several internet drugstore sites that I evaluated did not list repaglinide and gemfibrozil or rosiglitazone and gemfibrozil as potentially interacting drugs.

Adverse drug effects are very common and represent a large part of the reason that people visit doctors' offices, emergency rooms, and eventually hospitals. Don't hesitate to notify your doctor if you think you are experiencing a drug side effect or to ask about potential drug interactions. If you see different doctors for different medical conditions, one may not be aware of what the others have prescribed for you. Similarly, if you get different prescriptions filled at different pharmacies, no one pharmacist will have access to all of your information, and potential interactions may be missed. For this reason, it is recommended that people fill all their prescriptions at one pharmacy, if possible. In addition, maintain a list of all of your medicines and update it when one is added or removed. Review your list with your doctor or pharmacist regularly, particularly when you begin taking a new medicine.

Chapter 27

New Diabetes Drugs

Chapter Contents

Section 27.1

Incretins: Byetta, Symlin, and Januvia

Over the past three years, three diabetes treatments with entirely new modes of action were approved: Byetta® (for people with type 2 diabetes), Symlin® (as an add-on to insulin therapy for people with type 1 diabetes or type 2 diabetes), and Januvia® (also for people with type 2 diabetes). "New is not necessarily better, but these are additional weapons in the armament," says Nora Saul, M.S., C.D.E., R.D., L.D.N., who educates Joslin Diabetes Center patients on blood glucose management.

Some diabetes medications help the pancreas release more insulin (if you have type 2 diabetes), others help cells use insulin better, and others keep the liver from releasing too much glucose. The three new treatments focus action on hormones called "incretins." The two given by injection—Byetta and Symlin—have an added bonus of promoting weight loss.

With more options, treatments can be better tailored to an individual. Since type 2 diabetes is progressive, what works for some people for a period of time may lose effectiveness. For example, some people with type 2 diabetes may start treating the chronic disease with oral medications, and then subsequently discover that insulin would give them more control.

Here are the three new medical options that enhance blood glucose control for people with type 1 or type 2 diabetes.

Byetta (Generic: Exenatide)

- By injection twice a day at mealtime
- For those with type 2 diabetes who have been unable to control blood glucose with oral medicines

- Improves blood glucose control by mimicking incretin hormones, stimulating insulin, and slowing stomach emptying

- Leads to weight loss (feel full faster, so people feel satiated faster and stop eating)

- Can cause nausea

Symlin (Pramlintide Acetate)

- For those with type 1 or type 2 diabetes who use insulin

- By injection at mealtime

- Must never mix Symlin and insulin in one syringe; also means an additional injection

- Better control, reduces spikes in blood glucose, reduces food intake (leads to weight loss)

- Can cause nausea; hypoglycemia (dangerously low blood sugars)

Januvia (Sitagliptin)

- By pill once a day

- For type 2 diabetes

- Does not promote weight gain

- Often used in combination with metformin

- Very few, if any, side effects

- Slows the breakdown of incretins, so insulin is released over a longer period of time

Section 27.2

Dapagliflozin

A new drug, the first in its class, gives added blood sugar control to people with type 2 diabetes who are already taking the glucose-lowering medication metformin.

The new agent, dapagliflozin, which also helped patients lose weight, is novel in that it does not work directly on the body's insulin mechanisms, according to a study appearing in the June 26, 2010, issue of *The Lancet* and slated for presentation at the annual meeting of the American Diabetes Association (ADA) in Orlando, Florida.

"It will probably be used as an add-on therapy," said study author Clifford Bailey, a chemical pathologist and professor of clinical science at Aston University in Birmingham, U.K. "If you don't quite get to target with [the first therapy tried], this approach would offer you an opportunity hopefully to maintain improved control."

Bailey, who could not predict if or when the drug might get final approval from drug regulatory authorities, also pointed out that dapagliflozin is flexible, meaning it can be used with various other treatments and at more or less any stage in the disease.

"It's a good add-on," agreed Dr. Stanley Mirsky, an endocrinologist at Lenox Hill Hospital, and associate clinical professor of metabolic diseases at Mount Sinai Medical Center, New York City. "Is it a wonder drug? No. It may play a small role."

"This could be used at any time during the continuum of diabetes, whether beginning, middle, or towards the end of the lifespan of the patient," said Dr. Anupa Patel, senior clinical fellow in endocrinology at the Texas A&M Health Science Center College of Medicine and at Scott & White in Temple. "It could be added on at any time as an adjunct to therapy, [but] there should be some other type of therapy whether insulin or an oral agent."

Patel noted that there were statistically significant improvements in weight loss and blood sugar levels over time, especially at the two higher doses. Even at the end of one week, she said, "there was a significant decline in fasting plasma glucose in the two higher doses."

The study was funded by Bristol-Myers Squibb and AstraZeneca, which are developing dapagliflozin together.

Dapagliflozin works by stimulating the kidneys to eliminate more glucose from the body via urine.

In this study of 534 adult patients with type 2 diabetes who were already taking metformin, the highest dose of dapagliflozin (10 milligrams [mg] daily) was associated with a 0.84 percent decrease in HbA1c levels.

HbA1c is a measure of blood sugar control over time.

Participants taking 5 mg of the drug saw a 0.70 percent decrease in HbA1c levels, while those taking 2.5 mg showed a 0.67 percent decrease.

In the placebo group, the decrease in HbA1c was 0.3 percent, the study found.

Weight loss was also greater in volunteers taking the study drug: 2.2 kilograms (4.8 pounds) in the 2.5-mg group; 3 kilograms (6.6 pounds) in the 5-mg group; and 2.9 kilograms (6.4 pounds) in the 10-mg group.

Those in the placebo group lost 0.9 kilograms, or almost 2 pounds.

Much, though not all, of this loss was likely water weight, the authors stated.

There were more genital infections seen among those taking dapagliflozin, the team noted.

"One of the complications of the drug is an increase in urinary tract infections or yeast infections because you have high glucose levels in the urine," said Dr. Jacob Warman, chief of endocrinology at The Brooklyn Hospital Center in New York City. "That's a very good culture medium for yeast, so the endocrinologists aren't too happy about that."

On the other hand, he said, this drug appears to work without some of the kidney, liver, and muscle complications of other drugs, so "it would be excellent as an add-on to usual medications."

A second study, also simultaneously being presented at the ADA meeting and published in *The Lancet*, found that adding inhaled insulin before each meal and long-acting insulin glargine before going to bed worked just as well as conventional therapy.

The regular therapy consisted of taking biaspart insulin twice a day. This is a combination of short-acting insulin and intermediate-acting insulin.

The new regimen involved less weight gain, fewer episodes of low blood sugar, and was more convenient, according to the study, which was funded by MannKind, the maker of Technosphere®, the inhaled insulin featured in the trial.

A third study found that once-weekly injections of the drug ex-enatide (Byetta®) worked better at controlling blood sugar levels than long-acting insulin.

The practice thus far has been to give Byetta twice a day. This study, funded by Amylin Pharmaceuticals and Eli Lilly, looked at a new formulation of the drug.

Patients who got the once-a-week form also lost an average of 2.6 kilograms (5.7 pounds), the study found.

Section 27.3

Rituximab

"Cancer and Arthritis Therapy May Be Promising Treatment for Diabetes," December 17, 2007, reprinted with permission from the Yale University Office of Public Affairs and Communications. © 2007 Yale University.

An antibody used to treat certain cancers and rheumatoid arthritis appears to greatly delay type 1 diabetes in mice, Yale School of Medicine researchers report in the *Journal of Clinical Investigation*.

"Even better, the beneficial effects of the antibody continue to be observed long after the antibody is no longer administered," the researchers said.

The antibody, rituximab (anti-CD20), depletes B cells. Experimental evidence in mutant mice indicates that B cells play a role in autoimmune diseases by interacting with T cells of the immune system. It is T cells that destroy insulin-producing cells directly in the pancreas, leading to type 1 diabetes.

"Our paper shows, for the first time, that after successful B cell depletion, regulatory cells emerge that can continue to suppress the inflammatory and autoimmune response even after the B cells return," said Li Wen, senior research scientist in the division of endocrinology. "Even more strikingly, we found that these regulatory cells include both B and T cells."

To determine if B cell depletion would work as a therapy for type 1 diabetes, Wen and her colleague at Yale, Mark Shlomchik, M.D., professor of laboratory medicine and immunobiology, developed a mouse model. They engineered mice that were predisposed to diabetes and had the human version of CD20, the molecule rituximab targets, on the surface of their B cells.

The researchers tested a mouse version of the drug to deplete B cells in mice either before diabetes onset, or within days of diagnosis with diabetes. The drug treatment significantly delayed diabetes onset in pre-diabetic mice. This translated to a ten- to fifteen-week delay in developing diabetes compared to mice given a "sham" treatment. The equivalent period for humans would be approximately ten to fifteen years. Of the fourteen mice that already had diabetes, five stopped needing insulin for two to five months while all the sham-treated mice remained diabetic.

"These studies suggest that B cells can have dual roles in diabetes and possibly other autoimmune diseases. The B cells might promote disease initially, but after being reconstituted following initial depletion with rituximab, they actually block further disease," Shlomchik added. "This means that multiple rounds of medication to deplete the B cells might not be necessary or even advisable."

Chapter 28

Aspirin Therapy for Diabetics

The Facts

If you have type 2 diabetes, your chance of heart attack or stroke is higher than it is for most other people. In fact, you have the same risk as someone who already has heart disease! So take steps to reduce your risk.

To get your diabetes in control, work with your healthcare provider to get on a program that includes a healthy diet and physical activity. These changes will also help reduce your risk of heart disease and stroke.

Another step may be to use aspirin. Aspirin also helps prevent heart attacks and strokes.

All about Aspirin

Most heart attacks and strokes occur when the blood supply to a part of your heart muscle or brain is blocked. This usually starts with atherosclerosis, a process in which deposits of fatty substances, cholesterol, cellular waste products, calcium, and other substances build up in the inner lining of an artery. This buildup is called plaque.

Plaque usually affects large and medium-sized arteries. Plaques can grow large enough to significantly reduce the blood's flow through an artery. But most of the damage occurs when a plaque becomes fragile and ruptures. Plaques that rupture cause blood clots to form that can

---

block blood flow or break off and travel to another part of the body. This is called an embolism:

- If a blood clot blocks a blood vessel that feeds the heart, it causes a heart attack.

- If a blood clot blocks a blood vessel that feeds the brain, it causes a stroke.

Aspirin "thins" the blood and helps prevent blood clots from forming. So it helps prevent heart attack and stroke.

Who Should Take Aspirin?

Healthcare providers suggest aspirin usage for people who have had a previous stroke or heart attack. Recent studies show that aspirin also helps prevent heart attack and stroke in those people who are at high risk for cardiovascular disease—like those with diabetes. Aspirin is recommended for:

- people with type 2 diabetes who also have a history of:

  - **Myocardial infarction:** This is another name for a heart attack.

  - **Bypass surgery:** This surgery uses a graft artery to create a detour around a diseased artery.

  - **Angina:** Angina is chest pain or discomfort that occurs when your heart doesn't get as much blood and oxygen as it needs.

  - **Transient ischemic attack (TIA):** A TIA is a "warning stroke" or "mini-stroke" that produces stroke-like symptoms but usually produces no lasting damage.

  - **Peripheral artery disease (PAD):** PAD is the term for atherosclerosis (plaque buildup) in the arteries outside the heart and brain, such as in the legs.

- People with type 2 diabetes also may have other risk factors such as:

  - increased age (above forty);

  - family history of cardiovascular disease;

  - high blood pressure;

  - smoking;

- high cholesterol levels, specifically high low-density lipoprotein (LDL) levels.

The best way to know if you're a candidate for aspirin therapy is to ask your healthcare provider. You should not start aspirin on your own.

Baby Aspirin or Full Aspirin?

Most of the dosages in clinical trials have ranged from 81 mg to 325 mg. The American Heart Association generally recommends doses of 75–162 mg per day (or about a baby aspirin to half of an adult aspirin). This dose works as well as higher doses. A lower dosage is better because higher doses tend to result in more side effects and risks.

Know the Risks

Because aspirin thins the blood, it can cause several complications. Talk to your doctor if any of these situations apply to you. You should not take aspirin if you:

- have an aspirin allergy or intolerance;

- are at risk for gastrointestinal bleeding or hemorrhagic stroke;

- drink alcohol regularly;

- are undergoing any simple medical or dental procedures.

Using Aspirin during a Heart Attack or Stroke

The most important thing to do if any heart attack warning signs occur is to call 9-1-1 immediately. Don't do anything before calling 9-1-1. In particular, don't take an aspirin, then wait for it to relieve your pain. Aspirin won't treat a heart attack by itself.

After you call 9-1-1, the operator may tell you to take an aspirin. He or she can make sure that you don't have an allergy to aspirin or a condition that makes using it too risky. If the 9-1-1 operator doesn't talk to you about taking an aspirin, the emergency medical technicians or the physician in the Emergency Department will give you an aspirin if it's right for you. Research shows that taking aspirin early in treating a heart attack can significantly improve your chances of survival (along with other treatments).

Don't take aspirin during a stroke, because not all strokes are caused by blood clots. Some are caused by ruptured blood vessels. Taking aspirin could make these bleeding strokes more severe.

Chapter 29

Alternative and Complementary Therapies for Diabetes

Chapter Contents

Section 29.1

Dietary Supplements

Excerpted from "Diabetes and CAM: A Focus on Dietary Supplements,"
National Center for Complementary and Alternative Medicine, National
Institutes of Health, NCCAM Publication No. D416, June 2009.

Diabetes is a chronic condition affecting millions of Americans.
Conventional medical treatments are available to control diabetes
and its complications. However, some people also try complementary
and alternative medicine (CAM) therapies, including dietary supplements. This section summarizes scientific research on the effectiveness and safety of selected supplements that people with diabetes
sometimes use.

Key Points

• In general, there is not enough scientific evidence to prove that
dietary supplements have substantial benefits for type 2 diabetes or its complications.

• It is very important not to replace conventional medical therapy
for diabetes with an unproven CAM therapy.

• Tell your healthcare providers about any complementary and
alternative practices you use. Give them a full picture of what
you do to manage your health. This will help ensure coordinated
and safe care. Medicines for diabetes and other health conditions may need to be adjusted if a person is also using a dietary
supplement.

Dietary Supplements and Type 2 Diabetes

Some people with diabetes use CAM therapies for their health condition. For example, they may try acupuncture or biofeedback to help
with painful symptoms. Some use dietary supplements in efforts to
improve their blood glucose control, manage symptoms, and lessen the
risk of developing serious complications such as heart problems.

This section addresses what is known about a few of the many supplements used for diabetes, with a focus on some that have been studied in clinical trials, such as alpha-lipoic acid, chromium, and polyphenols.

Alpha-Lipoic Acid

Alpha-lipoic acid (ALA, also known as lipoic acid or thioctic acid) is an antioxidant—a substance that protects against cell damage. ALA is found in certain foods, such as liver, spinach, broccoli, and potatoes. Some people with type 2 diabetes take ALA supplements in the hope of lowering blood glucose levels by improving the body's ability to use insulin; others use ALA to prevent or treat diabetic neuropathy (a nerve disorder). Supplements are marketed as tablets or capsules.

ALA has been researched for its effect on insulin sensitivity, glucose metabolism, and diabetic neuropathy. Some studies have found benefits, but more research is needed. (There are some studies, reported from outside the United States, of ALA delivered intravenously; however, this research is outside the scope of this section.)

Because ALA might lower blood sugar too much, people with diabetes who take it must monitor their blood sugar levels very carefully.

Chromium

Chromium is an essential trace mineral—that is, the body requires small amounts of it to function properly. Some people with diabetes take chromium in an effort to improve their blood glucose control. Chromium is found in many foods, but usually only in small amounts; relatively good sources include meat, whole grain products, and some fruits, vegetables, and spices. In supplement form (capsules and tablets), it is sold as chromium picolinate, chromium chloride, and chromium nicotinate.

Chromium supplementation has been researched for its effect on glucose control in people with diabetes. Study results have been mixed. Some researchers have found benefits, but many of the studies have not been well designed. Additional, high-quality research is needed.

At low doses, short-term use of chromium appears to be safe for most adults. However, people with diabetes should be aware that chromium might cause blood sugar levels to go too low. High doses can cause serious side effects, including kidney problems—an issue of special concern to people with diabetes.

Omega-3 Fatty Acids

Omega-3 fatty acids are polyunsaturated fatty acids that come from foods such as fish, fish oil, vegetable oil (primarily canola and soybean), walnuts, and wheat germ. Omega-3 supplements are available as capsules or oils (such as fish oil). Omega-3s are important in a number of bodily functions, including the movement of calcium and other substances in and out of cells, the relaxation and contraction of muscles, blood clotting, digestion, fertility, cell division, and growth. In addition, omega-3s are thought to protect against heart disease, reduce inflammation, and lower triglyceride levels.

Omega-3 fatty acids have been researched for their effect on controlling glucose and reducing heart disease risk in people with type 2 diabetes. Studies show that omega-3 fatty acids lower triglycerides, but do not affect blood glucose control, total cholesterol, or high-density lipoprotein (HDL, or "good") cholesterol in people with diabetes. In some studies, omega-3 fatty acids also raised low-density lipoprotein (LDL, or "bad") cholesterol. Additional research, particularly long-term studies that look specifically at heart disease in people with diabetes, is needed.

Omega-3s appear to be safe for most adults at low to moderate doses. Safety questions have been raised about fish oil supplements, because some species of fish can be contaminated by substances such as mercury, pesticides, or polychlorinated biphenyls (PCBs). In high doses, fish oil can interact with certain medications, including blood thinners and drugs used for high blood pressure.

Polyphenols

Polyphenols—antioxidants found in tea and dark chocolate, among other dietary sources—are being studied for possible effects on vascular health (including blood pressure) and on the body's ability to use insulin.

Laboratory studies suggest that epigallocatechin gallate (EGCG), a polyphenol found in green tea, may protect against cardiovascular disease and have a beneficial effect on insulin activity and glucose control. However, a few small clinical trials studying EGCG and green tea in people with diabetes have not shown such effects.

No adverse effects of EGCG or green tea were discussed in these studies. Green tea is safe for most adults when used in moderate amounts. However, green tea contains caffeine, which can cause, in some people, insomnia, anxiety, or irritability, among other effects. Green tea also has small amounts of vitamin K, which can make anticoagulant drugs, such as warfarin, less effective.

Other Supplements

Other supplements are also being studied for diabetes-related effects. For example:

- Preliminary research has explored the use of garlic for lowering blood glucose levels, but findings have not been consistent.

- Studies of the effects of magnesium supplementation on blood glucose control have had mixed results, although researchers have found that eating a diet high in magnesium may lower the risk of diabetes.

- There is not enough evidence to evaluate the effectiveness of coenzyme Q10 supplementation as a CAM therapy for diabetes; studies of its ability to affect glucose control have had conflicting findings.

- Researchers are studying whether the herb ginseng and the trace mineral vanadium might help control glucose levels.

- Some people with diabetes may also try botanicals such as prickly pear cactus, gurmar, *Coccinia indica*, aloe vera, fenugreek, and bitter melon to control their glucose levels. However, there is limited research on the effectiveness of these botanicals for diabetes.

If You Have Diabetes and Are Thinking About Using a Dietary Supplement

Tell your healthcare providers about any complementary and alternative practices you use. Give them a full picture of what you do to manage your health. This will help ensure coordinated and safe care. Medicines for diabetes and other health conditions may need to be adjusted if a person is also using a dietary supplement.

Women who are pregnant or nursing, or people who are thinking of using supplements to treat a child, should consult their healthcare provider before using any dietary supplement.

Do not replace scientifically proven treatments for diabetes with CAM treatments that are unproven. The consequences of not following one's prescribed medical regimen for diabetes can be very serious.

Be aware that the label on a dietary supplement bottle may not accurately reflect what is inside. For example, some tests of dietary supplements have found that the contents did not match the dose on the label, and some herbal supplements have been found to be contaminated.

Section 29.2

Chinese Herbal Medicine

"Chinese Herbal Medicine May Benefit People with Pre-Diabetes, but Evidence Is Inconclusive," National Center for Complementary and Alternative Medicine, National Institutes of Health, November 3, 2009.

People with pre-diabetes have higher than normal levels of blood glucose, a form of sugar the body uses for energy. Pre-diabetes, also called impaired fasting glucose or impaired glucose tolerance, can lead to type 2 diabetes, heart disease, and stroke. Preventive measures include weight loss, behavior modification, and glucose-lowering drugs. In China and other Asian countries, Chinese herbal medicines have long been used to prevent or delay the onset of diabetes, and there is anecdotal evidence regarding efficacy for this purpose. A recent review, funded in part by the National Center for Complementary and Alternative Medicine (NCCAM), examined related clinical trials to see whether scientific evidence supports recommending Chinese herbal medicine as a treatment option for people with pre-diabetes.

The review looked at sixteen clinical trials involving 1,391 participants with pre-diabetes, fifteen different herbal formulations, and various comparisons (i.e., lifestyle modification, drug interventions, placebo). Study duration ranged from four weeks to two years (average nine months). No adverse events were reported. Analysis of data from eight trials that included lifestyle modification as a comparison found that lifestyle modification combined with Chinese herbs was twice as effective as lifestyle modification alone in normalizing blood sugar levels. Participants who received herbal formulations were also less likely to develop full-blown diabetes during the study period.

A number of factors make it impossible to draw firm conclusions from this analysis. The trials tested different herbal formulations and had methodological problems (e.g., lack of details about lifestyle modifications, unclear methods of randomization, poor reporting) that increase the risk of bias. The reviewers concluded that although their findings are promising, further, well-designed trials are needed to clarify the potential role of Chinese herbal medicines in glucose control and diabetes prevention.

Reference

Grant SJ, Bensoussan A, Chang D, et al. Chinese herbal medicines for people with impaired glucose tolerance or impaired fasting blood glucose. *Cochrane Database of Systematic Reviews*. 2009(4):CD00066690.

Part Four

Dietary and Other
Lifestyle Issues Important
for Diabetes Control

Chapter 30

Diabetes Meal Planning

Chapter Contents

Section 30.1

Meal Planning: An Overview

Excerpted from "Your Guide to Diet and Diabetes: General Overview of Diabetes and Food," reprinted with permission from the University of Illinois Extension. © 2009 University of Illinois.

The purpose of meal planning is to help you reach your personal blood glucose or weight goals. These goals should be discussed with your healthcare provider. How these goals are achieved will be different for everyone. Some may reach their goals by spacing their food intake and limiting portion sizes. Others benefit from a more specific meal plan. Serving sizes are always important when you plan your meals. Day-to-day variation in meals and snacks leads to uneven glucose pattern.

Four commonly used methods of meal planning include:

- the plate method;
- the Food Guide Pyramid (MyPyramid.com);
- exchange lists;
- carbohydrate counting.

The Plate Method

The plate method is one way that meals can be planned. For breakfast, starch should take up half of the plate, and meat or non-meat protein may take up one-quarter of the plate, if desired. In the lunch and dinner plate method, vegetables should take up half of the plate, starch should take up one-quarter of the plate, and meat or non-meat protein should take up another one-quarter of the plate. One serving of fruit and a cup of low-fat milk may accompany your meal. Although the plate method is relatively easy, portion sizes are still critical. The amount of food on your plate should vary according to the number of calories that you need each day. A recommended plate size is about nine inches across (nine-inch diameter). Try measuring your plates!

Starchy foods include: bread, rolls, rice, pasta, potatoes, yams, corn, lima beans, and cereals.

Vegetables include: lettuce, tomatoes, mushrooms, spinach, green beans, and broccoli.

Meat and non-meat protein foods include: chicken, beef, pork, fish, cheese, beans, tofu, and soy products that resemble meat or chicken.

Fruits include: oranges, applesauce, grapes, and peaches.

Food Guide Pyramid

The Food Guide Pyramid is a tool used to show the type and the amount of food that you need daily. Recently modified to take into consideration the new Dietary Guidelines for Americans, the new Food Guide Pyramid was renamed MyPyramid, and now has six colored bands which represent food groups, and steps up the side to emphasize physical activity. Listed below are the food groups that the colored bands of the pyramid represent:

- **Orange:** Grains
- **Green:** Vegetables
- **Red:** Fruit
- **Yellow:** Oils
- **Blue:** Milk
- **Purple:** Meat and beans

MyPyramid suggests that you:

- make half your grains whole grains;
- vary your veggies;
- focus on fruit;
- get your calcium-rich foods;
- go lean with protein;
- find your balance between food and physical activity.

Exchange Lists

(Adapted from the American Dietetic Association and the American Diabetes Association.)

The Diabetic Exchange List is a program that was developed by the American Dietetics Association and the American Diabetes Association. Exchange lists are used to balance the amount of calories, carbohydrate, protein, and fat eaten each day. The exchange list book can be ordered from the American Diabetes Association website. To use the exchange lists, individuals must first talk with their doctor or dietitian about their dietary requirements and the number of calories that they need each day. Then the doctor or dietitian can explain how many servings from each group are needed to meet these daily requirements. Individuals can then use the exchange lists to determine what foods and in what amounts they need to eat each day.

There are six different exchange list groups, including the starch group, the fruit group, the milk group, the non-starchy vegetable group, the meat and meat substitutes group, and the fat group. Each serving of food within an exchange group has about the same amount of carbohydrate, protein, fat, and calories as the other foods in that group. For this reason, foods within an exchange list group can be substituted for each other, but foods on one group list cannot be substituted for foods on another group list. For example, you may substitute eating a small apple for a small orange, because they are both one serving in the fruit group. However, you could not substitute eating a small apple for one slice of bread, because these foods are in different groups.

The amount and type of exchanges recommended each day are based on individual calorie needs, weight goals, and the amount of physical activity performed daily.

Exchange List Groups

The following are the six groups of the Diabetic Exchange Lists:

Starches List (Includes Breads, Cereals, Grains and Starchy Vegetables)

One exchange from this group has 15 grams of carbohydrates, 3 grams of protein, and 0 to 1g of fat for a total of 80 calories per serving.

Examples of one serving from this group include one slice of bread, one-third cup cooked rice, or one-third cup cooked pasta.

Fruit List

One exchange from this group has 15 grams of carbohydrates for a total of 60 calories per serving. Foods in the fruit list do not contain any protein or fat.

Examples of one serving from this group include one small apple, seventeen small grapes, or one-half cup of orange juice.

Non-Starchy Vegetable List

One exchange from this group has 2 grams of carbohydrates and 5 grams of protein for a total of 25 calories per serving. Non-starchy vegetables contain no fat.

Examples of one serving from this group include one-half cup cooked green beans, one cup raw lettuce, or one-half cup vegetable juice.

Milk List

Items on the milk list are divided into fat-free/low-fat milk, reduced-fat milk, and whole milk categories.

One fat-free/low-fat milk exchange has 12 grams of carbohydrates, 8 grams of protein, and 0 to 3g of fat for a total of 90 calories per serving. One reduced-fat milk exchange has 12 grams of carbohydrates, 8 grams of protein, and 5g of fat for a total of 120 calories per serving. One whole milk exchange has 12 grams of carbohydrates, 8 grams of protein, and 8g of fat for a total of 150 calories per serving.

Examples of one serving from the fat-free/low-fat milk exchange are one cup of non-fat skim or 1 percent milk, or two-thirds cup (or six ounces) of fat-free plain yogurt.

Meat and Meat Substitutes List

Meats are divided into very lean, lean, medium-fat, and high-fat lists based on the amount of fat they contain. High-fat exchanges should be eaten a maximum of three times a week.

One very lean meat exchange has 7 grams of protein and 0 to 1 gram of fat for a total of 35 calories per serving. Examples of one very lean meat exchange are one ounce white meat chicken or turkey with no skin.

One lean meat exchange has 7 grams of protein and 3 grams of fat for a total of 55 calories per serving. Examples of one lean meat exchange are one ounce lean beef or lean pork.

One medium-fat meat exchange has 7 grams of protein and 5 grams of fat for a total of 75 calories per serving. Examples of one medium-fat meat exchange are one ounce dark meat chicken with skin, one egg, or one ounce of fried fish.

One high-fat meat exchange has 7 grams of protein and 8 grams of fat for a total of 100 calories per serving. Examples of one high-fat meat exchange are one ounce pork sausage, one ounce American cheese, or one ounce of a hot dog.

Whereas one exchange from this list only refers to a one-ounce portion of meat or meat substitute, a serving refers to two- to three-ounce portions of the foods in this list. A serving is often used in referring to the foods in this group because most people eat more than one ounce of meat or meat substitute at a time.

Fat List

One exchange from this group has 5 grams of fat for a total of 45 calories per serving. Most items in the fat exchange list do not contain protein or carbohydrate.

Examples of one serving from this group include one teaspoon oil, one teaspoon butter, one teaspoon mayonnaise, or one tablespoon salad dressing.

Carbohydrate Counting

The carbohydrate counting method is similar to the exchange list method in that they both use food groups. However, when you use carbohydrate counting, you keep track or "count" servings equal to 15 grams or 1 unit of carbohydrate The food groups that have carbohydrate and are counted are:

- the starch and starchy vegetables group;

- the fruit group;

- the milk group.

One serving from any of these three groups would count as one carbohydrate unit. For example if you ate two pieces of buttered toast and an eight-ounce glass of milk for breakfast, you would count that breakfast as having three carbohydrate units.

Carbohydrate counting differs from the exchange list in that the amount of protein and fats in foods is not taken into consideration. So the butter on the toast consumed at breakfast would not be counted, because butter is in the fat group and does not contain carbohydrate.

Some examples of one carbohydrate unit would be:

- **Starch and starchy vegetables group:** one slice of bread, one-third cup of cooked rice or pasta, one half of a small bagel

- **Milk group:** one cup milk, two-thirds cup fat-free-yogurt, three-quarters cup low-fat yogurt

- **Fruit group:** one small piece of fruit, three-quarters cup berries, one-half cup apple juice

If you are planning to use the carbohydrate counting method, you and your healthcare provider should decide how many servings of carbohydrate you should consume each day and at each meal for optimal health.

Section 30.2

Diabetes Food Pyramid

Excerpted from "What I Need to Know about Eating and Diabetes,"
National Institute of Diabetes and Digestive and Kidney Diseases,
National Institutes of Health, NIH Publication No. 08-5043, October 2007.

The diabetes food pyramid can help you make wise food choices. It divides foods into groups, based on what they contain. Eat more from the groups at the bottom of the pyramid, and less from the groups at the top. Foods from the starches, fruits, vegetables, and milk groups are highest in carbohydrate. They affect your blood glucose levels the most.

How Much Should I Eat Each Day?

Have about 1,200 to 1,600 calories a day if you are a:

- small woman who exercises;
- small or medium-sized woman who wants to lose weight;
- medium-sized woman who does not exercise much.

Choose this many servings from these food groups to have 1,200 to 1,600 calories a day:

- 6 starches
- 2 milks
- 3 vegetables
- 4 to 6 ounces meat and meat substitutes
- 2 fruits
- up to 3 fats

Have about 1,600 to 2,000 calories a day if you are a:

- large woman who wants to lose weight;
- small man at a healthy weight;
- medium-sized man who does not exercise much;
- medium-sized or large man who wants to lose weight.

Choose this many servings from these food groups to have 1,600 to 2,000 calories a day:

- 8 starches
- 2 milks
- 4 vegetables
- 4 to 6 ounces meat and meat substitutes
- 3 fruits
- up to 4 fats

Have about 2,000 to 2,400 calories a day if you are a:

- medium-sized or large man who exercises a lot or has a physically active job;
- large man at a healthy weight;
- medium-sized or large woman who exercises a lot or has a physically active job.

Choose this many servings from these food groups to have 2,000 to 2,400 calories a day:

- 10 starches
- 2 milks
- 4 vegetables
- 5 to 7 ounces meat and meat substitutes
- 4 fruits
- up to 5 fats

Talk with your diabetes teacher about how to make a meal plan that fits the way you usually eat, your daily routine, and your diabetes medicines. Then make your own plan.

Starches

Starches are bread, grains, cereal, pasta, and starchy vegetables like corn and potatoes. They provide carbohydrate, vitamins, minerals, and fiber. Whole-grain starches are healthier because they have more vitamins, minerals, and fiber.

Eat some starches at each meal. Eating starches is healthy for everyone, including people with diabetes.

Examples of starches are as follows:

- Bread
- Corn
- Potatoes
- Crackers
- Tortillas
- Yams

- Pasta
- Pretzels
- Rice
- Cereal
- Beans
- Lentils

How Much Is a Serving of Starch?

Examples of one serving: one slice of bread, one small potato, one-half cup cooked cereal, three-quarters cup dry cereal flakes, or one six-inch tortilla.

Examples of two servings: one small potato and one small ear of corn, or two slices of bread.

Examples of three servings: one small roll plus one-half cup of peas plus one small potato or one cup of rice.

If your plan includes more than one serving at a meal, you can choose different starches or have several servings of one starch.

What Are Healthy Ways to Eat Starches?

- Buy whole-grain breads and cereals.

- Eat fewer fried and high-fat starches such as regular tortilla chips and potato chips, French fries, pastries, or biscuits. Try pretzels, fat-free popcorn, baked tortilla chips or potato chips, baked potatoes, or low-fat muffins.

- Use low-fat or fat-free plain yogurt or fat-free sour cream instead of regular sour cream on a baked potato.

- Use mustard instead of mayonnaise on a sandwich.

- Use low-fat or fat-free substitutes such as low-fat mayonnaise or light margarine on bread, rolls, or toast.

- Eat cereal with fat-free (skim) or low-fat (1 percent) milk.

Vegetables

Vegetables provide vitamins, minerals, and fiber. They are low in carbohydrate.

Examples of vegetables are as follows:

- Lettuce
- Broccoli

- Vegetable juice
- Spinach

- Peppers
- Carrots

- Green beans
- Tomatoes

- Celery
- Chilies

- Greens
- Cabbage

How Much Is a Serving of Vegetables?

Examples of one serving: one-half cup cooked carrots, one-half cup cooked green beans, or one cup salad.

Examples of two servings: one-half cup cooked carrots plus one cup salad or one-half cup vegetable juice plus one-half cup cooked green beans.

Examples of three servings: one-half cup cooked greens plus one-half cup cooked green beans and one small tomato or one-half cup broccoli plus one cup tomato sauce.

If your plan includes more than one serving at a meal, you can choose several types of vegetables or have two or three servings of one vegetable.

What Are Healthy Ways to Eat Vegetables?

- Eat raw and cooked vegetables with little or no fat, sauces, or dressings.

- Try low-fat or fat-free salad dressing on raw vegetables or salads.

- Steam vegetables using water or low-fat broth.

- Mix in some chopped onion or garlic.

- Use a little vinegar or some lemon or lime juice.

- Add a small piece of lean ham or smoked turkey instead of fat to vegetables when cooking.

- Sprinkle with herbs and spices.

- If you do use a small amount of fat, use canola oil, olive oil, or soft margarines (liquid or tub types) instead of fat from meat, butter, or shortening.

Fruits

Fruits provide carbohydrate, vitamins, minerals, and fiber. Examples of fruits include the following;

- Apples
- Strawberries
- Grapefruit
- Raisins
- Watermelon
- Mango
- Papaya
- Canned fruit

- Fruit juice
- Dried fruit
- Bananas
- Oranges
- Peaches
- Guava
- Berries

How Much Is a Serving of Fruit?

Examples of one serving: one small apple, one-half cup juice, or one-half grapefruit.

Examples of two servings: one banana, one-half cup orange juice, or one and a quarter cups whole strawberries.

If your plan includes more than one serving at a meal, you can choose different types of fruit or have several servings of one fruit.

What Are Healthy Ways to Eat Fruits?

- Eat fruits raw or cooked, as juice with no sugar added, canned in their own juice, or dried.

- Buy smaller pieces of fruit.

233

- Choose pieces of fruit more often than fruit juice. Whole fruit is more filling and has more fiber.

- Save high-sugar and high-fat fruit desserts such as peach cobbler or cherry pie for special occasions.

Milk

Milk provides carbohydrate, protein, calcium, vitamins, and minerals.

How Much Is a Serving of Milk?

Examples of one serving: one cup fat-free or low-fat yogurt or one cup fat-free (skim) or low-fat (1 percent) milk.

Note: If you are pregnant or breastfeeding, have four to five servings of milk each day.

What Are Healthy Ways to Have Milk?

- Drink fat-free (skim) or low-fat (1 percent) milk.

- Eat low-fat or fat-free fruit yogurt sweetened with a low-calorie sweetener.

- Use low-fat plain yogurt as a substitute for sour cream.

Meat and Meat Substitutes

The meat and meat substitutes group includes meat, poultry, eggs, cheese, fish, and tofu. Eat small amounts of some of these foods each day.

Meat and meat substitutes provide protein, vitamins, and minerals.

Examples of meat and meat substitutes include the following:

• Chicken	• Beef
• Fish	• Canned tuna or other fish
• Eggs	• Peanut butter
• Tofu	• Cottage cheese
• Cheese	• Pork
• Lamb	• Turkey

How Much Is a Serving of Meat and Meat Substitutes?

Meat and meat substitutes are measured in ounces. Here are examples.

Examples of a one-ounce serving: one egg or two tablespoons of peanut butter.

Examples of a two-ounce serving: one slice (one ounce) of turkey plus one slice (one ounce) of low-fat cheese.

Examples of a three-ounce serving: three ounces of cooked lean meat, chicken, or fish (three ounces of meat [after cooking] is about the size of a deck of cards).

What Are Healthy Ways to Eat Meat and Meat Substitutes?

- Buy cuts of beef, pork, ham, and lamb that have only a little fat on them. Trim off the extra fat.

- Eat chicken or turkey without the skin.

- Cook meat and meat substitutes in low-fat ways:

  - Broil

  - Grill

  - Stir-fry

  - Roast

  - Steam

  - Microwave

- To add more flavor, use vinegars, lemon juice, soy sauce, salsa, ketchup, barbecue sauce, herbs, and spices.

- Cook eggs using cooking spray or a nonstick pan.

- Limit the amount of nuts, peanut butter, and fried foods you eat. They are high in fat.

- Check food labels. Choose low-fat or fat-free cheese.

Fats and Sweets

Limit the amount of fats and sweets you eat. Fats and sweets are not as nutritious as other foods. Fats have a lot of calories. Sweets can be high in carbohydrate and fat. Some contain saturated fats, trans fats, and cholesterol that increase your risk of heart disease. Limiting these foods will help you lose weight and keep your blood glucose and blood fats under control.

Examples of fats include the following:

- Salad dressing
- Oil
- Cream cheese
- Butter
- Margarine
- Mayonnaise
- Avocado
- Olives
- Bacon

Examples of sweets include the following:

- Cake
- Ice cream
- Pie
- Syrup
- Cookies
- Doughnuts

How Much Is a Serving of Sweets?

Examples of one serving: one three-inch cookie, one plain cake doughnut, or one tablespoon maple syrup.

How Much Is a Serving of Fat?

Examples of one serving: one strip of bacon or one teaspoon oil.

Examples of two servings: one tablespoon regular salad dressing or two tablespoons reduced-fat salad dressing plus one tablespoon reduced-fat mayonnaise.

How Can I Satisfy My Sweet Tooth?

Try having sugar-free popsicles, diet soda, fat-free ice cream or frozen yogurt, or sugar-free hot cocoa mix.

Other tips:

- Share desserts in restaurants.

- Order small or child-size servings of ice cream or frozen yogurt.

- Divide homemade desserts into small servings and wrap each individually. Freeze extra servings.

Remember, fat-free and low-sugar foods still have calories. Talk with your diabetes teacher about how to fit sweets into your meal plan.

Alcoholic Drinks

Alcoholic drinks have calories but no nutrients. If you have alcoholic drinks on an empty stomach, they can make your blood glucose level go too low. Alcoholic drinks also can raise your blood fats. If you want to have alcoholic drinks, talk with your doctor or diabetes teacher about how much to have.

Section 30.3

Carbohydrate Counting

Carbohydrate counting can be used to track and balance the amount of carbohydrates in your diet. You can have better blood glucose control by keeping the amount of carbohydrates you eat consistent and spaced throughout the day.

What Are the Basics of Carbohydrate Counting?

- Foods are made up of three components: carbohydrate, protein, and fat.

- Carbohydrate is the portion of food that affects blood glucose levels the most.

- By using food labels and estimating portion sizes of foods, you can count the grams of carbohydrate in your diet.

What Foods Contain Carbohydrates?

- Foods from the starch, fruit, and milk groups.

- Almost all dessert and snack foods.

- Starchy vegetables such as potatoes, corn, and peas.

How Much Carbohydrate Do I Need?

The amount of carbohydrate you need will vary based on such things as your height, weight, and activity level. In general to promote weight loss:

- women need about 45 grams per meal or three servings of carbohydrate per meal;

- men need about 60 grams per meal or four servings of carbohydrate per meal.

15 grams of carbohydrate = 1 serving

Carbohydrate Serving Sizes

Starch group—one serving equals:

- one slice of bread;
- half a hamburger bun;
- half a cup of mashed potatoes
- one-third cup rice or pasta;
- one-half cup corn;
- approximately three-quarters cup cereal (check food label on box).

Fruit group—one serving equals:

- one small piece of fruit;
- one-half cup orange juice;
- one-half cup canned fruit;
- one cup cut up melon;
- one-quarter cup dried fruit;
- three-quarters cup berries;
- one cup grapes.

Milk group—one serving equals:

- one cup milk;
- two-thirds to three-quarters cup yogurt (check food label on carton).

Other Carbohydrates

- This group includes sweets and other carbohydrates including cookies, candies, cake, and chips.

- Try to limit the amount of these foods in the diet because they are a concentrated source of calories and fat. These foods are also very high in carbohydrates.

Food Groups That Do Not Increase Blood Glucose

Non-Starchy Vegetable Group

- Foods in this category should not be limited.
- Each serving of vegetables contain 5 grams of carbohydrate.

Meat Group

- Try to choose low-fat meats such as skinless chicken breast, turkey, or fish.
- Avoid meats that are high in saturated fat such as bacon and sausage.

Fat Group

- Choose monounsaturated or polyunsaturated fats which are found in foods such as olives, olive oil, canola oil, fish, nuts, and other vegetable oils such as corn, safflower, and soy.
- Avoid saturated fats which are found in foods such as butter and high-fat animal products.

Fiber

- A high-fiber diet can help you control your blood sugar. Choose whole grains that are high in fiber as well as fruits, vegetables, beans, and lentils. Your registered dietitian (RD) can help you increase the fiber in your diet.

Menu Examples

Sample Breakfast

Three-quarters cup unsweetened cereal or one slice of toast = 15 grams

One cup milk or one tablespoon jelly = 15 grams
One small banana or One small orange = 15 grams
Total = 45 grams

Sample Lunch

Three ounces tuna fish or one tablespoon peanut butter = 0
One-half bagel (two ounces) or two slices bread = 30 grams
One tablespoon light mayo or one ounce cheese = 0
One-half cup cooked broccoli or one cup celery sticks = 0
One-half cup fruit cocktail or one small cookie = 15 grams
Total = 45 grams

Sample Dinner

One medium baked potato (six ounces) or two small dinner rolls = 30 grams
Four ounces grilled chicken or four ounces steak = 0
One tablespoon sour cream or one tablespoon salad dressing = 0
One cup California mixed vegetables or 1 cup salad = 0
One-half cup sugar-free pudding or one and one-quarter cup strawberries = 15 grams
Total = 45 grams
Talk to your doctor or others on your healthcare team if you have questions.

Section 30.4

Exchange Lists

Excerpted from "Diabetes Diet," © 2010 A.D.A.M., Inc.
Reprinted with permission.

Diabetic Exchange Lists

The objective of using diabetic exchange lists is to maintain the proper balance of carbohydrates, proteins, and fats throughout the day. Patients should meet with a dietician or diabetes nutrition expert for help in learning this approach.

In developing a menu, patients must first establish their individual dietary requirements, particularly the optimal number of daily calories and the proportion of carbohydrates, fats, and protein. The exchange lists should then be used to set up menus for each day that fulfill these requirements.

The following are some general rules:

- The diabetic exchanges are six different lists of foods grouped according to similar calorie, carbohydrate, protein, and fat content; these are starch/bread, meat, vegetables, fruit, milk, and fat. A person is allowed a certain number of exchange choices from each food list per day.

- The amount and type of these exchanges are based on a number of factors, including the daily exercise program, timing of insulin injections, and whether or not an individual needs to lose weight or reduce cholesterol or blood pressure levels.

- Foods can be substituted for each other within an exchange list but not between lists even if they have the same calorie count.

- In all lists (except in the fruit list) choices can be doubled or tripled to supply a serving of certain foods. (For example three starch choices equal one and a half cups of hot cereal or three meat choices equal a three-ounce hamburger.)

- On the exchange lists, some foods are "free." These contain fewer than twenty calories per serving and can be eaten in any amount spread throughout the day unless a serving size is specified.

Table 30.1. Number of Exchanges per Day for Various Calories Levels

Calories	1,200	1,500	1,800	2,000	2,200
Starch/Bread	5	8	10	11	13
Meat	4	5	7	8	8
Vegetable	2	3	3	4	4
Fruit	3	3	3	3	3
Milk	2	2	2	2	2
Fat	3	3	3	4	5

Exchange List Categories

The following are the categories on exchange lists:

- **Starches and bread:** Each exchange under starches and bread contains about 15 grams of carbohydrates, 3 grams of protein, and a trace of fat for a total of 80 calories. A general rule is that a half-cup of cooked cereal, grain, or pasta equals one exchange. One ounce of a bread product is one serving.

- **Meat and cheese:** The exchange groups for meat and cheese are categorized by lean meat and low-fat substitutes, medium-fat meat and substitutes, and high-fat meat and substitutes. Use high-fat exchanges a maximum of three times a week. Fat should be removed before cooking. Exchange sizes on the meat list are generally one ounce and based on cooked meats (three ounces of cooked meat equals four ounces of raw meat).

- **Vegetables:** Exchanges for vegetables are one-half cup cooked, one cup raw, and one-half cup juice. Each group contains 5 grams of carbohydrates, 2 grams of protein, and 2 to 3 grams of fiber. Vegetables can be fresh or frozen; canned vegetables are less desirable because they are often high in sodium. They should be steamed or cooked in a microwave without added fat.

- **Fruits and sugar:** Sugars are included within the total carbo-hydrate count in the exchange lists. Sugars should not be more than 10 percent of daily carbohydrates. Each exchange contains about 15 grams of carbohydrates for a total of 60 calories.

- **Milk and substitutes:** The milk and substitutes list is catego-rized by fat content similar to the meat list. A milk exchange is usually one cup or eight ounces. Those who are on weight-loss or low-cholesterol diets should follow the skim and very low-fat milk lists—while avoiding the whole milk group. Others should use the whole milk list very sparingly. All people with diabetes should avoid artificially sweetened milks.

- **Fats:** A fat exchange is usually one teaspoon, but it may vary. People, of course, should avoid saturated and trans fatty acids and choose polyunsaturated or monounsaturated fats instead.

Section 30.5

The Plate Method

"The Idaho Plate Method for Diabetes Management,"
by Laura L. Sant, MS, RD, University of Idaho Extension
Educator. © 2010 University of Idaho. Reprinted with permission.

The Idaho Plate Method is a visual guide for healthy eating with diabetes. All foods can fit into the Idaho Plate Method. It encourages you to eat a variety of different foods and includes servings from all food groups in each meal. The meal plan is designed to provide approximately 1,400 calories for the entire day. Each meal has 45 grams of carbohydrate or 3 carbohydrate choices. The foods that provide these carbohydrates are starches, fruits, and dairy.

To eat according to the Idaho Plate Method, begin with a nine-inch plate. This may be considered a small plate by some people's standards, but a nine-inch plate allows for just the right size in food portions. Even if you have only a nine-inch plate, you may be thinking that you can stack a lot of food on that plate. Well, in order to take control of your diabetes, you do not want to go overboard with the food. The

243

Idaho Plate Method suggests that your food should be no greater than one-inch high on the plate.

Below lists what to eat if you want to follow the Idaho Plate Method:

- Fill half of the plate (approximately one cup) with nonstarchy vegetables:

  - Lettuce, cabbage, cucumbers, peppers, mushrooms, onions, garlic, beets, green beans, broccoli, celery, carrots, cauliflower, and/or tomatoes

- Fill one-quarter of the plate with high-protein foods:

  - Three ounces meat, poultry, fish, or tofu

  - One to two eggs

  - Two tablespoons peanut butter

  - One-third cup nuts

  - Two ounces cheese

- Fill one-quarter of the plate with starchy foods:

  - One slice of bread

  - One-half cup cooked or three-quarters cup dry nonsweetened cereal

  - One-third cup cooked pasta or rice

  - Six-inch tortillas

  - One-half cup dried beans or lentils

  - One-half cup potatoes, corn, or peas

- Add a small serving of fruit:

  - A small piece of fruit (similar in size to a tennis ball)

  - One-half cup fresh, frozen, or canned fruit

  - Two tablespoons dried fruit

- Add a serving of dairy:

  - One cup milk

  - Six to eight ounces light yogurt

  - One-half cup sugar-free pudding

You may be thinking that you will not always want to eat according to the Idaho Plate Method. The Idaho Plate Method is flexible and allows you to substitute one type of carbohydrate for another. For example if you want two starches at one meal, you would then omit the fruit or dairy to make up for the addition. However, eating according to the original method gives you the most variety and nutrition.

What about dessert? Dessert may occasionally be substituted for the fruit serving. However, because desserts often contain a lot of sugar and fat, eat them in moderation. Moderation means eating small portions every once in a while, like one or two times a week.

Chapter 31

Components of the Diabetic Diet

Carbohydrates

Compared to fats and protein, carbohydrates have the greatest impact on blood sugar (glucose). Except for dietary fiber, which is not digestible, carbohydrates are eventually broken down by the body into glucose. Carbohydrate types are either complex (as in starches) or simple (as in fruits and sugars).

One gram of carbohydrates provides four calories. The current general recommendation is that carbohydrates should provide between 45 and 65 percent of the daily caloric intake. Carbohydrate intake should not fall below 130 grams/day.

Complex carbohydrates are broken down more slowly by the body than simple carbohydrates. They are more likely to provide other nutritional components and fiber:

- Vegetables, fruits, whole grains, and beans are good sources of carbohydrates. Whole-grain foods provide more nutritional value than pasta, white bread, and white potatoes. Brown rice is a better choice than white rice.

- Patients should try to consume a minimum of 20 to 35 grams of fiber daily (ideally 50 grams/day), from vegetables, fruits, whole-grain cereals, breads, nuts, and seeds.

Excerpted from "Diabetes Diet," © 2010 A.D.A.M., Inc. Reprinted with permission.

- Whole grains specifically are extremely important for people with diabetes or at risk for it.

Simple carbohydrates, or sugars (either as sucrose or fructose), add calories, increase blood glucose levels quickly, and provide little or no other nutrients:

- Sucrose (table sugar) is the source of most dietary sugar, found in sugar cane, honey, and corn syrup.

- Fructose, the sugar found in fruits, may produce a slower increase in blood sugar than sucrose. Dark-colored fruits are rich in important vitamins and other nutrients. Other fruits, such as apples and grapes, also have important beneficial food chemicals.

- People with diabetes should avoid products listing more than 5 grams of sugar per serving, and some doctors recommend limiting fruit intake. If specific amounts are not listed, patients should avoid products with either sucrose or fructose listed as one of the first four ingredients on the label.

The Carbohydrate Counting System

Some people plan their carbohydrate intake using a system called carbohydrate counting. It is based on two premises:

- All carbohydrates (either from sugars or starches) will raise blood sugar to a similar degree. In general, 1 gram of carbohydrates raises blood sugar by 3 points in people who weigh 200 pounds, 4 points for people who weigh 150 pounds, and 5 points for 100 pounds.

- Carbohydrates have the greatest impact on blood sugar; fats and protein play only minor roles.

In other words, the amount of carbohydrates eaten (rather than fats or proteins) will determine how high blood sugar levels will rise. There are two options for counting carbohydrates: advanced and simple. Both rely on collaboration with a doctor, dietitian, or both. Once the patient learns how to count carbohydrates and adjust insulin doses to their meals, many find it more flexible, more accurate in predicting blood sugar increases, and easier to plan meals than other systems.

The basic goal is to balance insulin with the amount of carbohydrates eaten in order to control blood glucose levels after a meal. The steps to the plan are as follows.

The patient must first carefully record a number of factors that are used to determine the specific requirements for a meal plan based on carbohydrate grams:

- Multiple blood glucose readings (taken several times a day)
- The time of meals
- Amount in grams of all the carbohydrates eaten
- Time, type, and duration of exercise
- The time, type, and dose of insulin or oral medications
- Other relevant factors, such as menstruation, illness, and stress

The patient works with the dietitian for two or three forty-five- to ninety-minute sessions to plan how many grams of carbohydrates are needed. There are three carbohydrate groups:

- Bread/starch
- Fruit
- Milk

One serving from each group should contain twelve to fifteen carbohydrate grams. (Patients can find the amount of carbohydrates in foods from labels on commercial foods and from a number of books and websites.)

The dietitian creates a meal plan that accommodates the patient's weight and needs, as determined by the patient's record, and makes a special calculation called the carbohydrate-to-insulin ratio. This ratio determines the number of carbohydrate grams that a patient needs to cover the daily pre-meal insulin needs. Eventually, patients can learn to adjust their insulin doses to their meals.

Patients who choose this approach must still be aware of protein and fat content in foods. These food groups may add excessive calories and saturated fats. Patients must still follow basic healthy dietary principles.

The Glycemic Index

The glycemic index helps determine which carbohydrate-containing foods raise blood glucose levels more or less quickly after a meal. The index uses a scale of numbers for specific foods that reflect greatest to least delay in producing an increase in blood sugar after a meal.

The lower the index number, the better the impact on glucose levels. Some evidence suggests that the benefit of foods with a low glycemic index is due to their ability to increase insulin levels quickly (thus removing blood sugar) rather than their ability to slow the release of blood sugar itself.

There are two indices in use. One uses a scale of 1 to 100 with 100 representing a glucose tablet, which has the most rapid effect on blood sugar. The other common index uses a scale with 100 representing white bread (so some foods will be above 100).

Choosing foods with low glycemic index scores often has a significant effect on controlling the surge in blood sugar after meals. Many of these foods are also high in fiber and so have heart benefits as well. Substituting low- for high-glycemic-index foods may also help prevent weight gain.

One easy way to improve glycemic index is to simply replace starches and sugars with whole grains and legumes (dried peas, beans, and lentils). However, there are many factors that affect the glycemic index of foods, and maintaining a diet with low glycemic load is not straightforward.

No one should use the glycemic index as a complete dietary guide, since it does not provide nutritional guidelines for all foods. It is simply an indication of how the metabolism will respond to certain carbohydrates.

The Glycemic Index of Some Foods

The following list assumes 100 = a glucose tablet:

- Breads:
  - Pumpernickel: 49
  - Sourdough: 54
  - Rye: 64
  - White: 69
  - Whole wheat: 72
- Grains:
  - Barley: 22
  - Sweet corn: 58
  - Brown rice: 66
  - White rice: 72

- Beans:
    - Soy: 14
    - Red lentils: 27
    - Kidney (dried and boiled, not canned): 29
    - Chickpeas: 36
    - Baked: 43
- Dairy products:
    - Milk: 30
    - Ice cream: 60
- Cereals:
    - Oatmeal: 53
    - All bran: 54
    - Swiss muesli: 60
    - Shredded wheat: 70
    - Corn flakes: 83
    - Puffed rice: 90
- Pasta:
    - Spaghetti-protein enriched: 28
    - Spaghetti (boiled five minutes): 33
    - Spaghetti (boiled fifteen minutes): 44
- Fruit:
    - Strawberries: 32
    - Apple: 38
    - Orange: 43
    - Orange juice: 49
    - Banana: 61
- Potatoes:
    - Sweet: 50
    - Yams: 54

- New: 58
- Mashed: 72
- Instant mashed: 86
- White: 87

- Snacks:
  - Potato chips: 56
  - Oatmeal cookies: 57
  - Corn chips: 72

- Sugars:
  - Fructose: 22
  - Refined sugar: 64
  - Honey: 91

Note: These numbers are general values, but they may vary widely depending on other factors, including if and how they are cooked and foods they are combined with.

Low-Carbohydrate Diets

Low-carb diets generally restrict the amount of carbohydrates but do not restrict protein sources. Popular low-carb diet plans include Atkins, South Beach, The Zone, and Sugar Busters:

- The Atkins diet restricts complex carbohydrates in vegetables and fruits that are known to protect against heart disease. The Atkins diet also can cause excessive calcium excretion in urine, which increases the risk for kidney stones and osteoporosis.

- Low-carb diets such as South Beach, The Zone, and Sugar Busters rely on the glycemic index. Foods on the lowest end of the index take longer to digest. Slow digestion wards off hunger pains. It also helps stabilize insulin levels. Foods high on the glycemic index include bread, white potatoes, and pasta while low-glycemic foods include whole grains, fruit, lentils, and soybeans.

According to the American Diabetes Association (ADA), low-carb diets may help reduce weight in the short term (up to one year). However, because these diets tend to include more fat and protein, the ADA recommends that people on these diet plans have their blood lipids, including cholesterol and triglycerides, regularly monitored. Patients who have kidney problems need to be careful about protein consumption, as high-protein diets can worsen this condition.

Whole Grains, Nuts, and Fiber-Rich Foods

Fiber is an important component of many complex carbohydrates. It is found only in plant foods such as vegetables, fruits, whole grains, nuts, and legumes (dried beans, peanuts, and peas). Fiber cannot be digested. Instead, it passes through the intestines, drawing water with it, and is eliminated as part of feces content. The following are specific advantages from high-fiber diets (up to 55 grams a day):

- Insoluble fiber (found in wheat bran, whole grains, seeds, nuts, legumes, and fruit and vegetable peels) may help achieve weight loss. Consuming whole grains on a regular basis appears to provide many important benefits, especially for people with type 2 diabetes. Whole grains may even lower the risk for type 2 diabetes in the first place. Of special note, nuts, such as almonds, macadamia, and walnuts, may be highly heart protective, independent of their fiber content. However, nuts are high in calories.

- Soluble fiber (found in dried beans, oat bran, barley, apples, citrus fruits, and potatoes) has important benefits for the heart, particularly for achieving healthy cholesterol levels and possibly reducing blood pressure as well.

- Soluble fiber supplements, such as those that contain psyllium or glucomannan, may be beneficial. Psyllium is taken from the husk of a seed grown in India. It is found in laxatives (Metamucil®), breakfast cereals (Bran Buds®), and other products. Psyllium can increase sodium so people who increase their levels of soluble fiber should also drink more fluids (especially water).

Fat Substitutes and Artificial Sweeteners

Replacing fats and sugars with substitutes may help some people who have trouble maintaining weight.

Fat Substitutes

Fat substitutes added to commercial foods or used in baking deliver some of the desirable qualities of fat, but do not add as many calories. They cannot be eaten in unlimited amounts. Fat substitutes include:

- Plant substances known as sterols, and their derivatives called stanols, reduce cholesterol by blocking its absorption in the intestinal tract. Margarines containing sterols are available.

- Olestra (Olean®) passes through the body without leaving behind any calories from fat. However, it can cause cramps and diarrhea, and even small amounts of olestra may deplete the body of certain vitamins and nutrients.

- Beta-glucan is a soluble fiber found in oats and barley.

Artificial Sweeteners

Artificial sweeteners use chemicals to mimic the sweetness of sugar. These products do not contain calories and do not affect blood sugar. Artificial sweeteners approved by the U.S. Food and Drug Administration (FDA) include:

- Aspartame (NutraSweet®, Equal®). Aspartame is generally considered safe, but people with phenylketonuria (PKU), a rare genetic condition, should not use it.

- Saccharin (Sweet'N Low®). Saccharin is the oldest artificial sweetener. Although early studies in rats indicated a potential risk for cancer, subsequent research has shown that saccharin does not cause cancer.

- Sucralose (Splenda®). Sucralose has no bitter aftertaste and works well in baking, unlike other artificial sweeteners. It is made from real sugar by replacing hydroxyl atoms with chlorine atoms.

- Rebiana (Truvia®, PureVia®) is an extract derived from stevia, a South American plant. (Stevia is also sold in health food stores as a dietary supplement.) Approved in 2008, rebiana is used in table sweeteners and soft drinks

- Acesulfame potassium, also known as Acesulfame-K (Sweet One®, Sunette®).

- Neotame (Neotame®). Neotame is structurally similar to aspartame. Unlike other artificial sweeteners, Neotame is not available as a table sweetener. It is only used as a general-purpose sweetener in commercial food products such as baked goods and soft drinks.

Sugar alcohols (which include xylitol, mannitol, and sorbitol) are often used in sugar-free products, such as cookies, hard candies, and chewing gum. Sugar alcohols can slightly increase blood sugar levels.

The American Diabetes Association recommends against consuming large amounts of sugar alcohol as it can cause gas and diarrhea, especially in children.

Protein

Protein intake in diabetes is complicated and depends on various factors. These factors include whether a patient has type 1, type 2, or pre-diabetes. There are additional guidelines for patients who show signs of kidney damage (diabetic nephropathy).

In general, diabetes dietary guidelines recommend that proteins should provide 12 to 20 percent of total daily calories. This daily amount poses no risk to the kidney in people who do not have kidney disease. Protein is important for strong muscles and bone. Some doctors recommend a higher proportion of protein (20 to 30 percent) for patients with pre- or type 2 diabetes. They think that eating more protein helps people feel more full and thus reduces overall calories. In addition, protein consumption helps the body maintain lean body mass during weight loss.

Patients with diabetic kidney problems need to limit their intake of protein. A typical protein-restricted diet limits protein intake to no more than 10 percent of total daily calories. Patients with kidney damage also need to limit their intake of phosphorus, a mineral found in dairy products, beans, and nuts. (However, patients on dialysis need to have more protein in their diets.) Potassium and phosphorus restriction is often necessary as well.

One gram of protein provides four calories. Protein is commonly recommended as part of a bedtime snack to maintain normal blood sugar levels during the night, although studies are mixed over whether it adds any protective benefits against nighttime hypoglycemia. If it does, only small amounts (14 grams) may be needed to stabilize blood glucose levels.

Good sources of protein include fish, skinless chicken or turkey, nonfat or low-fat dairy products, soy (tofu), and legumes (kidney beans, black beans, chick peas, lentils).

Fish

Fish is probably the best source of protein. Evidence suggests that eating moderate amounts of fish (twice a week) may improve triglycerides and help lower the risks for death from heart disease, dangerous heart rhythms, blood pressure, a tendency for blood clots, and the risk for stroke.

The most healthy fish are oily fish such as salmon, mackerel, or sardines, which are high in omega-3 fatty acids. Three capsules of fish oil (preferably as supplements of DHA-EPA) are about equivalent to one serving of fish.

Women who are pregnant (or planning on becoming pregnant) or nursing should avoid fish that contains a high amount of mercury. These high-mercury fish include swordfish, tuna, bass, and mackerel.

Soy

Soy is an excellent food. It is rich in both soluble and insoluble fiber, omega-3 fatty acids, and provides all essential proteins. Soy proteins have more vitamins and minerals than meat or dairy proteins. They also contain polyunsaturated fats, which are better than the saturated fat found in meat. The best sources of soy protein are soy products (tofu, soy milk, soybeans). Soy sauce is not a good source. It contains only a trace amount of soy and is very high in sodium.

For many years, soy was promoted as a food that could help lower cholesterol and improve heart disease risk factors. Recent studies have found that soy protein and isoflavone supplement pills do not have major effects on cholesterol or heart disease prevention. The American Heart Association still encourages patients to include soy foods as part of an overall heart healthy diet, but does not recommend using isoflavone supplements.

Meat and Poultry

Lean cuts of meat are the best choice for heart health and diabetes control. Saturated fat in meat is the primary danger to the heart. The fat content of meat varies depending on the type and cut. For patients with diabetes, skinless chicken or turkey is a better choice than red meat. (Fish is an even better choice.)

Dairy Products

A high intake of dairy products may lower risk factors related to type 2 diabetes and heart disease (insulin resistance, high blood pressure, obesity, and unhealthy cholesterol). Some researchers suggest the calcium in dairy products may be partially responsible for these benefits. However, because many dairy products are high in saturated fats and calories, it's best to choose low-fat and nonfat dairy items.

Fats and Oils

Some fat is essential for normal body function. Fats can have good or bad effects on health, depending on their chemistry. New research suggests that the type of fat is more important than the total amount of fat when it comes to reducing heart disease. Monounsaturated fatty acids (MUFA) and polyunsaturated fatty acids (PUFA) are good fats that help promote heart health, and should be the main type of fats consumed. Saturated fats and trans fats (trans fatty acids) are bad fats that can contribute to heart disease, and should be avoided or limited.

Current dietary guidelines for diabetes and heart health recommend that:

- Total fat from all fat sources should be 25 to 35 percent of total daily calories.

- Monounsaturated fatty acids (found in olive oil, canola oil, peanut oil, nuts, and avocados) and omega-3 polyunsaturated fatty acids (found in fish, shellfish, flaxseed, and walnuts) should be the first choice for fats.

- Omega-6 polyunsaturated fatty acids (corn, safflower, sunflower, and soybean oils and nuts and seeds) are the second choice and should account for 5 to 10 percent of total calories as part of total fat intake. Linoleic acid, the main omega-6 fatty acid found in food, has anti-inflammatory properties. Higher intakes of omega-6 fatty acids may help improve insulin resistance, reduce diabetes risk, and lower blood pressure.

- Limit saturated fat (found predominantly in animal products, including meat and full fat dairy products, as well as coconut and palm oils) to less than 7 percent of total daily calories.

- Limit trans fats (found in margarine, commercial baked goods, snack and fried foods) to less than 1 percent of total calories.

All fats, good or bad, are high in calories compared to proteins and carbohydrates. In order to calculate daily fat intake, multiply the number of fat grams eaten by nine (one fat gram provides nine calories, whether it's oil or fat) and divide by the number of total daily calories desired. One teaspoon of oil, butter, or other fats contains about five grams of fat. All fats, no matter what the source, add the same calories. The American Heart Association recommends

257

that fats and oils have fewer than two grams of saturated fat per tablespoon.

Try to replace saturated fats and trans fatty acids with unsaturated fats from plant and fish oils. Omega-3 fatty acids, which are found in fish and a few plant sources, are a good source of unsaturated fats. Generally, two servings of fish per week provide a healthful amount of omega-3 fatty acids. Fish oil dietary supplements are another option. Fish and fish oil supplements contain docosahexaenoic (DHA) and eicosapentaenoic (EPA) acids, which have significant benefits for the heart. Discuss with your doctor whether you should consider taking fish oil supplements.

Low-Fat Diets

The American Diabetes Association states that low-fat diets can help reduce weight in the short term (up to one year). Low-fat diets that are high in fiber, whole grains, legumes, and fresh produce can offer health advantages for cholesterol control. These foods are also lower on the glycemic index than high-glycemic foods such as white bread, white potatoes, and pasta.

Dietary Cholesterol

The story on cholesterol found in the diet is not entirely straightforward. The body produces cholesterol naturally and obtains it through meals. Animal-based food products contain cholesterol. High amounts occur in meat, dairy products, egg yolks, and shellfish. (Plant foods, such as fruits, nuts, and grains, do not contain cholesterol.) The American Heart Association recommends no more than 300 mg of dietary cholesterol per day for the general population and no more than 200 mg daily for those with high cholesterol or heart disease.

Vitamins and Supplements

Research on the effects of vitamin supplements on heart disease and diabetes has been mixed. Because of the lack of scientific evidence for benefit, the American Diabetes Association does not recommend regular use of vitamin supplements, except for people who have vitamin deficiencies.

Patients with type 2 diabetes who take metformin (Glucophage®) should be aware that this drug can interfere with vitamin B_{12} absorption. Calcium supplements may help counteract metformin-associated vitamin B_{12} deficiency.

Salt (Sodium)

It is a good idea for everyone to restrict their salt intake to less than 2,300 mg (about one teaspoon) a day. People with existing high blood pressure may need to reduce sodium intake to less than 1,500 mg daily. Limiting or avoiding consumption of processed foods can go a long way to reducing salt intake. Simply eliminating table and cooking salt is also beneficial.

Salt substitutes, such as Nu-Salt® and Mrs. Dash® (which contain mixtures of potassium, sodium, and magnesium), are available, but they can be risky for people with kidney disease or those who take blood pressure medication that causes potassium retention. Similarly, while eating more potassium-rich foods is helpful for achieving healthy blood pressure, patients with diabetes should check with their doctors before increasing the amount of potassium in their diets.

Other Minerals

Calcium

Calcium supplements may be important in older patients with diabetes to help reduce the risk for osteoporosis, particularly if their diets are low in dairy products.

Potassium and Phosphorus

Potassium-rich foods, and potassium supplements, can help lower systolic and diastolic blood pressure. Current guidelines support the use of potassium supplements or enough dietary potassium to achieve 3,500 mg per day for people with normal or high blood pressure (who have no risk factors for excess potassium levels). This goal is particularly important in people who have high sodium intake.

The best source of potassium is from the fruits and vegetables that contain them. Potassium-rich foods include bananas, oranges, pears, prunes, cantaloupes, tomatoes, dried peas and beans, nuts, potatoes, and avocados. No one should take potassium supplements without consulting a doctor. Kidney problems can cause potassium overload, and medications commonly used in diabetes (such as angiotensin-converting enzyme [ACE] inhibitors or potassium-sparing diuretics) also limit the kidney's ability to excrete potassium. Patients with diabetic nephropathy (kidney disease) and kidney failure need to restrict dietary potassium, as well as phosphorus. Phosphorus-rich foods that should be avoided include meats, dairy products, beans, whole foods, and nuts. In addition, many processed and fast foods contain high amounts of phosphorus additives.

Magnesium

Magnesium deficiency may have some role in insulin resistance and high blood pressure. Research indicates that magnesium-rich diets may help lower type 2 diabetes risk. Whole-grain breads and cereals, nuts (almonds, cashews, soybeans), and certain fruits and vegetables (spinach, avocados, beans) are excellent dietary sources of magnesium. Dietary supplements do not provide any benefit. Persons who live in soft water areas, who use diuretics, or who have other risk factors for magnesium deficiency may require more dietary magnesium than others.

Chromium

Most studies have indicated that chromium supplements have little or no effect on glucose metabolism and may cause adverse side effects.

Selenium

Selenium, a trace mineral, does not reduce diabetes risk. In fact, it may increase it. An average healthy diet supplies adequate amounts of selenium. There is no need to take dietary supplements.

Zinc

Many patients with type 2 diabetes are also deficient in zinc. More studies are needed to establish the benefits or risks of taking supplements. Zinc has some toxic side effects, and some studies have associated high zinc intake with prostate cancer.

Alcohol and Coffee

Alcohol

The American Diabetes Association recommends limiting alcoholic beverages to one drink per day for nonpregnant adult women and two drinks per day for adult men.

Coffee

Many studies have noted an association between coffee consumption (both caffeinated and decaffeinated) and reduced risk for developing type 2 diabetes. Researchers are still not certain if coffee protects against diabetes.

Chapter 32

Alcohol and Tobacco Can Increase Diabetes Problems

Chapter Contents

Section 32.1

Alcohol and Diabetes: A Dangerous Mix

Excerpted from "Generation D: A Young Adult's Guide to Diabetes Self-Management," © 2010 Canadian Diabetes Association (www.diabetes.ca). All rights reserved. Reprinted with permission.

What Do I Need to Know about Alcohol and Managing My Diabetes?

It's likely that members of your healthcare team have told you to not consume alcohol. Unfortunately, they are right. Diabetes and alcohol do not mix well together. However, just because someone has told you about the dangers of alcohol and diabetes doesn't mean you will decide to abstain for life.

First and foremost, know the legal drinking age in your state. If you are caught breaking the law, there are serious consequences. Remember that alcohol jeopardizes your safety and your health.

A few things to think about:

- There is sugar/carbohydrates in all types of alcohol—some types have more sugar than others.

- You will still consume a lot of sugar even if you drink diet soda with hard liquor.

- You may need insulin to cover these carbohydrates.

- Alcohol can have a delayed effect on your blood glucose level.

- All bodies treat alcohol as a poison.

- If you consume too much alcohol, you may not be able to keep an eye on your blood glucose level.

- If you forget to take your insulin or miscalculate how much you need, who will be watching your blood glucose level?

- It can be hard to maintain a healthy blood glucose level when you drink.

- You can have one or two standard alcoholic drinks with food, without subtracting food from the usual meal plan.

The Party Scene

If you understand your diabetes and are in control, going to a party should not be an issue. If the party involves a meal, be sure you have an idea what kind of food will be served as well as when it will be served. Parties usually mean late nights, which can lead to late mornings. Be sure you figure out in advance how you'll manage your need for food and insulin in the morning.

It's important to ensure that if you do decide to consume alcohol you are with someone who knows you have diabetes and will be able to react and keep you safe if needed. Wearing a medical alert bracelet can also be a good idea.

Table 32.1. Steps to Reduce Your Risk of Hypoglycemia with Alcohol Consumption

Before Drinking	While Drinking	After Drinking
Eat regular meals	Eat carbohydrate-rich foods	Tell someone you trust you've been drinking
Take your medication	Eat additional carbohydrates if dancing or doing other physical activity	Eat a carbohydrate-rich snack if your blood glucose is low
Check your blood glucose level	Pour your own drinks	Check your blood glucose before going to sleep
Get low blood glucose treatment (such as Life-Savers, pop, glucose tablets)	Avoid fortified beverages (i.e., brandy, port, ice wine, liqueurs)	Set alarms to wake you up throughout the night
Tell someone what your symptoms are like and how to treat them	Use less alcohol and stretch your drinks with sugar-free mixes or diet soda	Know that a delayed low blood glucose level can happen up to 24 hours after drinking
Know that glucagon will not work with alcohol in your body	Alternate alcoholic drinks with diet soda or water	Wake up at your regular time to eat, take medication or insulin
Wear diabetes identification (such as Medi-cAlert®)	Drink slowly	Don't ever encourage your friends to let you "sleep it off"
Keep a fast-acting carbohydrate with you at all times	Don't get drunk	Don't drink and drive

The *Canadian Diabetes Association 2008 Clinical Practice Guidelines for the Prevention and Management of Diabetes in Canada* recommend that:

- People using insulin should be aware that delayed hypoglycemia (low blood glucose) can occur up to twenty-four hours after drinking alcohol.

- People with type 1 diabetes should be aware of the risk of morning hypoglycemia if alcohol is consumed two to three hours after the previous evening's meal.

If you are going to drink alcohol, the following steps reduce your risk of experiencing low blood glucose.

Section 32.2

Smoking and Diabetes

"Smoking and Risk of Diabetes," © 2010 Virginia Department of Health (www.vahealth.org). Reprinted with permission.

Smoking and Risk of Diabetes

The nicotine in cigarette smoke can raise your blood glucose (sugar) level, which can lead to insulin resistance (a pre-diabetic condition where glucose levels are above normal).[1]

People who never smoked but were exposed to secondhand smoke are also at increased risk for developing glucose intolerance in young adulthood.[1]

Twelve percent of diabetes cases in the United States are attributable to smoking.[2]

Based on a review of twenty-five studies, current smokers have a 44 percent greater chance of developing diabetes than nonsmokers. The risk is greatest for heavy smokers.[3]

Current smokers were two to three times more likely than never smokers to develop Type 2 diabetes within five years. The risk was highest (fivefold) among adults who smoked a pack per day for twenty years or more (greater than or equal to twenty "pack years").[4]

It appears to be a modifiable risk factor: the risk of developing diabetes among former smokers was similar to that of never smokers.

Smoking, Diabetes, and Related Health Problems

Smoking aggravates certain health problems that people with diabetes already face:[3,5,6]

- High blood pressure

- High blood cholesterol levels, which can lead to heart attack and stroke

- Reduced oxygen levels in the blood, which increases risk of heart attack and stroke

- Reduced blood circulation and impaired ability to heal wounds, which can lead to infection

- Difficulty controlling blood glucose levels and managing your diabetes

- Neuropathy or nerve damage (pain, tingling, numbness, weakness), especially in the feet and hands, that can lead to infection and limb amputation

- Impotence

- Kidney disease

- Eye problems (retinopathy) that can lead to impaired vision or blindness

- Periodontal (teeth) problems like bleeding gums and ulcers

- Premature death: diabetics who smoke have triple the risk of death from heart disease of nonsmokers

- Increased body fat (especially in the abdomen or stomach area), body inflammation, oxidative stress, and impaired endothelial function

Smoking, Pregnancy and Diabetes

Women who smoked heavily during pregnancy increased by almost fivefold the likelihood of their offspring later developing early adult onset of Type 2 diabetes.[7]

Benefits of Quitting Smoking

People with diabetes who quit regain control over their blood glucose levels and achieve better A1c levels over time. Other benefits: less insulin resistance, fewer diabetes complications, better blood circulation, lower blood pressure, lower blood cholesterol levels, and subsequently lower risk for heart disease.[8]

Former smokers reduce their risk of diabetes to that of never smokers after five years for women and after ten years for men.[9]

Barriers to Quitting

Healthcare providers do not frequently ask their diabetic patients if they smoke[9] nor advise them to quit.[10]

Patients think that quitting smoking is less important than avoiding certain foods or limiting intake of alcohol.[11]

Because smoking suppresses appetite for some, people with diabetes may view smoking as a strategy for controlling their weight and better managing their diabetes. People with diabetes are concerned about possible weight gain associated with quitting.[12]

People with diabetes are at greater risk for depression.[13] Because nicotine is a mood-altering drug (acts as a sedative and alleviates anxiety when it first reaches the brain), smokers with diabetes may be using cigarettes as a way of coping with their depression.

Notes

1. Houston TK, Person SD, Pletcher MJ, Liu K, Iribarren C, Kiefe CI. Active and passive smoking and development of glucose intolerance among young adults in a prospective cohort: CARDIA study. *BMJ* 2006 (June 3); 332(7549): 1064–69.

2. Ding EL, Hu FB. Smoking and Type 2 diabetes (editorial). *JAMA* 2007; 298(22): 2675–76.

3. Willi C, et al. Active smoking and the risk of Type 2 diabetes. *JAMA* 2007; 298(22): 2654–64.

4. Foy CG, Bell FA, Farmer DR, Goff DC, Wagenknect LE. Smoking and incidence of diabetes among U.S. adults. *Diabetes Care* 2005 (October); 28(10): 2501–7. Assuming twenty cigarettes in a pack, a "pack-year" is defined as the number of cigarettes smoked daily divided by twenty (assuming twenty cigarettes per pack) and multiplied by the number of years smoked.

5. American Diabetes Association (ADA; http://www.diabetes.org/), "Smoking" fact sheet (accessed June 30, 2009).

6. Haire-Joshu D, Glasgow RE, Tibbs TL. Smoking and diabetes. *Diabetes Care* 1999 (November); 22(11): 1887–98.

7. Montgomery SM, Ekbom A. Smoking during pregnancy and diabetes mellitus in a British longitudinal birth cohort. *British Medical Journal* 2002; 324: 26–27.

8. Will JC, Galuska DA, Ford ES, Mokdad A, Calle EE. Cigarette smoking and diabetes mellitus: Evidence of a positive association from a large prospective cohort study. *International Journal of Epidemiology* 2001; 30: 540–46.

9. Robinson M, Laurent S, Little JJ. Including smoking status as a new vital sign: It works. *Journal of Family Practice* 1995; 40: 556–63.

10. Centers for Disease Control and Prevention. Physician and other health care professional counseling of smokers to quit—United States, 1991. *MMWR* 1993; 42(44): 854–57.

11. Glasgow R, Hampson S, Strycker L, Ruggiero L. Personal-model beliefs and social-environmental barriers related to diabetes self-management. *Diabetes Care* 1997; 20: 556–61.

12. Haire-Joshu D, Heady S, Thomas L, Schechtman K, Fisher EB Jr. Beliefs about smoking and diabetes care. *Diabetes Education* 1994; 20: 410–15.

13. Lustman P, Griffith L, Gavard J, Clouse R. Depression in adults with diabetes. *Diabetes Care* 1992; 15: 1631–39.

Chapter 33

Physical Activity and Diabetes

How Can I Take Care of My Diabetes?

Diabetes means your blood glucose, also called blood sugar, is too high. Your body uses glucose for energy. But having too much glucose in your blood can hurt you.

When you take care of your diabetes, you'll feel better. You'll reduce your risk for problems with your kidneys, eyes, nerves, feet and legs, and teeth. You'll also lower your risk for a heart attack or a stroke. You can take care of your diabetes by doing the following things:

- Being physically active

- Following a healthy meal plan

- Taking medicines, if prescribed by your doctor

What Can a Physically Active Lifestyle Do For Me?

Research has shown that physical activity can do the following things:

- Lower your blood glucose and your blood pressure

- Lower your bad cholesterol and raise your good cholesterol

"What I Need to Know about Physical Activity and Diabetes," National Institute of Diabetes and Digestive and Kidney Diseases, National Institutes of Health, NIH Publication No. 08-5180, March 2008.

- Improve your body's ability to use insulin
- Lower your risk for heart disease and stroke
- Keep your heart and bones strong
- Keep your joints flexible
- Lower your risk of falling
- Help you lose weight
- Reduce your body fat
- Give you more energy
- Reduce your stress levels

Physical activity also plays an important part in preventing type 2 diabetes. A major government study, the Diabetes Prevention Program (DPP), showed that modest weight loss of 5 to 7 percent—for example, ten to fifteen pounds for a two-hundred-pound person—can delay and possibly prevent type 2 diabetes. People in the study used diet and exercise to lose weight.

What Kinds of Physical Activity Can Help Me?

Four kinds of activity can help. You can do the following things:

- Be extra active every day
- Do aerobic exercise
- Do strength training
- Stretch

Be Extra Active Every Day

Being extra active can increase the number of calories you burn. Try these ways to be extra active, or think of other things you can do:

- Walk around while you talk on the phone.
- Play with the kids.
- Take the dog for a walk.
- Get up to change the TV channel instead of using the remote control.
- Work in the garden or rake leaves.

- Clean the house.

- Wash the car.

- Stretch out your chores. For example, make two trips to take the laundry downstairs instead of one.

- Park at the far end of the shopping center parking lot and walk to the store.

- At the grocery store, walk down every aisle.

- At work, walk over to see a co-worker instead of calling or emailing.

- Take the stairs instead of the elevator.

- Stretch or walk around instead of taking a coffee break and eating.

- During your lunch break, walk to the post office or do other errands.

Do Aerobic Exercise

Aerobic exercise is activity that requires the use of large muscles and makes your heart beat faster. You will also breathe harder during aerobic exercise. Doing aerobic exercise for thirty minutes a day at least five days a week provides many benefits. You can even split up those thirty minutes into several parts. For example, you can take three brisk ten-minute walks, one after each meal.

If you haven't exercised lately, see your doctor first to make sure it's ok for you to increase your level of physical activity. Talk with your doctor about how to warm up and stretch before you exercise and how to cool down after you exercise. Then start slowly with 5 to 10 minutes a day. Add a little more time each week, aiming for at least 150 minutes per week. Try the following:

- Walking briskly

- Hiking

- Climbing stairs

- Swimming or taking a water-aerobics class

- Dancing

- Riding a bicycle outdoors or a stationary bicycle indoors

- Taking an aerobics class

- Playing basketball, volleyball, or other sports

- In-line skating, ice skating, or skateboarding
- Playing tennis
- Cross-country skiing

Do Strength Training

Doing exercises with hand weights, elastic bands, or weight machines three times a week builds muscle. When you have more muscle and less fat, you'll burn more calories because muscle burns more calories than fat, even between exercise sessions. Strength training can help make daily chores easier, improving your balance and coordination, as well as your bones' health. You can do strength training at home, at a fitness center, or in a class. Your healthcare team can tell you more about strength training and what kind is best for you.

Stretch

Stretching increases your flexibility, lowers stress, and helps prevent muscle soreness after other types of exercise. Your healthcare team can tell you what kind of stretching is best for you.

Can I Exercise Any Time I Want?

Your healthcare team can help you decide the best time of day for you to exercise. Together, you and your team will consider your daily schedule, your meal plan, and your diabetes medicines.

If you have type 1 diabetes, avoid strenuous exercise when you have ketones in your blood or urine. Ketones are chemicals your body might make when your blood glucose level is too high and your insulin level is too low. Too many ketones can make you sick. If you exercise when you have ketones in your blood or urine, your blood glucose level may go even higher.

If you have type 2 diabetes and your blood glucose is high but you don't have ketones, light or moderate exercise will probably lower your blood glucose. Ask your healthcare team whether you should exercise when your blood glucose is high.

Are There Any Types of Physical Activity I Shouldn't Do?

If you have diabetes complications, some kinds of exercise can make your problems worse. For example, activities that increase the pressure in the blood vessels of your eyes, such as lifting heavy weights, can make diabetic eye problems worse. If nerve damage from diabetes has made your feet numb, your doctor may suggest that you try swimming instead of walking for aerobic exercise.

When you have numb feet, you might not feel pain in your feet. Sores or blisters might get worse because you don't notice them. Without proper care, minor foot problems can turn into serious conditions, sometimes leading to amputation. Make sure you exercise in cotton socks and comfortable, well-fitting shoes designed for the activity you are doing. After you exercise, check your feet for cuts, sores, bumps, or redness. Call your doctor if any foot problems develop.

Can Physical Activity Cause Low Blood Glucose?

Physical activity can cause low blood glucose, also called hypoglycemia, in people who take insulin or certain types of diabetes medicines. Ask your healthcare team whether your diabetes medicines can cause low blood glucose.

Low blood glucose can happen while you exercise, right afterward, or even up to a day later. It can make you feel shaky, weak, confused, grumpy, hungry, or tired. You may sweat a lot or get a headache. If your blood glucose drops too low, you could pass out or have a seizure.

However, you should still be physically active. The following steps can help you be prepared for low blood glucose.

Before exercise:

- Ask your healthcare team whether you should check your blood glucose level before exercising.

- If you take diabetes medicines that can cause low blood glucose, ask your health care team whether you should change the amount you take before you exercise or have a snack if your blood glucose level is below 100.

During exercise:

- Wear your medical identification (ID) bracelet or necklace or carry your ID in your pocket.

- Always carry food or glucose tablets so you'll be ready to treat low blood glucose.

- If you'll be exercising for more than an hour, check your blood glucose at regular intervals. You may need snacks before you finish.

273

After exercise:

- Check to see how exercise affected your blood glucose level.

Treating Low Blood Glucose

If your blood glucose is below 70, have one of the following right away:

- Three or four glucose tablets
- One serving of glucose gel—the amount equal to fifteen grams of carbohydrate
- One-half cup (four ounces) of any fruit juice
- One-half cup (four ounces) of a regular—not diet—soft drink
- One cup (eight ounces) of milk
- Five or six pieces of hard candy
- One tablespoon of sugar or honey

After fifteen minutes, check your blood glucose again. If it's still too low, have another serving. Repeat until your blood glucose is 70 or higher. If it will be an hour or more before your next meal, have a snack as well.

What Should I Do Before I Start a Physical Activity Program?

Check with your doctor. Always talk with your doctor before you start a new physical activity program. Ask about your medicines—prescription and over-the-counter—and whether you should change the amount you take before you exercise. If you have heart disease, kidney disease, eye problems, or foot problems, ask which types of physical activity are safe for you.

Decide exactly what you'll do and set some goals. Choose the following things:

- The type of physical activity you want to do
- The clothes and items you'll need to get ready
- The days and times you'll add activity
- The length of each session
- Your plan for warming up, stretching, and cooling down for each session

- A backup plan, such as where you'll walk if the weather is bad
- Your measures of progress

Find an exercise buddy. Many people find they are more likely to do something active if a friend joins them. If you and a friend plan to walk together, for example, you may be more likely to do it.

Keep track of your physical activity. Write down when you exercise and for how long in your blood glucose record book. You'll be able to track your progress and see how physical activity affects your blood glucose.

Decide how you'll reward yourself. Do something nice for yourself when you reach your activity goals. For example, treat yourself to a movie or buy a new plant for the garden.

What Can I Do to Make Sure I Stay Active?

One of the keys to staying on track is finding some activities you like to do. If you keep finding excuses not to exercise, think about why. Are your goals realistic? Do you need a change in activity? Would another time be more convenient? Keep trying until you find a routine that works for you. Once you make physical activity a habit, you'll wonder how you lived without it.

Chapter 34

Weight Management and Diabetes

It's hard to flip through a magazine or surf a health website without getting the lowdown on weight. The general idea: Being active and eating healthy are the best ways to manage weight.

This advice works for everybody, but it can be particularly helpful for people with diabetes. That's because weight can influence diabetes, and diabetes can influence weight. This relationship may be different for both type 1 and type 2 diabetes, but the end advice is the same: Managing weight can really make a difference in a person's diabetes management plan.

Weight and Type 1 Diabetes

If a person has type 1 diabetes but hasn't been treated yet, he or she often loses weight. In type 1 diabetes, the body can't use glucose (pronounced: gloo-kose) properly because the pancreas no longer produces insulin that's needed to get glucose into the cells.

Then the body flushes the unusable glucose (and the calories) out of the body in urine, or pee. As a result, the person can lose weight. After treatment for type 1 diabetes, though, a person usually returns to a healthy weight.

"Weight and Diabetes," July 2009, reprinted with permission from www.kids health.org. Copyright © 2009 The Nemours Foundation. This information was provided by KidsHealth, one of the largest resources online for medically reviewed health information written for parents, kids, and teens. For more articles like this one, visit www.KidsHealth.org, or www.TeensHealth.org.

Sometimes, though, people with type 1 diabetes can be overweight, too. They may be overweight when they find out they have diabetes or they may become overweight after they start treatment. Being overweight can make it harder for people with type 1 diabetes to keep their blood sugar levels under control.

Weight and Type 2 Diabetes

Most people are overweight when they're diagnosed with type 2 diabetes. Being overweight or obese increases a person's risk for developing type 2 diabetes.

People with type 2 diabetes have a condition called insulin resistance. People with insulin resistance are able to make insulin, but the body can't use it properly to move glucose into the cells. As a result, the amount of glucose in the blood rises. The pancreas then makes more insulin to try to overcome the problem.

Eventually, the pancreas can wear out from working overtime and may no longer be able to produce enough insulin to keep blood glucose levels within a normal range. At this point, a person has type 2 diabetes.

People who don't have diabetes may also have insulin resistance. People with insulin resistance are at high risk for developing type 2 diabetes if they don't already have it.

People with insulin resistance are often overweight and don't exercise very much. But weight loss, eating healthier foods and portion sizes, and getting exercise can actually reverse insulin resistance.

For people with type 2 diabetes, reversing insulin resistance makes it easier to get blood sugar levels into a healthier range. For people who have insulin resistance but not diabetes, reversing insulin resistance can reduce the risk that they'll develop diabetes.

Managing Your Weight

Getting to and staying at a healthy weight helps you feel better and have more energy, and being at a healthy weight also reduces the risk of heart disease and other health problems. Reaching and maintaining a healthy weight may also help you reduce diabetes symptoms and control your blood sugar levels.

Your doctor will let you know if you should lose weight to control your diabetes. Doctors usually use your weight and height to calculate your body mass index (BMI), which helps them judge whether your weight is healthy. Your doctor can talk to you about the weight range that is right for you and help you create a meal and exercise plan to stay within that range. Even if your weight is healthy, eating right and exercising regularly can make your diabetes easier to control and prevent problems down the road.

If you're overweight, don't feel bad about it or guilty about your diabetes (lots of people who don't have diabetes need to lose weight, too). Instead, take action. Use your meal plan, exercise, and medications to reach and maintain a healthier weight. It won't happen overnight.

Learning how to eat right and exercise to get to a healthy weight can be challenging for most people—those who don't have diabetes, too—because it takes time.

Weight management offers special challenges for people with diabetes. Here are some tips:

- **Forget fad diets:** The latest fad in losing pounds—whether it involves starving yourself or cutting out food groups—can cause major problems when it comes to controlling your blood sugar. Instead, follow your meal plan—it's tailored just for you and your unique needs.

- **Stick to the insulin schedule:** It's very important that people with diabetes don't skip insulin injections to lose weight. Putting off or skipping injections can lead to very high blood sugar levels and even a dangerous condition called diabetic ketoacidosis (pronounced: keh-toe-as-ih-doe-sis), which can lead to coma.

- **Watch the snacking:** Some people may eat too many snacks because they're afraid that their blood sugar levels will get too low. This can lead to weight gain. Follow your diabetes plan and take your medications at the right times to avoid these problems.

- **Turn the table on cravings:** Everyone has cravings now and then. But when people with diabetes sneak extra candy or sweets, it can push blood sugar levels up. Then when you take more insulin to bring your sugar back down, it can lead to gaining extra body fat. Talk to your doctor or a parent if you feel like you don't get to eat sweets or other foods as much as you like. And try some tricks for managing cravings, such as taking a walk or brushing your teeth.

If you need more info about diabetes and how it affects your weight, or if you're worried about it, talk to a member of your diabetes healthcare team. Your team can help you learn healthy ways to make it easier to manage your weight, so don't hesitate to take advantage of their knowledge and expertise. When your weight is on track, you'll feel like you're more in control of your diabetes, your body, and your health.

279

Chapter 35

Diabetes and Daily Challenges

Chapter Contents

Section 35.1

Driving

Excerpted from "Driving When You Have Diabetes," National Highway Traffic Safety Administration, U.S. Department of Transportation, November 2003. Revised by David A. Cooke, MD, FACP, February 2011.

Driving When You Have Diabetes

For most people, driving represents freedom, control, and independence. Driving enables most people to get to the places they want or need to go. For many people, driving is important economically—some drive as part of their job or to get to and from work.

Driving is a complex skill. Our ability to drive safely can be affected by changes in our physical, emotional, and mental condition. This section is designed to give you the information you need to talk to your healthcare team about driving and diabetes.

How Can Having Diabetes Affect My Driving?

In the short term, diabetes can make your blood glucose (sugar) levels too high or too low. As a result, diabetes can make you:

- feel sleepy or dizzy;

- feel confused;

- have blurred vision;

- lose consciousness or have a seizure.

In the long run, diabetes can lead to problems that affect driving. Diabetes may cause nerve damage in your hands, legs, and feet, or eyes. In some cases, diabetes can cause blindness or lead to amputation.

Can I Still Drive with Diabetes?

Yes, people with diabetes are able to drive unless they are limited by certain complications of diabetes. These include severe low blood glucose levels or vision problems. If you are experiencing diabetes-related complications, you should work closely with your diabetes healthcare team to find out if diabetes affects your ability to drive. If it does, discuss whether there are actions you can take to continue to drive safely.

People who drive professionally and need a commercial driver's license (CDL) may be a different situation. State and federal laws may bar some diabetics from having a CDL, but this is usually determined on a case-by-case basis. If you are diabetic and drive professionally, you should discuss this with your doctor and licensing agency.

What Can I Do to Ensure That I Can Drive Safely with Diabetes?

Insulin and some oral medications can cause blood glucose levels to become dangerously low (hypoglycemia). Do not drive if your blood glucose level is too low. If you do, you might not be able to make good choices, focus on your driving, or control your car. Your healthcare team can help you determine when you should check your blood glucose level before driving and how often you should check while driving.

Make sure you always carry your blood glucose meter and plenty of snacks (including a quick-acting source of glucose) with you. Pull over as soon as you feel any of the signs of a low blood glucose level. Check your blood glucose.

If your glucose level is low, eat a snack that contains a fast-acting sugar such as juice, soda with sugar (not diet), hard candy, or glucose tablets. Wait fifteen minutes, and then check your blood glucose again. Treat again as needed. Once your glucose level has risen to your target range, eat a more substantial snack or meal containing protein. Do not continue driving until your blood glucose level has improved.

Most people with diabetes experience warning signs of a low blood glucose level. However, if you experience hypoglycemia without advance warning, you should not drive. Talk to your healthcare team about how glycemic awareness training might help you sense the beginning stages of hypoglycemia.

In extreme situations, high blood glucose levels (hyperglycemia) also may affect driving. Talk to your healthcare team if you have a history of very high glucose levels to determine at what point such levels might affect your ability to be a safe driver.

The key to preventing diabetes-related eye problems is good control of blood glucose levels, good blood pressure control, and good eye care. A yearly exam with an eye care professional is essential.

If you are experiencing long-term complications of diabetes such as vision or sensation problems, or if you have had an amputation, your diabetes healthcare team can refer you to a driving specialist. This specialist can give you on- and off-road tests to see if, and how, your diabetes is affecting your driving. The specialist also may offer training to improve your driving skills.

Improving your driving skills could help keep you and others around you safe. To find a driver rehabilitation specialist near you go to www. aota.org/olderdriver to find the name of a specialist in your state. You also can call hospitals and rehabilitation facilities to find an occupational therapist who can help with the driving skills assessment and remediation. Depending on where you live, you may need to travel to nearby communities to find these services.

What If I Have to Cut Back or Give Up Driving?

You can keep your independence even if you have to cut back or give up on your driving. It may take planning ahead on your part, but planning will help get you to the places you need to go and to the people you want to see. Consider the following:

- Rides with family and friends

- Taxi cabs

- Shuttle buses or vans

- Public buses, trains, and subways

- Walking

Also, senior centers and religious and other local service groups often offer transportation services for older adults in the community.

Wear Your Safety Belt

Always wear your safety belt when you are driving or riding in a car. Make sure that every person who is riding with you also is buckled up. Wear your safety belt even if your car has air bags.

Section 35.2

Eating Out

Whether it's the local pizza joint after a game, the food court at the mall, or barbecued ribs on your best friend's back porch, eating out is probably a part of your social scene.

You don't want to miss out on these activities just because you have to watch what you eat, and the good news is you don't have to. You can pretty much eat the same foods as your friends and family—you just have to keep track of what you eat and eat certain foods in moderation.

Which restaurant should I choose?

If you're choosing where to eat, think about the places that offer you the most options—even fast-food places have healthy choices on their menus. Whenever possible, look for nutritional facts on the meal you plan to order—like calorie, carbohydrate, and fat content. This information is available in many chain restaurants (you may need to ask for it) or online. Or ask your server what's in the food you're eating.

Don't worry—you're not limited to places that serve only soy burgers and carrot sticks. If you can order a meal that includes a good balance of proteins, fats, and carbohydrates, you're doing ok. But if you find that certain restaurants don't offer many vegetable choices or that they only serve fried food that's covered in cheese, you might want to pick a place that offers more options.

You might find that there are more healthy breakfast choices—like yogurt, fresh fruit, and scrambled eggs—for you at the diner than at the coffeehouse, so convincing your friends to chow down on diner food is one option. But if your friends prefer the coffeehouse, one alternative is to buy something to drink and bring a snack in your backpack or purse that's easy to eat discreetly, like pretzels or raisins. Some people may be embarrassed or worried that the manager might give them a hard time, though. If you think you may get caught in a situation like this, you can talk about what to do with your doctor or dietitian and how to adjust your meal plan or insulin doses.

What should I order?

When it's time to order, follow the same rules for food content and portion sizes that you follow at home. Your meal plan probably calls for you to eat a good balance of proteins, fats, and carbs. Usually, you can get all of the nutrients you need at a restaurant, too.

These tips can help:

- **Change and rearrange:** To get a well-balanced meal in a restaurant, feel free to substitute certain ingredients or side orders (for example, you could substitute salad for fries). Don't feel weird about it—people ask for substitutions all the time. You can also ask for a different preparation, like having your chicken broiled instead of fried.

- **Watch the sides:** Avoid foods with sauces or gravy, and ask for low-fat salad dressings on the side.

- **Pick your own portion:** Restaurant portions often offer enough food to feed your entire crew, but try to eat the same portion of food that you'd eat at home. Either eat only part of your order and take the rest home or split it with a friend.

- **Master menu lingo:** Watch out for words like "jumbo," "super-size," "deluxe," or "value" when eating at your favorite fast-food joint or the food court at the mall. Instead, order junior- or regular-sized sandwiches and sides.

- **Split with a friend:** Are you hungry for some fries? Order a healthy sandwich and side salad for yourself and sneak a few of your friend's fries instead of ordering your own. And dividing an entrée or sandwich between friends also helps keep portion sizes under control.

- **Go light on buns and crusts:** Choose thin-crust pizza over the deep-dish pie and skip double burgers and extra-long hot dogs to keep carb intake under control. And keep in mind that English muffins, bread, and small buns often contain fewer calories and fat than croissants and biscuits.

The same tips apply to eating at your school cafeteria. To be a healthy eater at school, make sure you pick a variety of healthy foods and stop to think about when you're getting full.

What should I bring with me?

When you go out to eat, you should bring the things you take with you everywhere, like testing supplies, snacks, and medications. A quick-reference guide to food content and portions can make choosing healthy foods a little easier. (If you don't have one, you can get one from your doctor or dietitian.) If you use things like artificial sweeteners or fat-free spreads, bring them along, too.

If you take insulin, there's no need to stay home if you have to eat later than usual—in most cases you can just make a few simple adjustments to your medicine schedule.

Do you have questions about how to make eating out even easier? Talk to your doctor or dietitian.

Section 35.3

Sick Days

Whether your head feels like it's stuffed with cotton because you have a cold or you're spending a lot of time on the toilet because of a stomach bug, being sick is no fun for anyone.

For people with diabetes, being sick can also affect blood sugar levels. The good news is that taking a few extra precautions can help you keep your blood sugar levels under control.

How Illness Affects Blood Sugar Levels

When you get sick—whether it's a minor illness like a sore throat or cold or a bigger problem like dehydration or surgery—the body perceives the illness as stress. To relieve the stress, the body fights the illness. This process requires more energy than the body normally uses.

On one hand, this is good because it helps supply the extra fuel the body needs. On the other hand, in a person with diabetes, this can lead to high blood sugar levels. Some illnesses cause the opposite problem, though. If you don't feel like eating or have nausea or vomiting, and you're taking the same amount of insulin you normally do, you can develop blood sugar levels that are too low.

Blood sugar levels can be very unpredictable when you're sick. Because you can't be sure how the illness will affect your blood sugar levels, it's important to check blood sugar levels often on sick days and adjust your insulin doses as needed.

Planning for Sick Days

Your diabetes management plan will help you know what to do when you're sick. The plan might tell you:

- how to monitor your blood glucose levels and ketones when you're sick;

- which medicines are ok to take;

- what changes you might make to your food and drink and diabetes medications;

- when to call your doctor.

In addition, people with diabetes should get the pneumococcal vaccine, which protects against some serious infections. You should also get a flu shot every year. These vaccines may help you keep your diabetes under better control and cut down on the number of sick days you have.

What to Do When You're Sick

Your doctor will give you specific advice when you're sick. But here are some general guidelines:

- **Stay on track:** Unless your doctor tells you to make a change, keep taking the same diabetes medications. You need to keep taking insulin when you're sick, even if you're not eating as much as you usually do. That's because your liver makes and releases glucose into your blood—even when you're stuck channel surfing on the couch—so you always need insulin. Some people with diabetes need more insulin than usual on sick days. Even some people with type 2 diabetes who don't usually take insulin may need some on sick days.

- **Check blood sugar and ketone levels often:** Your doctor will tell you how often to check your blood sugar and ketone levels—usually you'll need to check more frequently while you're sick.

- **Pay special attention to nausea and vomiting:** People with diabetes sometimes catch a bug that causes nausea or vomiting. But nausea and vomiting are also symptoms of ketoacidosis. If you feel sick to your stomach or are throwing up, it's important to keep a close eye on your blood glucose and ketone levels and seek medical help according to the guidelines in your diabetes management plan. The best approach is to stick to your insulin schedule, check ketones regularly, and follow your doctor's advice about when to get help.

- **Prevent dehydration:** Be sure to drink plenty of fluids, even if you have nausea or vomiting. Your doctor can recommend the types and amounts of fluids to drink that can help you manage both your illness and your blood sugar levels.

- **Use over-the-counter (OTC) medications wisely:** People sometimes take OTC medications for illnesses like the cold or flu. But these have ingredients that can raise or lower blood sugar or cause symptoms that look similar to high or low blood sugar. Follow your doctor's advice about taking an OTC medication. Your doctor might even include common medications that are ok for you in your diabetes management plan, and can also explain the things to check for on medication labels.

- **Take notes:** Your doctor might have a lot of questions about your illness and the symptoms you've had. You can answer these questions more easily if you write down your symptoms, medications and doses, what food and drink you had, and whether you kept the food down. Also, tell the doctor if you've lost weight or had a fever and have the record of your blood sugar and ketone level test results handy.

- **Get some rest:** People need rest when they're sick. It helps your body focus its energy on fighting illness. If you think you need to, let a parent take over managing your diabetes for a day or two. Your mom or dad can keep track of your blood sugar levels and figure out the best insulin dosage—and you can get some sleep!

When to Call Your Doctor

Your diabetes management plan will explain when you may need medical help. It will tell you what to do and whom to call. Here are some general reasons for calling the doctor:

- All the same reasons you normally would call about diabetes management, as well as for any questions you have about being sick

- If you have no appetite or you can't eat or drink

- If your blood sugar level is low because you haven't been eating much—but remember to take steps at home to bring your blood sugar back up

- If you keep vomiting or having diarrhea

- If your blood sugar levels are high for several checks or don't decrease when you take extra insulin

- If you have moderate or large amounts of ketones in the urine

- If you think you might have ketoacidosis

- If you can't eat or drink because you're having a medical test like an x-ray, surgery, or a dental procedure

Any time you have questions or concerns, ask your doctor for advice.

Section 35.4

Sleep Problems

Sleep complaints are common among those with diabetes, according to Elizabeth Bashoff, M.D., clinic physician, at Joslin Diabetes Center. "The important thing to do first is to pinpoint why you are not sleeping."

There are a wide variety of reasons for disrupted sleep in people with diabetes. Some of the causes of sleep problems can include:

- **Sleep apnea:** Sleep apnea is increasingly common for everyone, but is more frequent among those with type 2 diabetes. Sleep apnea is also linked to obesity, a risk factor for diabetes. Symptoms include daytime fatigue and exhaustion, and nighttime snoring or irregular breathing. Weight loss is by far the most effective treatment, Bashoff says.

- **Neuropathy and leg pain:** Leg pain due to neuropathy is a very common reason people with diabetes have sleep problems. "There are many medications to treat neuropathy, some of which can also have a beneficial sedative effect," Bashoff suggests.

- **Nighttime lows:** Another reason some with diabetes might have disrupted sleep is nighttime hypoglycemia. People with type 1, and those with type 2 who are being treated with insulin or sulfonylurea, are at risk. Symptoms include waking up

291

suddenly with a feeling of impending doom, nightmares, night sweats, or morning headaches. Sometimes the only symptom is a high fasting blood glucose.

Women going through menopause may also experience drenching night sweats, which can be confused with nighttime hypoglycemia. Bashoff says it's important to find out if the cause is menopause or a low blood glucose reaction.

Healthy Habits Help

There may be a link between sleep and blood glucose levels. "Clinically, we see that people who keep regular sleep schedules seem to maintain better blood sugar control," Bashoff says. "It is more of a challenge if sleep is disrupted." There is also some evidence that disrupted sleep affects insulin resistance and may contribute to the development of type 2 diabetes.

When it comes to diabetes and good sleep, healthy habits always help. There is some evidence that those who exercise have better quality and quantity of sleep (as long as you don't exercise right before bedtime). Getting enough sleep and creating healthy sleep patterns are prescriptions for good diabetes health.

Section 35.5

Depression

Symptoms of depression are common in people with diabetes compared with the general population, and major depression is present in approximately 15 percent of people with diabetes. Depression is associated with poorer self-care behavior, poorer blood glucose management, health complications, decreased quality of life and psychological wellbeing, increased family problems, and higher healthcare costs.

The association between depression and diabetes is unclear. Depression may develop because of stress but also may result from the metabolic effects of diabetes on the brain. Studies suggest that people with diabetes who have a history of depression are more likely to develop diabetic complications than those without depression.

Despite the enormous advances in brain research in the past twenty years, depression often goes undiagnosed and untreated. It often takes a mental health professional to recognize these symptoms, inquire about their duration and severity, diagnose the disorder, and suggest appropriate treatment.

Research shows that depression leads to poorer physical and mental functioning, so a person is less likely to follow a required meal or medication plan. Treating depression with psychotherapy ("talk" therapy), medication, or a combination of these treatments can improve a patient's wellbeing and ability to manage diabetes. In people who have diabetes and depression, scientists report that psychotherapy and antidepressant medications have positive effects on both mood and blood glucose management.

Prescription antidepressant medications are generally well tolerated and safe for people with diabetes. Specific types of psychotherapy can also relieve depression. However, recovery from depression takes time. Antidepressant medications can take several weeks to work and may need to be combined with ongoing psychotherapy. Not everyone responds to treatment in the same way. Prescriptions and dosing may need to be adjusted.

Therefore, treatment for depression in the context of diabetes should be managed by a mental health professional, such as a psychiatrist, psychologist, or clinical social worker who is in close communication with the physician providing diabetes care. This is especially important when antidepressant medication is needed or prescribed, so that potentially harmful drug interactions can be avoided.

In some cases, a mental health professional who specializes in treating individuals with depression and co-occurring physical illnesses, such as diabetes, may be available. People with diabetes who develop depression, as well as people in treatment for depression who subsequently develop diabetes, should make sure to tell any physician they visit about the full range of medications they are taking.

Use of herbal supplements of any kind should be discussed with a physician before they are tried. Recently, scientists have discovered that St. John's wort, an over-the-counter herbal remedy promoted as a treatment for mild depression, can have harmful interactions with some other medications.

It is important to remember that depression is a disorder of the brain that can be treated in addition to whatever other illnesses a person might have, including diabetes. If you think you may be depressed or know someone who is, don't lose hope. Seek help for depression.

Anxiety

It's normal to feel anxious or worried at times. Everyone does. In fact, a moderate amount of anxiety can be good. It helps you respond appropriately to real danger, and it can help motivate you to excel at work and at home.

But if you often feel anxious without reason and your worries disrupt your daily life, you may have an anxiety disorder. Anxiety disorders cause excessive or unrealistic anxiety and worry about life circumstances, usually without a readily identifiable cause.

Little is known about the relationship between diabetes and anxiety. Recent evidence suggests that the rate of anxiety disorders is elevated in people with type 1 diabetes. Anxiety disorders appear to be increased in individuals with diabetes compared with the general population (14 vs. 3 to 4 percent, respectively). As many as 40 percent of people have at least some anxiety symptoms, and fear of hypoglycemia is not uncommon in those with diabetes. Recent studies suggest that anxiety disorders in people with type 1 and 2 diabetes is associated with poor blood sugar control.

Signs and Symptoms

The signs and symptoms of generalized anxiety disorder can vary in combination or severity. They may include:

- restlessness;
- feeling of being keyed up or on edge;
- feeling a lump in your throat;
- difficulty concentrating;
- fatigue;
- irritability;
- impatience;
- being easily distracted;
- muscle tension;
- trouble falling or staying asleep (insomnia);
- excessive sweating;
- shortness of breath;
- stomachache;
- diarrhea;
- headache.

The two main treatments for anxiety disorders are medication (anti-anxiety drugs and/or anti-depressants) and psychotherapy ("talk therapy"), either alone or in combination.

If you have difficulty controlling your worries, or if anxiety interferes with your daily life, speak with your doctor, diabetes healthcare team, or mental health professional.

Eating Disorders

Adolescent females and young women with type 1 diabetes have about twice the risk of developing eating disorders as their peers without diabetes. This may be because of the weight changes that can occur with insulin therapy and good metabolic control and the extra attention people with diabetes must pay to what they eat.

Researchers estimate that 10 to 20 percent of girls in their midteen years and 30 to 40 percent of late teenaged girls and young adult women with diabetes skip or alter insulin doses to control their weight. Studies of eating disorders and diabetes also show a higher rate of bulimia in girls with diabetes compared with healthy controls.

In people with diabetes, eating disorders can lead to poor metabolic control and repeated hospitalizations for dangerously high or low blood sugar. Chronic poor blood sugar control leads to long-term complications, such as eye, kidney, and nerve damage.

Early Warning Signs

- Extremely high A1C test results
- Frequent bouts of and hospitalizations for poor blood sugar control
- Anxiety about or avoidance of being weighed
- Frequent requests to switch meal-planning approaches
- Frequent severe low blood sugar
- Widely fluctuating blood sugar levels without obvious reason
- Delay in puberty or sexual maturation or irregular or no menses
- Binging with food or alcohol at least twice a week for three months
- Exercise more than is necessary to stay fit
- Severe family stress

If you think that you or a loved one has an eating disorder, talk to your doctor or diabetes healthcare team. They will recommend a mental health professional who will work with the diabetes team to help you and your family deal with this problem. It is important to be nonjudgmental and supportive. It is also extremely important to seek evaluation and treatment.

Section 35.6

Stress

What Is Stress?

Stress is any feeling that bothers you or puts a strain on the body or mind. Some people describe stress as an uncomfortable feeling of tension. Others describe it as a feeling of excitement and challenge. Stress is a part of everyday life and everyone has it. Life is not perfect and many of its challenges can be stressful.

Stress can be both good and bad. Examples of "good" stress may include getting married, the birth of a grandchild, or a promotion. These types of good stress can add interest and excitement to your life.

Examples of "bad" stress could be a traffic ticket, doing poorly on a test in school, going through a divorce, or the death of a loved one. These types of stress can be upsetting and hard to deal with.

How Can Stress Be Dangerous?

The body's normal response to stress is to release hormones made by the endocrine glands. The body responds to stress with a rise in pulse, blood pressure, and blood sugar (glucose). You may have heard this reaction called the "fight or flight" response. Release of these hormones gives a quick source of energy for coping with stress.

These body changes can be harmful for anyone, but high blood sugars can be especially dangerous for persons with diabetes. Stress can easily upset the balance of medicine, diet, and exercise a person uses to control diabetes. Uncontrolled diabetes may lead to diabetes emergencies or complications over time.

What Are Some Signs of Stress?

High blood sugars caused by stress usually result in physical warning signs. Since your body can show signs of stress in many ways, you must be able to identify them. Recognizing stress is the first step in dealing with it. Do any of these signs of stress sound familiar?

- Frequent or prolonged boredom
- Crying spells
- Sweating
- Constant tiredness
- Feeling discouraged
- Problems sleeping (insomnia)
- Tight mouth or jaw
- Headaches
- Clenched teeth
- Rapid and/or shallow breathing
- Upset stomach
- Hunched, tight shoulders
- Rapid heartbeat
- Apathy
- Emptiness
- Nervous laughter
- Twitching
- Frequent self-criticism
- Neck stiffness or tightness
- Prolonged frustration
- Tightened fists
- Diarrhea
- Feeling helpless
- Avoiding people

You may have only a few or several symptoms of stress. It is important for you to learn to recognize your personal stress symptoms.

Diabetes and Stress

Life's everyday challenges can be stressful. There always seems to be too much to do in a given day when trying to balance work, families, community, church, and homes. It is rare to have everything done or caught up. Adding diabetes to your daily routine can be an added challenge.

Having a routine or schedule may be boring, but it is important in living well with diabetes. A successful diabetes routine includes seeing yourself and your health as a priority. Many people with diabetes have shared that their illness helps them live a healthier lifestyle because they do not take their health for granted. They work hard to maintain and improve it.

A successful diabetes routine includes the following:

- Taking medicines as prescribed.

- Checking and keeping a record of daily glucoses (blood sugars). Check your blood sugars more often when you feel stressed and look for patterns of low or high glucoses. Learn to adjust your insulin with help from your diabetes team. If you have Type 1 diabetes, check for urine ketones if your glucose is more than 250 mg/dl or more than 200 mg/dl during pregnancy.

- Following a healthy meal plan.

- Exercising regularly three to seven times a week for a minimum of thirty minutes each time.

- Seeing a diabetes specialist and other doctors regularly.

- Continuing to learn about diabetes.

- Being an active partner in managing all aspects of diabetes.

- Having a plan for recognizing and managing stress.

Following a diabetes routine can be time-consuming and sometimes overwhelming. Take time to find out what works best for you. Diabetes affects everyone differently, so every person with diabetes should have a specific plan. A certified diabetes educator (usually a nurse or dietitian who specializes in diabetes) can help you with your diabetes plan.

It is common to feel overwhelmed about managing diabetes with everything else that is going on in your life. You may feel your body is no longer under your control. It is natural to sometimes feel angry, guilty, depressed, frustrated, and helpless about having diabetes and managing it day-by-day.

Your thoughts, feelings, and attitudes about diabetes and taking care of yourself have a powerful effect on your body. A good place to start is to accept diabetes as a challenge.

How Do I Manage or Cope with Stress?

A plan on how to live well with diabetes and manage stress should include the following:

- Good nutrition
- Exercise
- A way to improve one's attitude
- Training on relaxation techniques and stress management
- A commitment to lifelong learning

You may want some help to learn how to deal with stress. Challenge yourself to learn how to relax using stress management techniques and exercises (meditation, guided imagery, etc.). Begin by reading more about any of these topics at your public library. Many communities offer courses on a variety of stress or behavior modification topics.

Finally, the best way to live with stress is to prevent it. When that is not possible, learn to reduce it as well as control how you respond to it.

Section 35.7

Traveling

"Have Diabetes, Will Travel,"
National Diabetes Education Program, May 2010.

Heading out of town? Leaving your troubles behind? Off on an important business trip? Whenever you travel, your diabetes comes along with you. And while having diabetes shouldn't stop you from traveling in style, you will have to do some careful planning. Here are some helpful diabetes travel tips from the National Diabetes Education Program.

Plan ahead. Make sure you do the following:

- Get all your immunizations. Find out what's required for where you're going, and make sure you get the right shots, on time.

- Control your ABCs: A1C, blood pressure, and cholesterol. See your healthcare provider for a check-up four to six weeks before your trip to make sure your ABCs are under control and in a healthy range before you leave.

- Ask your healthcare provider for a prescription and a letter explaining your diabetes medications, supplies, and any allergies. Carry this with you at all times on your trip. The prescription should be for insulin or diabetes medications and could help in case of an emergency.

- Wear identification that explains you have diabetes. The identification should be written in the languages of the places you are visiting.

- Plan for time zone changes. Make sure you'll always know when to take your diabetes medicine, no matter where you are. Remember: eastward travel means a shorter day. If you inject insulin, less may be needed. Westward travel means a longer day, so more insulin may be needed.

- Find out how long the flight will be and whether meals will be served. However, you should always carry enough food to cover

301

the entire flight time in case of delays or unexpected schedule changes.

Pack properly:

- Take twice the amount of diabetes medication and supplies that you'd normally need. Better safe than sorry.
- Keep your insulin cool by packing it in an insulated bag with refrigerated gel packs.
- Keep snacks, glucose gel, or tablets with you in case your blood glucose drops.
- If you use insulin, make sure you also pack a glucagon emergency kit.
- Make sure you keep your medical insurance card and emergency phone numbers handy.
- Don't forget to pack a first aid kit with all the essentials.

Some things to keep in mind if you are flying:

- Plan to carry all your diabetes supplies in your carry-on luggage. Don't risk a lost suitcase.
- Have all syringes and insulin delivery systems (including vials of insulin) clearly marked with the pharmaceutical preprinted label that identifies the medications. The Federal Aviation Agency (FAA) recommends that patients travel with their original pharmacy-labeled packaging. Keep your diabetes medications and emergency snacks with you at your seat—don't store them in an overhead bin.
- If the airline offers a meal for your flight call ahead for a diabetic, low-fat, or low-cholesterol meal. Wait until your food is about to be served before you take your insulin. Otherwise, a delay in the meal could lead to low blood glucose.
- If no food is offered on your flight, bring a meal onboard yourself.
- If you plan on using the restroom for insulin injections, ask for an aisle seat for easier access.
- Don't be shy about telling the flight attendant that you have diabetes—especially if you are traveling alone.
- When drawing up your dose of insulin, don't inject air into the bottle (the air on your plane will probably be pressurized).

- Because prescription laws may be very different in other countries, write for a list of International Diabetes Federation groups: IDF, 1 rue Defaeqz, B-1000, Belgium or visit http://www.idf.org. You may also want to get a list of English-speaking foreign doctors in case of an emergency. Contact the American Consulate, American Express, or local medical schools for a list of doctors. Insulin in foreign countries comes in different strengths. If you purchase insulin in a foreign country, be sure to use the right syringe for the strength. An incorrect syringe may cause you to take too much or too little insulin.

Some things to keep in mind on a road trip:

- Don't leave your medications in the trunk, glove compartment, or near a window—they might overheat. If possible, carry a cooler in the car to keep medications cool. Bring extra food with you in the car in case you can't find a restaurant.

General traveling tips:

- Stay comfortable and reduce your risk for blood clots by moving around every hour or two.
- Always tell at least one person traveling with you about your diabetes.
- Protect your feet. Never go barefoot in the shower or pool.
- Check your blood glucose often. Changes in diet, activity, and time zones can affect your blood glucose in unexpected ways.

You may not be able to leave your diabetes behind, but you can manage it and have a relaxing, safe trip.

Chapter 36

Diabetes in the Workplace: Know Your Rights

Introduction

The Americans with Disabilities Act (ADA) is a federal law that prohibits discrimination against individuals with disabilities. Title I of the ADA covers employment by private employers with fifteen or more employees as well as state and local government employers. The Rehabilitation Act provides similar protections related to federal employment. In addition, most states have their own laws prohibiting employment discrimination on the basis of disability. Some of these state laws may apply to smaller employers and provide protections in addition to those available under the ADA.

The U.S. Equal Employment Opportunity Commission (EEOC) enforces the employment provisions of the ADA. This chapter explains how the ADA might apply to job applicants and employees with diabetes. In particular, this guide explains the following:

- When diabetes is a disability under the ADA

- When an employer may ask an applicant or employee questions about his or her diabetes

- What types of reasonable accommodations employees with diabetes may need

"Questions and Answers About Diabetes in the Workplace and the Americans with Disabilities Act (ADA)," U.S. Equal Employment Opportunity Commission, February 2, 2011.

- How an employer should handle safety concerns about applicants and employees with diabetes

General Information about Diabetes

Diabetes is becoming more common in the United States, with approximately one million new cases diagnosed each year.[1] Today, nearly seventeen million Americans age twenty years or older have diabetes, including individuals of nearly every race and ethnicity.[2] Diabetes occurs when the pancreas does not produce any insulin or produces very little insulin, or when the body does not respond appropriately to insulin. Insulin is a hormone that is needed to convert sugar, starches, and other food into energy. The process of turning food into energy is crucial because the body depends on this energy for every action, from pumping blood and thinking to running and jumping. Although diabetes cannot be cured, it can be managed. Some people control their diabetes by eating a balanced diet, maintaining a healthy body weight, and exercising regularly. Many individuals, however, must take oral medication and/or insulin to manage their diabetes.[3]

Individuals with diabetes successfully perform all types of jobs from heading major corporations to protecting public safety. Yet, many employers still automatically exclude them from certain positions based on myths, fears, or stereotypes. For example, some employers wrongly assume that anyone with diabetes will be unable to perform a particular job (e.g., one that requires driving) or will need to use a lot of sick leave. The reality is that, because many individuals with diabetes work with few or no restrictions, their employers do not know that they have diabetes. Some employees, however, tell their employers that they have diabetes because they need a "reasonable accommodation"—a change or adjustment in the workplace to better manage and control their condition. Most of the accommodations requested by employees with diabetes such as regular work schedules, meal breaks, a place to test their blood sugar levels, or a rest area do not cost employers anything to provide.

When is diabetes a disability under the ADA?

Diabetes is a disability when it substantially limits one or more of a person's major life activities. Major life activities are basic activities that an average person can perform with little or no difficulty, such as eating or caring for oneself. Diabetes also is a disability when it causes side effects or complications that substantially limit a major life activity. Even if diabetes is not currently substantially limiting because it is controlled by diet, exercise, oral medication, and/or insulin, and there are no serious side effects, the condition may be a disability because it was substantially limiting in the past (i.e., before it was diagnosed and adequately treated). Finally, diabetes is a disability when it does not significantly affect a person's everyday activities, but the employer treats the individual as if it does. For example, an employer may assume that a person is totally unable to work because he has diabetes. Under the ADA, the determination of whether an individual has a disability is made on a case-by-case basis.

Obtaining and Using Medical Information: Applicants

The ADA limits the medical information that an employer can seek from a job applicant. During the application stage, an employer may not ask questions about an applicant's medical condition or require an applicant to take a medical examination before it makes a conditional job offer. This means that an employer cannot ask:

- questions about whether an applicant has diabetes; or

- questions about an applicant's use of insulin or other prescription drugs.

After making a job offer, an employer may ask questions about an applicant's health (including asking whether the applicant has diabetes) and may require a medical examination as long as it treats all applicants the same.

May an employer ask any follow-up questions if an applicant reveals that he or she has diabetes?

If an applicant voluntarily tells an employer that she has diabetes, an employer may ask only two questions: whether she needs a reasonable accommodation and what type of accommodation.

Example. An individual applying at a grocery store for a cashier's position voluntarily discloses that she has diabetes and will need periodic breaks to take medication. The employer may ask the applicant questions about the reasonable accommodation, such as how often she will need breaks and how long the breaks need to be. Of course, the employer may not ask any questions about the condition itself, such as how long the applicant has had diabetes, whether she takes any medication, or whether anyone else in her family has diabetes.

What should an employer do when it learns that an appli-
cant has diabetes after he has been offered a job?

The fact that an applicant has diabetes may not be used to withdraw a job offer if the applicant is able to perform the fundamental
duties ("essential functions") of a job, with or without reasonable
accommodation, without posing a direct threat to safety. The employer, therefore, should evaluate the applicant's present ability
to perform the job effectively and safely. After an offer has been
made, an employer also may ask the applicant additional questions
about his condition. For example, following an offer, an employer
could ask the applicant how long he has had diabetes, whether he
takes any medication, and whether the condition is under control.
The employer also could send the applicant for a follow-up medical
examination. An employer may withdraw an offer from an applicant with diabetes only if it becomes clear that he cannot do the
essential functions of the job or would pose a direct threat (i.e., a
significant risk of substantial harm) to the health or safety of himself
or others.

Example. A qualified candidate for a police officer's position is
required to have a medical exam after he has been extended a job
offer. During the exam, he reveals that he has had diabetes for five
years. He also tells the doctor that since he started using an insulin
pump two years ago, his blood sugar levels have been under control.
The candidate also mentions that in his six years as a police officer
for another department, he never had an incident related to his
diabetes. Because there appears to be no reason why the candidate
could not safely perform the duties of a police officer, it would be
unlawful for the employer to withdraw the job offer.

Obtaining and Using Medical Information: Employees

The ADA strictly limits the circumstances under which an employer may ask questions about an employee's medical condition or
require the employee to have a medical examination. Generally, to
obtain medical information from an employee, an employer must
have a reason to believe that there is a medical explanation for
changes in the employee's job performance or must believe that the
employee may pose a direct threat to safety because of a medical
condition.

When may an employer ask an employee if diabetes, or some other medical condition, may be causing her performance problems?

If an employer has a legitimate reason to believe that diabetes, or some other medical condition, may be affecting an employee's ability to do her job, the employer may ask questions or require the employee to have a medical examination.

Example. Several times a day for the past month, a receptionist has missed numerous phone calls and has not been at her desk to greet clients. The supervisor overhears the receptionist tell a co-worker that she feels tired much of the time, is always thirsty, and constantly has to go to the bathroom. The supervisor may ask the receptionist whether she has diabetes or send her for a medical examination because he has a reason to believe that diabetes may be affecting the receptionist's ability to perform one of her essential duties sitting at the front desk for long periods of time.

May an employer obtain medical information from an employee known to have diabetes whenever he has performance problems?

No. Poor job performance often is unrelated to a medical condition and should be handled in accordance with an employer's existing policies concerning performance. Medical information can be sought only where an employer has a reasonable belief, based on objective evidence, that a medical condition may be the cause of the employee's performance problems.

Example. A normally reliable secretary with diabetes has been coming to work late and missing deadlines. The supervisor observed these changes soon after the secretary started going to law school in the evenings. The supervisor can ask the secretary why his performance has declined but may not ask him about his diabetes unless there is objective evidence that his poor performance is related to his medical condition.

Are there any other instances when an employer may ask an employee about diabetes?

An employer also may ask an employee about diabetes when an employee:

309

- has asked for a reasonable accommodation because of his diabetes;

- is participating in a voluntary wellness program that focuses on early detection, screening, and management of diseases such as diabetes.[4]

In addition, an employer may require an employee with diabetes to provide a doctor's note or other explanation to justify his use of sick leave, as long as it has a policy or practice of requiring all employees who use sick leave to do so.

Disclosure

With limited exceptions, an employer must keep confidential any medical information it learns about an applicant or employee. An employer, however, may disclose that an employee has diabetes under the following circumstances:

- To supervisors and managers in order to provide a reasonable accommodation or to meet an employee's work restrictions

- To first aid and safety personnel if an employee would need emergency treatment or require some other assistance because, for example, her blood sugar levels are too low[5]

- To individuals investigating compliance with the ADA and similar state and local laws

- Where needed for workers' compensation or insurance purposes (for example, to process a claim)

May an employer explain to other employees that their co-worker is allowed to do something that generally is not permitted (such as eat at his desk or take more breaks) because he has diabetes?

No. An employer may not disclose that an employee has diabetes. However, an employer certainly may respond to a question about why a co-worker is receiving what is perceived as "different" or "special" treatment by emphasizing that it tries to assist any employee who experiences difficulties in the workplace. The employer also may find it helpful to point out that many of the workplace issues encountered by employees are personal and that in these circumstances, it is the employer's policy to respect employee privacy. An employer may be able to make this point effectively by reassuring the employee asking the question that her privacy similarly would be respected if she ever had to ask the employer for some kind of workplace change for personal reasons.

An employer will benefit from providing information about reasonable accommodations to all of its employees. This can be done in a number of ways, such as through written reasonable accommodation procedures, employee handbooks, staff meetings, and periodic training. This kind of proactive approach may lead to fewer questions from employees who misperceive co-worker accommodations as "special treatment."

Accommodating Employees with Diabetes

The ADA requires employers to provide adjustments or modifications to enable people with disabilities to enjoy equal employment opportunities unless doing so would be an undue hardship (i.e., a significant difficulty or expense). Accommodations vary depending on the needs of the individual with a disability. Not all employees with diabetes will need an accommodation or require the same accommodation.

What types of reasonable accommodations may employees with diabetes need?

Some employees may need one or more of the following accommodations:

- A private area to test blood sugar levels or to take insulin
- A place to rest until blood sugar levels become normal[6]
- Breaks to eat or drink, take medication, or test blood sugar levels

Example. A manufacturing plant requires employees to work an eight-hour shift with just a one-hour break for lunch. An employee with diabetes needs to eat something several times a day to keep his blood sugar levels from dropping too low. Absent undue hardship, the employer could accommodate the employee by allowing him to take two fifteen-minute breaks each day and letting him make up the time by coming to work fifteen minutes earlier and staying fifteen minutes later.

- Leave for treatment, recuperation, or training on managing diabetes[7]
- Modified work schedule or shift change

311

Example. A nurse with insulin-treated diabetes rotated from working the 6 a.m. to 2 p.m. shift to the midnight to 8 a.m. shift. Her doctor wrote a note indicating that interferences in the nurse's sleep, eating routine, and schedule of insulin shots were making it difficult for her to manage her diabetes. Her employer eliminated her midnight rotation.

- Allowing a person with diabetic neuropathy (a nerve disorder caused by diabetes) to use a stool.

Although these are some examples of the types of accommodations commonly requested by employees with diabetes, other employees may need different changes or adjustments. Employers should ask the particular employee requesting an accommodation because of his diabetes what he needs that will help him do his job. There also are extensive public and private resources to help employers identify reasonable accommodations. For example, the website for the Job Accommodation Network (http://janweb.icdi.wvu.edu/media/diabetes.html) provides information about many types of accommodations for employees with diabetes.

How does an employee with diabetes request a reasonable accommodation?

There are no "magic words" that a person has to use when requesting a reasonable accommodation. A person simply has to tell the employer that she needs an adjustment or change at work because of her diabetes.

Example. A custodian tells his supervisor that he recently has been diagnosed with diabetes and needs three days off to attend a class on how to manage the condition. This is a request for reasonable accommodation.

A request for a reasonable accommodation also can come from a family member, friend, health professional, or other representative on behalf of a person with diabetes. If the employer does not already know that an employee has diabetes, the employer can ask the employee for verification from a healthcare professional.

Does an employer have to grant every request for a reasonable accommodation?

No. An employer does not have to provide a reasonable accommodation if doing so will be an undue hardship. Undue hardship means that providing the reasonable accommodation would result in significant difficulty or expense. If a requested accommodation is too difficult or expensive, an employer still would be required to determine whether there is another easier or less costly accommodation that would meet the employee's needs.

Is it a reasonable accommodation for an employer to make sure that an employee regularly checks her blood sugar levels and eats or takes insulin as prescribed?

No. Employers have no obligation to monitor an employee to make sure that she is keeping her diabetes under control. It may be a form of reasonable accommodation, however, to allow an employee sufficient breaks to check her blood sugar levels, eat a snack, or take medication.

Dealing with Safety Concerns on the Job

When it comes to safety concerns, an employer should be careful not to act on the basis of myths, fears, or stereotypes about diabetes. Instead, the employer should evaluate each individual on her skills, knowledge, experience, and how having diabetes affects her. In other words, an employer should determine whether a specific applicant or employee would pose a "direct threat" or significant risk of substantial harm to himself or others that cannot be reduced or eliminated through reasonable accommodation. This assessment must be based on objective, factual evidence, including the best recent medical evidence and advances to treat and control diabetes.

May an employer ask an employee questions about his diabetes or send him for a medical exam if it has safety concerns?

An employer may ask an employee about his diabetes when it has a reason to believe that the employee may pose a "direct threat" to himself or others. An employer should make sure that its safety concerns are based on objective evidence and not general assumptions.

Example. An ironworker works at construction sites hoisting iron beams weighing several tons. A rigger on the ground helps him load the beams, and several other workers help him to position them. During a break, the supervisor becomes concerned because the ironworker is sweating and shaking. The employee explains that he has diabetes and that his blood sugar has dropped too low. The supervisor may require the ironworker to have a medical exam or submit documentation from his doctor indicating that he can safely perform his job.

Example. The owner of a daycare center knows that one of her teachers has diabetes. She becomes concerned that the teacher might lapse into a coma when she sees the teacher eat a piece of cake at a child's birthday party. Although many people believe that individuals with diabetes should never eat sugar or sweets, this is a myth. The owner, therefore, cannot ask the teacher any questions about her diabetes because she does not have a reasonable belief, based on objective evidence, that the teacher is posing a direct threat to the safety of herself or others.

May an employer require an employee who has been on leave because of diabetes to submit to a medical exam or provide medical documentation before allowing him to return to work?

Yes, but only if the employer has a reasonable belief that the employee may be unable to perform his job or may pose a direct threat to himself or others. Any inquiries or examination must be limited to obtaining only the information needed to make an assessment of the employee's present ability to safely perform his job.

Example. A telephone repairman had a hypoglycemic episode right before climbing a pole and was unable to do his job. When the repairman explained that he recently had begun a different insulin regime and that his blood sugar levels occasionally dropped too low, his supervisor sent him home. Given the safety risks associated with the repairman's job, his change in medication, and his hypoglycemic reaction, the employer may ask him to submit to a medical exam or provide medical documentation indicating that he can safely perform his job without posing a direct threat before allowing him to return to work.

Example. A filing clerk, who was recently diagnosed with type 2 diabetes, took a week of approved leave to attend a class on diabetes management. Under these circumstances, the employer may not require the clerk to have a medical exam or provide medical documentation before allowing her to return to work because there is no indication that the employee's diabetes will prevent her from doing her job or will pose a direct threat.

What should an employer do when another federal law prohibits it from hiring anyone who takes insulin?

If a federal law prohibits an employer from hiring a person who takes insulin, the employer would not be liable under the ADA. The employer should be certain, however, that compliance with the law actually is required, not voluntary. The employer also should be sure that the law does not contain any exceptions or waivers. For example, the Department of Transportation has issued exemptions to certain insulin-treated diabetic drivers of commercial motor vehicles.

Conclusion

Although not everyone who has diabetes has a disability as defined by the ADA, it is in the employer's best interest to try to work with employees who have diabetes, or are at risk for the disease, to help improve productivity, decrease absenteeism, and generally promote healthier lifestyles. Employers also should avoid policies or practices that categorically exclude people with diabetes from certain jobs and, instead, should assess each applicant's and employee's ability to perform a particular job with or without reasonable accommodation.

Footnotes

1. National Diabetes Fact Sheet from the Centers for Disease Control, http://www.cdc.gov/diabetes/pubs/estimates.htm.

2. Id.

3. There are two basic types of diabetes: type 1 and type 2. Individuals with type 1 diabetes must take insulin. Some persons with type 2 diabetes control the disease with weight control, appropriate diet, and exercise. Many, but not all, individuals with type 2 diabetes take insulin and/or oral medication.

4. Employers must keep any medical records acquired as part of a wellness program confidential and separate from personnel records. Employers also may not use any information obtained from a voluntary wellness program to limit health insurance eligibility.

5. See footnote 6.

6. Insulin and some oral medications can sometimes cause blood sugar levels to go too low. A person experiencing hypoglycemia

(low blood sugar) may feel weak, shaky, confused, or faint. Most people with diabetes, however, recognize these symptoms and will immediately drink or eat something sweet. Many individuals with diabetes also carry a blood glucose monitoring kit with them at all times and test their blood sugar levels as soon as they feel minor symptoms such as shaking or sweating. It usually takes only a few minutes for a person's blood sugar to return to normal.

7. An employee with diabetes also may be entitled to leave under the Family and Medical Leave Act (FMLA), which provides for up to twelve weeks of unpaid leave for a serious health condition. The U.S. Department of Labor enforces the FMLA.

Chapter 37

Emergency Situations

Chapter Contents

Section 37.1

Diabetes Emergencies

"Handling Diabetes Emergencies," by David A. Cooke, M.D., © 2010.
This article originally appeared in *When Your Doctor Says Diabetes*,
edited by David A. Cooke, M.D. (Omnigraphics, 2010).

Although most diabetic problems develop over months, years, or even decades, some diabetes-related issues are more immediate. This section reviews diabetic problems that need urgent—or even emergency—treatment.

Some diabetic emergencies can kill if they aren't quickly recognized and treated. If you are diabetic, consider wearing a medical alert necklace or bracelet to let rescuers know about your condition. It is also wise to let family, friends, and close co-workers know you have diabetes and how to help if you are in trouble.

Hypoglycemia

A common misconception is that diabetes causes hypoglycemia, a condition when blood sugar drops below normal levels and the brain and other organs become starved for fuel. In fact, serious hypoglycemia is almost always a result of medications used to treat diabetes, not the disease itself. Medications are very important to prevent blood sugar from rising too high, but they can cause hypoglycemia if they lower sugars too far.

Some medications are more likely to cause hypoglycemia than others. Hypoglycemia is very rare with metformin, pioglitazone (Actos®), rosiglitazone (Avandia®), or sitagliptin (Januvia®). It is most common with sulfonylureas (glimepiride, glipizide, and glyburide), insulin, and pramlintide (Symlin®).

However, if hypoglycemia is frequent (generally more than once every one to two weeks) or severe, contact your physician.

Hypoglycemia is generally defined as a blood sugar less than 70 mg/dL (milligrams per deciliter). However, the level when symptoms develop varies considerably. Some diabetics have hypoglycemic symptoms with blood sugars in the 80–90 mg/dL range. Other diabetics may have hypoglycemic unawareness, where they do not feel ill until their sugars are critically low. A good rule is to treat if hypoglycemic symptoms occur when glucose is below 90 mg/dL. In addition, treat sugars below 75 mg/dL even without symptoms.

The first symptoms of hypoglycemia are usually nausea, sweating, shakiness, racing heartbeat, and light-headedness. Some people notice changes in their vision, and irritability is common. More severe hypoglycemia may cause confusion, slurred speech, stumbling, falling, and appearing drunk. If blood sugars become very low, especially into the 20–40 mg/dL range, seizures or unconsciousness may occur. Severe hypoglycemia can be fatal if it is not promptly treated.

If you feel hypoglycemic, check your blood sugar immediately. If your blood sugar is less than 90 mg/dL and you are having symptoms, you are probably hypoglycemic. If you can't check your sugar but feel hypoglycemic, assume you are and act accordingly.

The first step in treating hypoglycemia is to get more sugar into your bloodstream. Consuming high-sugar foods corrects hypoglycemia within a few minutes. Ideally, use an easy-to-absorb, high-sugar food. Good choices include fruit juice, regular (not diet) soda, and candy. Glucose tablets are sold over the counter and are easy to carry and use in these situations. Glucose paste is also available and may be more useful for a severe hypoglycemic episode. However, in an emergency, a candy bar, fruit, bread, or just about any carbohydrate-containing food can be used. Generally, about one cup of orange juice, two to three glucose tablets, or about 30 grams of carbohydrate will be sufficient to reverse hypoglycemia. Rechecking blood sugar after fifteen minutes is advisable to confirm that blood sugars are rising.

If your hypoglycemia is severe, you may need help getting sugar. Ask for help or call 911 if necessary. Do not try to drive, even to the doctor or hospital, as you could pass out behind the wheel.

If you are assisting a diabetic and he or she becomes unconscious or has a seizure, call 911 immediately. While you wait for emergency services to arrive, glucose paste, a crumbled glucose tablet, or powdered sugar can be rubbed on the inside of the patient's cheeks or gums. However, do not attempt to force down food or liquid, as this could cause choking.

If a seizure occurs, gently protect the patient's head with your hands and move objects and furniture away from the person to prevent him or her from injury. Do not try to put spoons or any other object into the patient's mouth; this is more dangerous than tongue biting. Roll the person onto his or her side with head tilted downward at the end of a seizure to help prevent breathing complications. If vomiting occurs,

319

keep the patient's mouth clear and open. Do not try to administer sugar during a seizure. You could seriously injure yourself or the person you are trying to help! Wait for the seizure to subside, and back away if another one starts.

Your doctor may prescribe a glucagon kit for use in hypoglycemic emergencies. Glucagon is a natural hormone that rapidly raises blood sugars. It is given by injection, usually in a premixed injector kit. If you do not understand the kit instructions, your pharmacist may be able to teach you how to use it. It may also be advisable to teach family, friends, housemates, or co-workers how to administer the injection in the event you cannot do so yourself. A crisis is not the time to learn how to use your kit!

Hyperglycemia

Hyperglycemia is excessively high blood sugar and is the result of inadequate diabetes control. Hyperglycemia may occur for a number of reasons, including overeating, missed medication doses, infections, or improperly dosed medications. In the short term, it can cause diabetic ketoacidosis or hyperglycemic hyperosmotic coma.

Generally speaking, a diabetic person's blood sugar should rarely exceed 200 mg/dL, even after a meal. Significant blood sugar elevations (greater than 200–250 mg/dL) persisting for more than one to two days in a type 1 diabetic should prompt medical evaluation to ensure ketoacidosis is not developing. In a type 2 diabetic, sugar levels greater than 350–400 mg/dL for days at a time should also be investigated. Any diabetic with an altered level of consciousness needs emergency medical evaluation.

Diabetic Ketoacidosis

Diabetic ketoacidosis is a serious state of metabolic imbalance caused by a combination of insulin deficiency, hyperglycemia, and dehydration. It occurs almost exclusively in type 1 diabetics and is usually triggered by acute illnesses or skipping insulin injections.

In a nondiabetic person, insulin is always present in the blood. Type 1 diabetics cannot produce insulin at all and must rely on insulin injections. If insulin injections are missed or inadequate, there may be almost no insulin in the blood. The physical stress of illness can increase the demand for insulin and can also lead to insulin deficiency.

Low insulin levels allow sugars to rise, and excess glucose in the blood spills into the urine. Sugar acts like a magnet for water, pulling water out of the body into the urine, resulting in increased urination, excessive fluid loss, and dehydration. Low insulin levels also signal the body to produce ketone bodies (often simply called ketones for short). Ketones are an emergency fuel produced to sustain brain cells under starvation conditions. However, very low insulin levels stimulate ketone production even when blood sugars are very high. High levels of ketones make the blood acidic and disrupt basic cell functions.

Diabetic ketoacidosis develops over a period of hours to days. Symptoms typically are fatigue, sleepiness, abdominal pain, and nausea. Excessive thirst and dry mouth are often present. Breathing may be rapid and shallow, and an unusual fruity odor may be noticeable on a person's breath. As ketoacidosis becomes more severe, unconsciousness, sometimes referred to as diabetic coma, may develop. Blood sugar is invariably elevated, usually more than 300 mg/dL. Your physician may prescribe urine strips that detect ketones in urine. Test strips that are strongly positive usually indicate ketoacidosis.

Untreated ketoacidosis may lead to kidney failure, heart rhythm abnormalities, and death. Seek care without delay if you suspect ketoacidosis. Treatment cannot wait more than a few hours, so don't wait for an appointment with your doctor. Ketoacidosis generally requires care at an emergency room or hospital admission and usually can't be treated in a doctor's office. Intravenous (IV) fluids and insulin are administered, and blood electrolytes need to be carefully monitored as rapid shifts can occur.

Hyperglycemic Hyperosmotic Coma

Hyperglycemic hyperosmotic coma is not the same disorder as diabetic ketoacidosis (diabetic coma), although there are some common features. Hyperglycemic hyperosmotic coma is seen almost exclusively in type 2 diabetics. Unlike type 1 diabetics, type 2 diabetics produce some insulin, so they don't develop the severe insulin deficiency that leads to ketoacidosis.

Prolonged hyperglycemia leads excess glucose to spill into the urine, drawing out water with it. Usually this triggers thirst, and drinking more water replaces the lost fluid. Most severe cases occur when a debilitated diabetic cannot get water without assistance. For this reason, hyperglycemic hyperosmotic coma is more rare than ketoacidosis.

Dehydration develops over days to weeks, concentrating the blood and driving sugars even higher. However, since ketoacidosis does not occur, very high sugars may be tolerated for some time. As dehydration worsens, sugars rise into the 500–1,000 mg/dL range, and fatigue and drowsiness progress to unconsciousness.

Once hyperglycemic hyperosmotic coma has been identified, it is treated with intravenous fluids and insulin. This always requires hospitalization, and it may take days to correct this degree of dehydration

While hyperglycemic hyperosmotic coma is not as immediately dangerous as hypoglycemia or ketoacidosis, unconsciousness is always an emergency as you may not be able to tell the cause.

Infections

High blood sugars interfere with the protective function of white blood cells. The cells effectively become drunk on the excess sugar, and they respond sluggishly when confronted with bacteria or viruses. This impaired immune function makes diabetics particularly prone to infections. Infections may spread more rapidly or widely than expected and can result in overwhelming infection and death.

Cellulitis is a rapidly spreading bacterial infection of the skin. It is most often seen on the arms or legs but can involve any part of the body. Small breaks in the skin allow bacteria to invade the deeper layers. Areas of cellulitis are bright red, hot to the touch, and usually quite painful. Often the borders are very sharply defined, and they may move over a period of hours to days. Fever may or may not be present. If cellulitis is suspected, immediate medical evaluation (within hours) is critical, as the condition can worsen very rapidly.

Urinary tract infections are common in both diabetic and nondiabetic people, especially women. However, they can be much more serious in diabetics and may lead to bloodstream infections or gas gangrene of the kidneys. Urinary infections typically result in burning during urination, increased urinary frequency, and sometimes blood in the urine. Pain or pressure in the lower abdomen and lower back may also be seen, as well as fever.

As with urinary infections, gallstones are not unique to diabetics. However, complications of gallstones can also be more severe in diabetics and may lead to life-threatening gangrene of the gallbladder. Gallstone disease typically causes pain in the upper abdomen that may radiate to the shoulder and generally lasts from thirty minutes to several hours at a time. Nausea and vomiting are also frequently present, and the presence of fever may be a sign of a very dangerous situation.

All these types of infections require treatment with antibiotics. If you have one of these problems and your physician cannot see you within twelve to twenty-four hours, go to an urgent care center or emergency room.

In addition to the aforementioned symptoms, fever in a person with diabetes should always be investigated. An unexplained sudden rise in blood sugars is often seen in infections and should also prompt evaluation

Emergency Action Guidelines

Call 911 if:

- a diabetic cannot be woken up;
- a seizure occurs;
- hypoglycemia does not correct with sugar;
- you are hypoglycemic and cannot get help;
- a diabetic is acting drunk without consuming alcohol.

Have someone take you to the emergency department immediately if:

- you suspect ketoacidosis;
- you have severe abdominal pain;
- you have severe low back pain;
- you cannot keep fluids down;
- you have rapidly spreading skin redness.

Call your doctor, even at night or on the weekend, if:

- you have a fever greater than 101 degrees Fahrenheit;
- you have a red, painful, hot area on your skin.

Call your doctor during his or her next regular office hours if:

- you have a new sore, wound, infection, or ulcer on your foot;
- you have urinary tract infection symptoms;
- you had recent abdominal pain that went away;
- your blood sugars are running much higher than usual.

Call to make an appointment with your doctor if:

- your sugars are above 200 mg/dL more than once or twice a week;
- you have hypoglycemia more than once or twice a week.

Talk to your doctor about these issues at your next regular visit:

- Is my sugar control adequate?
- Can my medications cause hypoglycemia?
- Do I need a glucagon kit?
- Am I at high risk for foot ulcers?

Foot Ulcers

Diabetic neuropathy predisposes patients to sores or ulcers on weight-bearing areas of the feet. A normal person feels pressure or pain from ill-fitting shoes or injuries. However, skin may be rubbed away without any pain when neuropathy is present. If neuropathy is severe, sharp objects such as broken glass, nails, or rocks may be stepped upon and become deeply embedded in the foot without pain.

People with diabetic neuropathy frequently have peripheral arterial disease, which reduces blood flow to the feet and toes. The combination of poor blood flow, lack of protective sensation, and poor immune function can lead to deep ulcerations in the foot, which may become infected. Bone may become exposed, which typically leads to very tenacious infections. If ulcers become sufficiently advanced, it may be necessary to amputate toes or even an entire foot due to intractable infection.

Paying close attention to their feet is important for diabetics, particularly those with diabetic neuropathy. A good habit is to check one's feet nightly before bed and make sure there are no cuts, sores, or red areas. If these are seen, clean the area carefully with soap and water and protect the injured area with padding and bandages. You should see your doctor within days. Prompt treatment of ulcers can prevent limb loss.

Summary

A high level of vigilance and care is required to prevent diabetic emergencies. It is important to be familiar with the symptoms and signs of the conditions discussed in this section and know how to take action if they appear. If in doubt, it is almost always better to check with a medical professional, as delaying care can lead to catastrophe.

Section 37.2

Importance of Wearing a Medical Alert Bracelet

Medical alert bracelets enable rapid identification of patients with a number of illnesses, including diabetes, which can make them unable to communicate their illness to others, according to Shamai Grossman, M.D., director of the Cardiac Emergency Center and Clinical Decision Unit at Beth Israel Deaconess Medical Center.

How They're Beneficial for People with Diabetes

Medical alert bracelets can be extremely important for people with diabetes. Should you have a low blood glucose reaction and suddenly become confused or unresponsive, the bracelet allows immediate identification of the problem to both bystanders and paramedics. The sooner the low blood glucose reactions can be identified, the sooner they can be treated.

Emergency department personnel also use medical alert bracelets to rapidly identify people with diabetes, particularly when they may not be able to express that they have diabetes on their own. On arrival to an emergency department, one of the routine parts of the evaluation of the critically ill, unconscious, or disoriented patients is to remove their clothing to inspect the body for a cause of their sudden alteration, Grossman says. In these situations, medical alert bracelets can be invaluable as a time saver.

Information People with Diabetes Should Put on a Medical Alert Bracelet

The message on your medical alert bracelet should be concise and to the point. "Diabetes" should be engraved boldly on one side. The other side of the bracelet can have other information such as "insulin

325

dependent" or "medication controlled," he says. Other important information can include:

- an emergency contact number;

- the name of your physician;

- a referral to another place for more information, for example "see wallet card for a full medical history."

Where to Purchase a Medical Alert Bracelet

Medical alert bracelets can be purchased online through multiple websites, or can be ordered through many surgical supply stores. Although attractive medical alert jewelry is now readily available, Grossman cautions that the more elaborate the setting, the more difficult it will be to inform people of your diabetes.

Part Five

Complications of Diabetes and Co-Occurring Disorders

Chapter 38

How to Prevent Diabetes Complications

Chapter Contents

Section 38.1

Controlling Glucose, Blood Pressure, and Cholesterol to Prevent Diabetes Complications

Excerpted from "2003 National Diabetes Fact Sheet: General," Centers for Disease Control and Prevention, March 12, 2010.

Diabetes can affect many parts of the body and can lead to serious complications such as blindness, kidney damage, and lower-limb amputations. Working together, people with diabetes and their healthcare providers can reduce the occurrence of these and other diabetes complications by controlling the levels of blood glucose, blood pressure, and blood lipids and by receiving other preventive care practices in a timely manner.

Glucose Control

Research studies in the United States and abroad have found that improved glycemic control benefits people with either type 1 or type 2 diabetes. In general, for every 1 percent reduction in results of A1C blood tests (e.g., from 8.0 percent to 7.0 percent), the risk of developing microvascular diabetic complications (eye, kidney, and nerve disease) is reduced by 40 percent.

Blood Pressure Control

Blood pressure control can reduce cardiovascular disease (heart disease and stroke) by approximately 33 to 50 percent and can reduce microvascular disease (eye, kidney, and nerve disease) by approximately 33 percent.

In general, for every ten millimeters of mercury (mm Hg) reduction in systolic blood pressure, the risk for any complication related to diabetes is reduced by 12 percent.

Control of Blood Lipids

Improved control of cholesterol or blood lipids (for example, high-density lipoprotein [HDL], low-density lipoprotein [LDL], and triglycerides) can reduce cardiovascular complications by 20 to 50 percent.

Preventive Care Practices for Eyes, Kidneys, and Feet

Detecting and treating diabetic eye disease with laser therapy can reduce the development of severe vision loss by an estimated 50 to 60 percent.

Comprehensive foot care programs can reduce amputation rates by 45 to 85 percent.

Detecting and treating early diabetic kidney disease by lowering blood pressure can reduce the decline in kidney function by 30 to 70 percent. Treatment with angiotensin-converting enzyme (ACE) inhibitors and angiotensin receptor blockers (ARBs) is more effective in reducing the decline in kidney function than other blood pressure–lowering drugs.

Section 38.2

Things You Can Do to Prevent Diabetes Complications

Excerpted from "Prevent Diabetes Problems: Keep Your Diabetes Under Control," National Institute of Diabetes and Digestive and Kidney Diseases, National Institutes of Health, NIH Publication No. 08-4349, February 2008.

Things to Do Every Day for Good Diabetes Care

- Follow the healthy eating plan that you and your doctor or dietitian have worked out.

- Be active a total of thirty minutes most days. Ask your doctor what activities are best for you.

- Take your medicines as directed.

- Check your blood glucose every day. Each time you check your blood glucose, write the number in your record book.

- Check your feet every day for cuts, blisters, sores, swelling, redness, or sore toenails.
- Brush and floss your teeth every day.
- Control your blood pressure and cholesterol.
- Don't smoke.

Things for Your Healthcare Provider to Look at Every Time You Have a Checkup

- **Your blood glucose records:** Show your records to your healthcare provider. Tell your healthcare provider if you often have low blood glucose or high blood glucose.
- **Your weight:** Talk with your healthcare provider about how much you should weigh. Talk about ways to reach your goal that will work for you.
- **Your blood pressure:** The goal for most people with diabetes is less than 130/80. Ask your healthcare provider about ways to reach your goal.
- **Your medicines:** Talk with your healthcare provider about any problems you have had with your medicines.
- **Your feet:** Ask your healthcare provider to check your feet for problems.
- **Your physical activity plan:** Talk with your healthcare provider about what you do to stay active.
- **Your meal plan:** Talk about what you eat, how much you eat, and when you eat.
- **Your feelings:** Ask your healthcare provider about ways to handle stress. If you are feeling sad or unable to cope with problems, ask about how to get help.
- **Your smoking:** If you smoke, talk with your healthcare provider about how you can quit.

Things for You or Your Healthcare Provider to Do at Least Once or Twice a Year

- **A1C test:** Have this blood test at least twice a year. Your result will tell you what your average blood glucose level was for the past two to three months.

- **Blood lipid (fats) lab tests:** Get a blood test to check your total cholesterol (aim for below 200), low-density lipoprotein (LDL—aim for below 100), high-density lipoprotein (HDL—aim for above 40 if you are a man, or above 50 if you are a woman), and triglycerides (aim for below 150). These test results will help you plan how to prevent heart attack and stroke.

- **Kidney function tests:** Once a year, get a urine test to check for protein. At least once a year, get a blood test to check for creatinine. The results will tell you how well your kidneys are working.

- **Dilated eye exam:** See an eye care professional once a year for a complete eye exam.

- **Dental exam:** See your dentist twice a year for a cleaning and checkup.

- **Foot exam:** Ask your healthcare provider to check your feet to make sure your foot nerves and your blood circulation are ok.

- **Flu shot:** Get a flu shot each year.

- **Pneumonia vaccine:** Get one; if you're over sixty-four and your shot was more than five years ago, get one more.

Chapter 39

Diabetes-Related Eye Disease

What are diabetes problems?

Too much glucose in the blood for a long time can cause diabetes problems. This high blood glucose, also called blood sugar, can damage many parts of the body, such as the heart, blood vessels, eyes, and kidneys. Heart and blood vessel disease can lead to heart attacks and strokes. You can do a lot to prevent or slow down diabetes problems.

What can I do to prevent diabetes eye problems?

You can do a lot to prevent diabetes eye problems:

- Keep your blood glucose and blood pressure as close to normal as you can.

- Have an eye care professional examine your eyes once a year. Have this exam even if your vision is ok. The eye care professional will use drops to make the black part of your eyes—pupils— bigger. This process is called dilating your pupil, which allows the eye care professional to see the back of your eye. Finding eye problems early and getting treatment right away will help prevent more serious problems later on.

Excerpted from "Prevent Diabetes Problems: Keep Your Eyes Healthy," National Institute of Diabetes and Digestive and Kidney Diseases, National Institutes of Health, NIH Publication No. 09-4279, November 2008.

- Ask your eye care professional to check for signs of cataracts and glaucoma.

- If you are planning to get pregnant soon, ask your doctor if you should have an eye exam.

- If you are pregnant and have diabetes, see an eye care professional during your first three months of pregnancy.

- Don't smoke.

How can diabetes hurt my eyes?

High blood glucose and high blood pressure from diabetes can hurt four parts of your eye:

- **Retina:** The retina is the lining at the back of the eye. The retina's job is to sense light coming into the eye.

- **Vitreous:** The vitreous is a jelly-like fluid that fills the back of the eye.

- **Lens:** The lens is at the front of the eye. The lens focuses light on the retina.

- **Optic nerve:** The optic nerve is the eye's main nerve to the brain.

How can diabetes hurt the retinas of my eyes?

Retina damage happens slowly. Your retinas have tiny blood vessels that are easy to damage. Having high blood glucose and high blood pressure for a long time can damage these tiny blood vessels.

First, these tiny blood vessels swell and weaken. Some blood vessels then become clogged and do not let enough blood through. At first, you might not have any loss of sight from these changes. Have a dilated eye exam once a year even if your sight seems fine.

One of your eyes may be damaged more than the other. Or both eyes may have the same amount of damage.

Diabetic retinopathy is the medical term for the most common diabetes eye problem.

What happens as diabetes retina problems get worse?

As diabetes retina problems get worse, new blood vessels grow. These new blood vessels are weak. They break easily and leak blood into the vitreous of your eye. The leaking blood keeps light from reaching the retina.

You may see floating spots or almost total darkness. Sometimes the blood will clear out by itself. But you might need surgery to remove it.

Over the years, the swollen and weak blood vessels can form scar tissue and pull the retina away from the back of the eye. If the retina becomes detached, you may see floating spots or flashing lights.

You may feel as if a curtain has been pulled over part of what you are looking at. A detached retina can cause loss of sight or blindness if you don't take care of it right away.

Call your eye care professional right away if you are having any vision problems or if you have had a sudden change in your vision.

What can I do about diabetes retina problems?

Keep your blood glucose and blood pressure as close to normal as you can.

Your eye care professional may suggest laser treatment, which is when a light beam is aimed into the retina of the damaged eye. The beam closes off leaking blood vessels. It may stop blood and fluid from leaking into the vitreous. Laser treatment may slow the loss of sight.

If a lot of blood has leaked into your vitreous and your sight is poor, your eye care professional might suggest you have surgery called a vitrectomy. A vitrectomy removes blood and fluid from the vitreous of your eye. Then clean fluid is put back into the eye. The surgery can make your eyesight better.

How do I know if I have retina damage from diabetes?

You may not have any signs of diabetes retina damage, or you may have one or more signs:

- Blurry or double vision

- Rings, flashing lights, or blank spots

- Dark or floating spots

- Pain or pressure in one or both of your eyes

- Trouble seeing things out of the corners of your eyes

What other eye problems can happen to people with diabetes?

You can get two other eye problems—cataracts and glaucoma. People without diabetes can get these eye problems, too. But people with diabetes get these problems more often and at a younger age.

A cataract is a cloud over the lens of your eye, which is usually clear. The lens focuses light onto the retina. A cataract makes everything you look at seem cloudy. You need surgery to remove the cataract. During surgery your lens is taken out and a plastic lens, like a contact lens, is put in. The plastic lens stays in your eye all the time. Cataract surgery helps you see clearly again.

Glaucoma starts from pressure building up in the eye. Over time, this pressure damages your eye's main nerve—the optic nerve. The damage first causes you to lose sight from the sides of your eyes. Treating glaucoma is usually simple. Your eye care professional will give you special drops to use every day to lower the pressure in your eyes. Or your eye care professional may want you to have laser surgery.

Chapter 40

Diabetes-Related Foot and Skin Disease

What are diabetes problems?

Too much glucose in the blood for a long time can cause diabetes problems. This high blood glucose, also called blood sugar, can damage many parts of the body, such as the heart, blood vessels, eyes, and kidneys. Heart and blood vessel disease can lead to heart attacks and strokes. You can do a lot to prevent or slow down diabetes problems.

How can diabetes hurt my feet?

High blood glucose from diabetes causes two problems that can hurt your feet:

- **Nerve damage:** One problem is damage to nerves in your legs and feet. With damaged nerves, you might not feel pain, heat, or cold in your legs and feet. A sore or cut on your foot may get worse because you do not know it is there. This lack of feeling is caused by nerve damage, also called diabetic neuropathy. Nerve damage can lead to a sore or an infection.

- **Poor blood flow:** The second problem happens when not enough blood flows to your legs and feet. Poor blood flow makes it hard for a sore or infection to heal. This problem is called

Excerpted from "Prevent Diabetes Problems: Keep Your Feet and Skin Healthy," National Institute of Diabetes and Digestive and Kidney Diseases, National Institutes of Health, NIH Publication No. 08-4282, May 2008.

peripheral vascular disease, also called PVD. Smoking when you have diabetes makes blood flow problems much worse.

These two problems can work together to cause a foot problem. For example, you get a blister from shoes that do not fit. You do not feel the pain from the blister because you have nerve damage in your foot. Next, the blister gets infected. If blood glucose is high, the extra glucose feeds the germs. Germs grow and the infection gets worse. Poor blood flow to your legs and feet can slow down healing. Once in a while a bad infection never heals. The infection might cause gangrene. If a person has gangrene, the skin and tissue around the sore die. The area becomes black and smelly.

To keep gangrene from spreading, a doctor may have to do surgery to cut off a toe, foot, or part of a leg. Cutting off a body part is called an amputation.

What can I do to take care of my feet?

Look at your feet every day to check for problems:

- Wash your feet in warm water every day. Make sure the water is not too hot by testing the temperature with your elbow. Do not soak your feet. Dry your feet well, especially between your toes.

- Look at your feet every day to check for cuts, sores, blisters, redness, calluses, or other problems. Checking every day is even more important if you have nerve damage or poor blood flow. If you cannot bend over or pull your feet up to check them, use a mirror. If you cannot see well, ask someone else to check your feet.

- If your skin is dry, rub lotion on your feet after you wash and dry them. Do not put lotion between your toes.

- File corns and calluses gently with an emery board or pumice stone. Do this after your bath or shower.

- Cut your toenails once a week or when needed. Cut toenails when they are soft from washing. Cut them to the shape of the toe and not too short. File the edges with an emery board.

- Always wear slippers or shoes to protect your feet from injuries.

- Always wear socks or stockings to avoid blisters. Do not wear socks or knee-high stockings that are too tight below your knee.

- Wear shoes that fit well. Shop for shoes at the end of the day when your feet are bigger. Break in shoes slowly. Wear them one to two hours each day for the first few weeks.

- Before putting your shoes on, feel the insides to make sure they have no sharp edges or objects that might injure your feet.

How can my doctor help me take care of my feet?

- Tell your doctor right away about any foot problems.

- Your doctor should do a complete foot exam every year.

- Ask your doctor to look at your feet at each diabetes checkup. To make sure your doctor checks your feet, take off your shoes and socks before your doctor comes into the room.

- Ask your doctor to check how well the nerves in your feet sense feeling.

- Ask your doctor to check how well blood is flowing to your legs and feet.

- Ask your doctor to show you the best way to trim your toenails. Ask what lotion or cream to use on your legs and feet.

- If you cannot cut your toenails or you have a foot problem, ask your doctor to send you to a foot doctor. A doctor who cares for feet is called a podiatrist.

What are common diabetes foot problems?

Anyone can have corns, blisters, and other foot problems. If you have diabetes and your blood glucose stays high, these foot problems can lead to infections.

Corns and calluses are thick layers of skin caused by too much rubbing or pressure on the same spot. Corns and calluses can become infected.

Blisters can form if shoes always rub the same spot. Wearing shoes that do not fit or wearing shoes without socks can cause blisters. Blisters can become infected.

Ingrown toenails happen when an edge of the nail grows into the skin. The skin can get red and infected. Ingrown toenails can happen if you cut into the corners of your toenails when you trim them. You can also get an ingrown toenail if your shoes are too tight. If toenail edges are sharp, smooth them with an emery board.

A bunion forms when your big toe slants toward the small toes and the place between the bones near the base of your big toe grows big. This spot can get red, sore, and infected. Bunions can form on one or both feet. Pointed shoes may cause bunions. Bunions often run in the family. Surgery can remove bunions.

Plantar warts are caused by a virus. The warts usually form on the bottoms of the feet.

Hammertoes form when a foot muscle gets weak. Diabetic nerve damage may cause the weakness. The weakened muscle makes the tendons in the foot shorter and makes the toes curl under the feet. You may get sores on the bottoms of your feet and on the tops of your toes. The feet can change their shape. Hammertoes can cause problems with walking and finding shoes that fit well. Hammertoes can run in the family. Wearing shoes that are too short can also cause hammertoes.

Dry and cracked skin can happen because the nerves in your legs and feet do not get the message to keep your skin soft and moist. Dry skin can become cracked. Cracks allow germs to enter and cause infection. If your blood glucose is high, it feeds the germs and makes the infection worse.

Athlete's foot is a fungus that causes itchiness, redness, and cracking of the skin. The cracks between the toes allow germs to get under the skin and cause infection. If your blood glucose is high, it feeds the germs and makes the infection worse. The infection can spread to the toenails and make them thick, yellow, and hard to cut.

Tell your doctor about any foot problem as soon as you see it.

How can special shoes help my feet?

Special shoes can be made to fit softly around your sore feet or feet that have changed shape. These special shoes help protect your feet. Medicare and other health insurance programs may pay for special shoes. Talk with your doctor about how and where to get them.

How can diabetes hurt my skin?

Diabetes can hurt your skin in two ways:

- If your blood glucose is high, your body loses fluid. With less fluid in your body, your skin can get dry. Dry skin can be itchy, causing you to scratch and make it sore. Also, dry skin can crack. Cracks allow germs to enter and cause infection. If your blood glucose is high, it feeds germs and makes infections worse. You may get dry skin on your legs, feet, elbows, and other places on your body.

- Nerve damage can decrease the amount you sweat. Sweating helps keep your skin soft and moist. Decreased sweating in your feet and legs can cause dry skin.

What can I do to take care of my skin?

- After you wash with a mild soap, make sure you rinse and dry yourself well. Check places where water can hide, such as under the arms, under the breasts, between the legs, and between the toes.

- Keep your skin moist by using a lotion or cream after you wash. Ask your doctor to suggest one.

- Drink lots of fluids, such as water, to keep your skin moist and healthy.

- Wear all-cotton underwear. Cotton allows air to move around your body better.

- Check your skin after you wash. Make sure you have no dry, red, or sore spots that might lead to an infection.

- Tell your doctor about any skin problems.

Chapter 41

Diabetes-Related Heart Disease, Vascular Disease, and Stroke

What are diabetes problems?

Too much glucose in the blood for a long time can cause diabetes problems. This high blood glucose, also called blood sugar, can damage many parts of the body, such as the heart, blood vessels, eyes, and kidneys. Heart and blood vessel disease can lead to heart attacks and strokes, the leading causes of death for people with diabetes. You can do a lot to prevent or slow down diabetes problems.

What do my heart and blood vessels do?

Your heart and blood vessels make up your circulatory system. Your heart is a muscle that pumps blood through your body. Your heart pumps blood carrying oxygen to large blood vessels, called arteries, and small blood vessels, called capillaries. Other blood vessels, called veins, carry blood back to the heart.

What can I do to prevent heart disease and stroke?

You can do a lot to prevent heart disease and stroke:

- **Keep your blood glucose under control:** You can see if your blood glucose is under control by having an A1C test at least

Excerpted from "Prevent Diabetes Problems: Keep Your Heart and Blood Vessels Healthy," National Institute of Diabetes, Digestive, and Kidney Diseases, National Institutes of Health, NIH Publication No. 09-4283, April 2009.

twice a year. The A1C test tells you your average blood glucose for the past two to three months. The target for most people with diabetes is below 7. In some people with heart disease or other special circumstances, their doctor may recommend slightly higher levels of A1C.

- **Keep your blood pressure under control:** Have it checked at every doctor visit. The target for most people with diabetes is below 130/80.

- **Keep your cholesterol under control:** Have it checked at least once a year. The targets for most people with diabetes are:

  - Low-density lipoprotein (LDL—bad cholesterol): below 100

  - High-density lipoprotein (HDL—good cholesterol): above 40 in men and above 50 in women

  - triglycerides (another type of fat in the blood): below 150

- **Make physical activity a part of your daily routine:** Aim for at least thirty minutes of exercise most days of the week. Check with your doctor to learn what activities are best for you. Take a half-hour walk every day. Or walk for ten minutes after each meal. Use the stairs instead of the elevator. Park at the far end of the lot.

- **Make sure the foods you eat are "heart-healthy":** Include foods high in fiber, such as oat bran, oatmeal, whole-grain breads and cereals, fruits, and vegetables. Cut back on foods high in saturated fat or cholesterol, such as meats, butter, dairy products with fat, eggs, shortening, lard, and foods with palm oil or coconut oil. Limit foods with trans fat, such as snack foods and commercial baked goods.

- **Lose weight if you need to:** If you are overweight, try to exercise most days of the week. See a registered dietitian for help in planning meals and lowering the fat and calorie content of your diet to reach and maintain a healthy weight.

- **If you smoke, quit:** Your doctor can tell you about ways to help you quit smoking.

- **Ask your doctor whether you should take an aspirin every day:** Studies have shown that taking a low dose of aspirin every day can help reduce your risk of heart disease and stroke.

- **Take your medicines as directed.**

How do my blood vessels get clogged?

Several things, including having diabetes, can make your blood cholesterol level too high. Cholesterol is a substance that is made by the body and used for many important functions. Cholesterol is also found in some food derived from animals. When cholesterol is too high, the insides of large blood vessels become narrowed or clogged. This problem is called atherosclerosis.

Narrowed and clogged blood vessels make it harder for enough blood to get to all parts of your body. This condition can cause problems.

What can happen when blood vessels are clogged?

When blood vessels become narrowed and clogged, you can have serious health problems:

- **Chest pain, also called angina:** When you have angina, you feel pain in your chest, arms, shoulders, or back. You may feel the pain more when your heart beats faster, such as when you exercise. The pain may go away when you rest. You also may sweat a lot and feel very weak. If you do not get treatment, chest pain may happen more often. If diabetes has damaged your heart nerves, you may not feel the chest pain. If you have chest pain with activity, contact your doctor.

- **Heart attack:** A heart attack happens when a blood vessel in or near your heart becomes blocked. Then your heart muscle can't get enough blood. When an area of your heart muscle stops working, your heart becomes weaker. During a heart attack, you may have chest pain along with nausea, indigestion, extreme weakness, and sweating. Or you may have no symptoms at all. If you have chest pain that persists, call 911. Delay in getting treatment may make a heart attack worse.

- **Stroke:** A stroke can happen when the blood supply to your brain is blocked. Then your brain can be damaged.

What are the warning signs of a heart attack?

You may have one or more of the following warning signs:

- Chest pain or discomfort
- Pain or discomfort in your arms, back, jaw, or neck
- Indigestion or stomach pain

- Shortness of breath
- Sweating
- Nausea
- Light-headedness

Or, you may have no warning signs at all. Warning signs may come and go. If you have any of these warning signs, call 911 right away. Getting prompt treatment can reduce damage to the heart.

How do narrowed blood vessels cause high blood pressure?

Narrowed blood vessels leave a smaller opening for blood to flow through. Having narrowed blood vessels is like turning on a garden hose and holding your thumb over the opening. The smaller opening makes the water shoot out with more pressure. In the same way, narrowed blood vessels lead to high blood pressure. Other factors, such as kidney problems and being overweight, also can lead to high blood pressure.

Many people with diabetes also have high blood pressure. If you have heart, eye, or kidney problems from diabetes, high blood pressure can make them worse.

You will see your blood pressure written with two numbers separated by a slash. For example, your reading might be 120/70, said as "120 over 70." For people with diabetes, the target is to keep the first number below 130 and the second number below 80.

If you have high blood pressure, ask your doctor how to lower it. Your doctor may ask you to take blood pressure medicine every day. Some types of blood pressure medicine can also help keep your kidneys healthy.

You may also be able to control your blood pressure by doing the following things:

- Eating more fruits and vegetables
- Eating less salt and fewer high-sodium foods
- Losing weight if you need to
- Being physically active
- Not smoking
- Limiting alcoholic drinks

What are the warning signs of a stroke?

A stroke happens when part of your brain is not getting enough blood and stops working. Depending on the part of the brain that is damaged, a stroke can cause the following problems:

- Sudden weakness or numbness of your face, arm, or leg on one side of your body

- Sudden confusion, trouble talking, or trouble understanding

- Sudden dizziness, loss of balance, or trouble walking

- Sudden trouble seeing in one or both eyes or sudden double vision

- Sudden severe headache

Sometimes, one or more of these warning signs may happen and then disappear. You might be having a "mini-stroke," also called a TIA or a transient ischemic attack. If you have any of these warning signs, call 911 right away. Getting care for a TIA may reduce or prevent a stroke. Getting prompt treatment for a stroke can reduce the damage to the brain and improve chances for recovery.

How can clogged blood vessels hurt my legs and feet?

Peripheral arterial disease, also called PAD, can happen when the openings in your blood vessels become narrow and your legs and feet don't get enough blood. You may feel pain in your legs when you walk or exercise. Some people also have numbness or tingling in their feet or legs or have sores that heal slowly.

What can I do to prevent or control PAD?

- Don't smoke.

- Keep blood glucose and blood pressure under control.

- Keep blood fats close to normal.

- Be physically active.

- Ask your doctor if you should take aspirin every day.

You also may need surgery to treat PAD.

Chapter 42

Diabetes-Related Kidney Disease

Diabetic nephropathy is kidney disease or damage that results as a complication of diabetes.

Causes

The exact cause of diabetic nephropathy is unknown, but it is believed that uncontrolled high blood sugar leads to the development of kidney damage, especially when high blood pressure is also present. In some cases, your genes or family history may also play a role. Not all persons with diabetes develop this condition.

Each kidney is made of hundreds of thousands of filtering units called nephrons. Each nephron has a cluster of tiny blood vessels called a glomerulus. Together these structures help remove waste from the body. Too much blood sugar can damage these structures, causing them to thicken and become scarred. Slowly, over time, more and more blood vessels are destroyed. The kidney structures begin to leak and protein (albumin) begins to pass into the urine.

Persons with diabetes who have the following risk factors are more likely to develop this condition:

- African American, Hispanic, or American Indian origin

- Family history of kidney disease or high blood pressure

- Poor control of blood pressure

"Diabetic Nephropathy," © 2010 A.D.A.M., Inc. Reprinted with permission.

- Poor control of blood sugars
- Type 1 diabetes before age twenty
- Smoking

Diabetic nephropathy generally goes along with other diabetes complications, including high blood pressure, retinopathy, and blood vessel changes.

Symptoms

Early stage diabetic nephropathy has no symptoms. Over time, the kidney's ability to function starts to decline. Symptoms develop late in the disease and may include:

- fatigue;
- foamy appearance or excessive frothing of the urine;
- frequent hiccups;
- general ill feeling;
- generalized itching;
- headache;
- nausea and vomiting;
- poor appetite;
- swelling of the legs;
- swelling, usually around the eyes in the mornings—general body swelling may occur with late-stage disease;
- unintentional weight gain (from fluid buildup).

Exams and Tests

The main sign of diabetic nephropathy is persistent protein in the urine. (Protein may appear in the urine for five to ten years before other symptoms develop.) If your doctor thinks you might have this condition, a microalbuminuria test will be done. A positive test often means you have at least some damage to the kidney from diabetes. Damage at this stage may be reversible. The test results can be high for other reasons, so it needs to be repeated for confirmation.

High blood pressure often goes along with diabetic nephropathy. You may have high blood pressure that develops rapidly or is difficult to control.

Laboratory tests that may be done include:

- blood urea nitrogen (BUN);
- serum creatinine.

The levels of these tests will increase as kidney damage gets worse. Other laboratory tests that may be done include:

- twenty-four-hour urine protein;
- blood levels of phosphorus, calcium, bicarbonate, parathyroid hormone (PTH), and potassium;
- hemoglobin;
- hematocrit;
- protein electrophoresis—urine.

A kidney biopsy confirms the diagnosis. However, your doctor can diagnose the condition without a biopsy if you meet the following three conditions:

- Persistent protein in the urine
- Diabetic retinopathy
- No other kidney or renal tract disease

A biopsy may be done, however, if there is any doubt in the diagnosis.

Treatment

The goals of treatment are to keep the kidney disease from getting worse and prevent complications. This involves keeping your blood pressure under control (under 130/80). Controlling high blood pressure is the most effective way of slowing kidney damage from diabetic nephropathy.

Your doctor may prescribe the following medicines to lower your blood pressure and protect your kidneys from damage:

- Angiotensin-converting enzyme (ACE) inhibitors
- Angiotensin receptor blockers (ARBs)

These drugs are recommended as the first choice for treating high blood pressure in persons with diabetes and for those with signs of kidney disease.

It is also very important to control lipid levels, maintain a healthy weight, and engage in regular physical activity.

You should closely monitor your blood sugar levels. Doing so may help slow down kidney damage, especially in the very early stages of the disease. Your can change your diet to help control your blood sugar.

Depending on how poorly your kidneys are working, your doctor may limit the amount of protein in your diet.

Your doctor may also prescribe medications to help control your blood sugar. Your dosage of medicine may need to be adjusted from time to time. As kidney failure gets worse, your body removes less insulin, so smaller doses may be needed to control glucose levels.

Urinary tract and other infections are common and can be treated with appropriate antibiotics.

Dialysis may be necessary once end-stage kidney disease develops. At this stage, a kidney transplant may be considered. Another option for patients with type 1 diabetes is a combined kidney-pancreas transplant.

Outlook (Prognosis)

Nephropathy is a major cause of sickness and death in persons with diabetes. It is the leading cause of long-term kidney failure and end-stage kidney disease in the United States, and often leads to the need for dialysis or kidney transplantation.

The condition slowly continues to get worse once large amounts of protein begin to appear in the urine or levels of creatinine in the blood begin to rise.

Complications due to chronic kidney failure are more likely to occur earlier, and get worse more rapidly, when it is caused by diabetes than other causes. Even after dialysis or transplantation, persons with diabetes tend to do worse than those without diabetes.

Possible Complications

Possible complications include:

- anemia;
- chronic kidney failure (rapidly gets worse);
- dialysis complications;
- end-stage kidney disease;
- hyperkalemia;

- severe hypertension;
- hypoglycemia;
- infections;
- kidney transplant complications;
- peritonitis (if peritoneal dialysis used).

When to Contact a Medical Professional

Call your healthcare provider if you have diabetes and a routine urinalysis shows protein.

Call your healthcare provider if you develop symptoms of diabetic nephropathy, or if new symptoms develop, including little or no urine output.

Prevention

All persons with diabetes should have a yearly checkup with their doctor to have their blood and urine tested for signs of possible kidney problems.

Persons with kidney disease should avoid contrast dyes that contain iodine, if possible. These dyes are removed through the kidneys and can worsen kidney function. Certain imaging tests use these types of dyes. If they must be used, fluids should be given through a vein for several hours before the test. This allows for rapid removal of the dyes from the body.

Commonly used nonsteroidal anti-inflammatory drugs (NSAIDs), including ibuprofen, naproxen, and prescription cyclooxygenase-2 (COX-2) inhibitors such as celecoxib (Celebrex®), may injure the weakened kidney. You should always talk to your healthcare provider before using any drugs.

Alternative Names

Kimmelstiel-Wilson disease; diabetic glomerulosclerosis; nephropathy—diabetic

References

American Diabetes Association. Standards of medical care in diabetes—2010. *Diabetes Care*. 2010 Jan;33 Suppl 1:S11–61.

Inzucchi SE, Sherwin RS. Diabetes Mellitus. In: Goldman L, Ausiello D, eds. *Cecil Textbook of Medicine. 23rd ed.* Philadelphia, Pa: Saunders Elsevier; 2007: chap 248.

American Diabetes Association (2004). Nephropathy in diabetes. Clinical Practice Recommendations 2004. *Diabetes Care.* 27(Suppl 1): S79–S83.

Parving H, Mauer M, Ritz E. Diabetic Nephropathy. In: Brenner BM. *Brenner and Rector's The Kidney. 8th ed.* Philadelphia, Pa: Saunders Elsevier; 2007: chap 36.

Chapter 43

Diabetes and Kidney Failure

Chapter Contents

Section 43.1

Kidney Failure in Diabetes

"Kidney Disease of Diabetes," National Institute of Diabetes and
Digestive and Kidney Diseases, National Institutes of Health,
NIH Publication No. 08-3925, September 2008.

The Burden of Kidney Failure

Each year in the United States, more than 100,000 people are diagnosed with kidney failure, a serious condition in which the kidneys fail to rid the body of wastes.[1] Kidney failure is the final stage of chronic kidney disease (CKD).

Diabetes is the most common cause of kidney failure, accounting for nearly 44 percent of new cases.[1] Even when diabetes is controlled, the disease can lead to CKD and kidney failure. Most people with diabetes do not develop CKD that is severe enough to progress to kidney failure. Nearly 24 million people in the United States have diabetes[2] and nearly 180,000 people are living with kidney failure as a result of diabetes.[1]

People with kidney failure undergo either dialysis, an artificial blood-cleaning process, or transplantation to receive a healthy kidney from a donor. Most U.S. citizens who develop kidney failure are eligible for federally funded care. In 2005, care for patients with kidney failure cost the United States nearly $32 billion.[1]

African Americans, American Indians, and Hispanics/Latinos develop diabetes, CKD, and kidney failure at rates higher than Caucasians. Scientists have not been able to explain these higher rates. Nor can they explain fully the interplay of factors leading to kidney disease of diabetes—factors including heredity, diet, and other medical conditions, such as high blood pressure. They have found that high blood pressure and high levels of blood glucose increase the risk that a person with diabetes will progress to kidney failure.

The Course of Kidney Disease

Diabetic kidney disease takes many years to develop. In some people, the filtering function of the kidneys is actually higher than normal in the first few years of their diabetes.

Over several years, people who are developing kidney disease will have small amounts of the blood protein albumin begin to leak into their urine. This first stage of CKD is called microalbuminuria. The kidney's filtration function usually remains normal during this period.

As the disease progresses, more albumin leaks into the urine. This stage may be called macroalbuminuria or proteinuria. As the amount of albumin in the urine increases, the kidneys' filtering function usually begins to drop. The body retains various wastes as filtration falls. As kidney damage develops, blood pressure often rises as well.

Overall, kidney damage rarely occurs in the first ten years of diabetes, and usually fifteen to twenty-five years will pass before kidney failure occurs. For people who live with diabetes for more than twenty-five years without any signs of kidney failure, the risk of ever developing it decreases.

Diagnosis of CKD

People with diabetes should be screened regularly for kidney disease. The two key markers for kidney disease are estimated glomerular filtration rate (eGFR) and urine albumin.

eGFR

eGFR stands for estimated glomerular filtration rate. Each kidney contains about one million tiny filters made up of blood vessels. These filters are called glomeruli. Kidney function can be checked by estimating how much blood the glomeruli filter in a minute. The calculation of eGFR is based on the amount of creatinine, a waste product, found in a blood sample. As the level of creatinine goes up, the eGFR goes down.

Kidney disease is present when eGFR is less than 60 milliliters per minute.

The American Diabetes Association (ADA) and the National Institutes of Health (NIH) recommend that eGFR be calculated from serum creatinine at least once a year in all people with diabetes.

Urine Albumin

Urine albumin is measured by comparing the amount of albumin to the amount of creatinine in a single urine sample. When the kidneys are healthy, the urine will contain large amounts of creatinine but almost no albumin. Even a small increase in the ratio of albumin to creatinine is a sign of kidney damage.

Kidney disease is present when urine contains more than 30 milligrams of albumin per gram of creatinine, with or without decreased eGFR.

The ADA and the NIH recommend annual assessment of urine albumin excretion to assess kidney damage in all people with type 2 diabetes and people who have had type 1 diabetes for five years or more.

If kidney disease is detected, it should be addressed as part of a comprehensive approach to the treatment of diabetes.

Effects of High Blood Pressure

High blood pressure, or hypertension, is a major factor in the development of kidney problems in people with diabetes. Both a family history of hypertension and the presence of hypertension appear to increase chances of developing kidney disease. Hypertension also accelerates the progress of kidney disease when it already exists.

Blood pressure is recorded using two numbers. The first number is called the systolic pressure, and it represents the pressure in the arteries as the heart beats. The second number is called the diastolic pressure, and it represents the pressure between heartbeats. In the past, hypertension was defined as blood pressure higher than 140/90, said as "140 over 90."

The ADA and the National Heart, Lung, and Blood Institute recommend that people with diabetes keep their blood pressure below 130/80.

Hypertension can be seen not only as a cause of kidney disease but also as a result of damage created by the disease. As kidney disease progresses, physical changes in the kidneys lead to increased blood pressure. Therefore, a dangerous spiral, involving rising blood pressure and factors that raise blood pressure, occurs. Early detection and treatment of even mild hypertension are essential for people with diabetes.

Preventing and Slowing Kidney Disease

Blood Pressure Medicines

Scientists have made great progress in developing methods that slow the onset and progression of kidney disease in people with diabetes. Drugs used to lower blood pressure can slow the progression of kidney disease significantly. Two types of drugs, angiotensin-converting enzyme (ACE) inhibitors and angiotensin receptor blockers (ARBs), have proven effective in slowing the progression of kidney disease. Many people require two or more drugs to control their blood pressure. In addition to an ACE inhibitor or an ARB, a diuretic can also be useful. Beta blockers, calcium channel blockers, and other blood pressure drugs may also be needed.

An example of an effective ACE inhibitor is lisinopril (Prinivil®, Zestril®), which doctors commonly prescribe for treating kidney disease of diabetes. The benefits of lisinopril extend beyond its ability to lower blood pressure: it may directly protect the kidneys' glomeruli. ACE inhibitors have lowered proteinuria and slowed deterioration even in people with diabetes who did not have high blood pressure.

An example of an effective ARB is losartan (Cozaar®), which has also been shown to protect kidney function and lower the risk of cardiovascular events.

Any medicine that helps patients achieve a blood pressure target of 130/80 or lower provides benefits. Patients with even mild hypertension or persistent microalbuminuria should consult a healthcare provider about the use of antihypertensive medicines.

Moderate-Protein Diets

In people with diabetes, excessive consumption of protein may be harmful. Experts recommend that people with kidney disease of diabetes consume the recommended dietary allowance for protein, but avoid high-protein diets. For people with greatly reduced kidney function, a diet containing reduced amounts of protein may help delay the onset of kidney failure. Anyone following a reduced-protein diet should work with a dietitian to ensure adequate nutrition.

Intensive Management of Blood Glucose

Antihypertensive drugs and low-protein diets can slow CKD. A third treatment, known as intensive management of blood glucose or glycemic control, has shown great promise for people with diabetes, especially for those in the early stages of CKD.

The human body normally converts food to glucose, the simple sugar that is the main source of energy for the body's cells. To enter cells, glucose needs the help of insulin, a hormone produced by the pancreas. When a person does not make enough insulin, or the body does not respond to the insulin that is present, the body cannot process glucose, and it builds up in the bloodstream. High levels of glucose in the blood lead to a diagnosis of diabetes.

Intensive management of blood glucose is a treatment regimen that aims to keep blood glucose levels close to normal. The regimen includes testing blood glucose frequently, administering insulin throughout the day on the basis of food intake and physical activity, following a diet and activity plan, and consulting a healthcare team regularly. Some people use an insulin pump to supply insulin throughout the day.

A number of studies have pointed to the beneficial effects of intensive management of blood glucose. In the Diabetes Control and Complications Trial supported by the National Institute of Diabetes and Digestive and Kidney Diseases (NIDDK), researchers found a 50 percent decrease in both development and progression of early diabetic kidney disease in participants who followed an intensive regimen for controlling blood glucose levels. The intensively managed patients had average blood glucose levels of 150 milligrams per deciliter—about 80 milligrams per deciliter lower than the levels observed in the conventionally managed patients. The United Kingdom Prospective Diabetes Study, conducted from 1976 to 1997, showed conclusively that, in people with improved blood glucose control, the risk of early kidney disease was reduced by a third. Additional studies conducted over the past decades have clearly established that any program resulting in sustained lowering of blood glucose levels will be beneficial to patients in the early stages of CKD.

Dialysis and Transplantation

When people with diabetes experience kidney failure, they must undergo either dialysis or a kidney transplant. As recently as the 1970s, medical experts commonly excluded people with diabetes from dialysis and transplantation, in part because the experts felt damage caused by diabetes would offset benefits of the treatments. Today, because of better control of diabetes and improved rates of survival following treatment, doctors do not hesitate to offer dialysis and kidney transplantation to people with diabetes.

Currently, the survival of kidneys transplanted into people with diabetes is about the same as the survival of transplants in people without diabetes. Dialysis for people with diabetes also works well in the short run. Even so, people with diabetes who receive transplants or dialysis experience higher morbidity and mortality because of coexisting complications of diabetes—such as damage to the heart, eyes, and nerves.

Good Care Makes a Difference

People with diabetes should do the following things:

- Have their healthcare provider measure their A1C level at least twice a year. The test provides a weighted average of their blood glucose level for the previous three months. They should aim to keep it at less than 7 percent.

- Work with their healthcare provider regarding insulin injections, medicines, meal planning, physical activity, and blood glucose monitoring.

- Have their blood pressure checked several times a year. If blood pressure is high, they should follow their healthcare provider's plan for keeping it near normal levels. They should aim to keep it at less than 130/80.

- Ask their healthcare provider whether they might benefit from taking an ACE inhibitor or ARB.

- Ask their healthcare provider to measure their eGFR at least once a year to learn how well their kidneys are working.

- Ask their healthcare provider to measure the amount of protein in their urine at least once a year to check for kidney damage.

- Ask their health care provider whether they should reduce the amount of protein in their diet and ask for a referral to see a registered dietitian to help with meal planning.

Points to Remember

- Diabetes is the leading cause of chronic kidney disease (CKD) and kidney failure in the United States.

- People with diabetes should be screened regularly for kidney disease. The two key markers for kidney disease are estimated glomerular filtration rate (eGFR) and urine albumin.

- Drugs used to lower blood pressure can slow the progression of kidney disease significantly. Two types of drugs, angiotensin-converting enzyme (ACE) inhibitors and angiotensin receptor blockers (ARBs), have proven effective in slowing the progression of kidney disease.

- In people with diabetes, excessive consumption of protein may be harmful.

- Intensive management of blood glucose has shown great promise for people with diabetes, especially for those in the early stages of CKD.

Hope through Research

The number of people with diabetes is growing. As a result, the number of people with kidney failure caused by diabetes is also growing. Some experts predict that diabetes soon might account for half the cases of kidney failure. In light of the increasing illness and death related to diabetes and kidney failure, patients, researchers, and healthcare professionals will continue to benefit by addressing the relationship between the two diseases. The NIDDK is a leader in supporting research in this area.

Several areas of research supported by the NIDDK hold great potential. Discovery of ways to predict who will develop kidney disease may lead to greater prevention, as people with diabetes who learn they are at risk institute strategies such as intensive management of blood glucose and blood pressure control.

Participants in clinical trials can play a more active role in their own health care, gain access to new research treatments before they are widely available, and help others by contributing to medical research.

Notes

1. United States Renal Data System. *USRDS 2007 Annual Data Report*. Bethesda, MD: National Institute of Diabetes and Digestive and Kidney Diseases, National Institutes of Health, U.S. Department of Health and Human Services; 2007.

2. National Institute of Diabetes and Digestive and Kidney Diseases. *National Diabetes Statistics, 2007*. Bethesda, MD: National Institutes of Health, U.S. Department of Health and Human Services, 2008.

Section 43.2

Steps to Prevent Diabetic Kidney Failure

Excerpted from "Prevent Diabetes Problems: Keep Your Kidneys Healthy," National Institute of Diabetes and Digestive and Kidney Diseases, National Institutes of Health, NIH Publication No. 08-4281, February 2008.

What are diabetes problems?

Too much glucose in the blood for a long time can cause diabetes problems. This high blood glucose, also called blood sugar, can damage many parts of the body, such as the heart, blood vessels, eyes, and kidneys. Heart and blood vessel disease can lead to heart attacks and strokes. You can do a lot to prevent or slow down diabetes problems.

What do my kidneys do?

The kidneys act as filters to clean the blood. They get rid of wastes and send along filtered fluid. The tiny filters in the kidneys are called glomeruli.

When kidneys are healthy, the artery brings blood and wastes from the bloodstream into the kidneys. The glomeruli clean the blood. Then wastes and extra fluid go out into the urine through the ureter. Clean blood leaves the kidneys and goes back into the bloodstream through the vein.

How can I prevent diabetes kidney problems?

- Keep your blood glucose as close to normal as you can. Ask your doctor what blood glucose numbers are healthy for you.

- Keep your blood pressure below 130/80 to help prevent kidney damage. Blood pressure is written with two numbers separated by a slash. For example, 120/70 is said as "120 over 70." Ask your doctor what numbers are best for you. If you take blood pressure pills every day, take them as your doctor tells you. Keeping your blood pressure under control will also slow down or prevent damage to your eyes, heart, and blood vessels.

- Ask your doctor if you should take pills to slow down kidney damage. Two kinds are available:

  - Angiotensin converting enzyme (ACE) inhibitor

  - Angiotensin receptor blocker (ARB)

- Follow the healthy eating plan you work out with your doctor or dietitian. If you already have kidney problems, your dietitian may suggest you cut back on protein, such as meat.

- Have your kidneys checked at least once a year by having your urine tested for small amounts of protein. This test is called the microalbumin test.

- Have your blood tested at least once a year for creatinine. The result of this test should be used to estimate your glomerular filtration rate (GFR), a measure of kidney function.

- Have any other kidney tests your doctor thinks you need.

- Avoid taking painkillers regularly. Daily use of pills like aspirin or acetaminophen can damage the kidneys. Taking a single dose of aspirin every day to protect the heart, however, should be safe. Taking acetaminophen for occasional pain should also be safe. But if you are dealing with chronic pain, such as arthritis, work with your doctor to find a way to control your pain without putting your kidneys at risk.

- See a doctor right away for bladder or kidney infections. You may have an infection if you have these symptoms:

  - Pain or burning when you urinate

  - A frequent urge to go to the bathroom

  - Urine that looks cloudy or reddish

  - Fever or a shaky feeling

  - Pain in your back or on your side below the ribs

How can my doctor protect my kidneys during special x-ray tests?

X-ray tests using a contrast agent pose a risk to your kidneys. If you need x-rays, your doctor can give you extra water before and after the x-rays to protect your kidneys. Or your doctor may decide to order a test that does not use a contrast agent.

How can diabetes hurt my kidneys?

When the kidneys are working well, the tiny filters in your kidneys, the glomeruli, keep protein inside your body. You need the protein to stay healthy.

High blood glucose and high blood pressure damage the kidneys' filters. When the kidneys are damaged, the protein leaks out of the kidneys into the urine. Damaged kidneys do not do a good job of cleaning out wastes and extra fluid. Wastes and fluid build up in your blood instead of leaving the body in urine.

Kidney damage begins long before you notice any symptoms. An early sign of kidney damage is when your kidneys leak small amounts of a protein called albumin into the urine. But the only way to know about this leakage is to have your urine tested.

With more damage, the kidneys leak more and more protein. This problem is called proteinuria. More and more wastes build up in the blood. This damage gets worse until the kidneys fail.

Diabetic nephropathy is the medical term for kidney problems caused by diabetes. Nephropathy affects both kidneys at the same time.

What can I do if I have kidney problems caused by diabetes?

Once you have kidney damage, you cannot undo it. But you can slow it down or stop it from getting worse by controlling your blood pressure, taking your ACE inhibitors or ARBs, and having your kidney function tested regularly. However, if you are pregnant, you should not take ACE inhibitors or ARBs.

How will I know if my kidneys fail?

At first, you cannot tell. Kidney damage from diabetes happens so slowly that you may not feel sick at all for many years. You will not feel sick even when your kidneys do only half the job of normal kidneys. You may not feel any signs of kidney failure until your kidneys have almost stopped working. However, getting your urine and blood checked every year can tell you how well your kidneys are working.

Once your kidneys fail, you may feel sick to your stomach and tired all the time. Your hands and feet may swell from extra fluid in your body.

What happens if my kidneys fail?

One way to treat kidney failure is with dialysis. Dialysis is a treatment that does some of the work your kidneys used to do. Two types of dialysis are available. You and your doctor will decide what type will work best for you:

- **Hemodialysis:** In hemodialysis, your blood flows through a tube from your arm to a machine that filters out the waste products and extra fluid. The clean blood flows back to your arm.

- **Peritoneal dialysis:** In peritoneal dialysis, your belly is filled with a special fluid. The fluid collects waste products and extra water from your blood. Then the fluid is drained from your belly and thrown away.

Another way to treat kidney failure is to have a kidney transplant. This operation gives you a new kidney. The kidney can be from a close family member, friend, or someone you do not know. You may be on dialysis for a long time. Many people are waiting for a new kidney. A new kidney must be a good match for your body.

Will I know if I start to have kidney problems?

No. You will know you have kidney problems only if your doctor checks your blood for creatinine and your urine for protein. Do not wait for signs of kidney damage to have your blood and urine checked.

How can I find out if I have kidney problems?

Two lab tests can tell you and your doctor how well your kidneys are working:

- Each year, make sure your doctor checks a sample of your urine to see if your kidneys are leaking small amounts of protein called microalbumin.

- At least once each year, your doctor should check your blood to measure the amount of creatinine. Creatinine is a waste product your body makes. If your kidneys are not cleaning waste products from your blood, they can build up and make you sick. Your doctor can use your creatinine level to check your GFR. GFR stands for glomerular filtration rate. Results of this test tell you how well your kidneys are removing wastes from the blood.

Section 43.3

Kidney Failure: Choosing a Treatment That's Right for You

Excerpted from "Kidney Failure: Choosing a Treatment That's Right for You," National Institute of Diabetes and Digestive and Kidney Diseases, National Institutes of Health, NIH Publication No. 08-2412, November 2007.

Introduction

Your kidneys filter wastes from your blood and regulate other functions of your body. When your kidneys fail, you need treatment to replace the work your kidneys normally perform.

Developing kidney failure means you have some decisions to make about your treatment. You may choose to forgo treatment. If you choose to receive treatment, your choices include hemodialysis, which requires a machine used to filter your blood outside your body; peritoneal dialysis, which uses the lining of your belly to filter your blood inside the body; and kidney transplantation, in which a new kidney is placed in your body. Each treatment has advantages and disadvantages. Your choice of treatment will have a big impact on your day-to-day lifestyle, such as being able to keep a job if you are working. You are the only one who can decide what means most to you. Reading this information is a good way to learn about your options so you can make an informed choice. And, if you find that your choice is not a good fit for your life, you can change treatments. With the help of your healthcare team, family, and friends, you can lead a full, active life.

When Your Kidneys Fail

Healthy kidneys clean your blood by removing excess fluid, minerals, and wastes. They also make hormones that keep your bones strong and your blood healthy. When your kidneys fail, harmful wastes build up in your body, your blood pressure may rise, and your body may retain excess fluid and not make enough red blood cells. When this happens, you need treatment to replace the work of your failed kidneys.

369

Treatment Choice: Hemodialysis

Purpose

Hemodialysis cleans and filters your blood using a machine to temporarily rid your body of harmful wastes, extra salt, and extra water. Hemodialysis helps control blood pressure and helps your body keep the proper balance of important chemicals such as potassium, sodium, calcium, and bicarbonate.

Dialysis can replace part of the function of your kidneys. Diet, medications, and fluid limits are often needed as well. Your diet, fluids, and the number of medications you need will depend on which treatment you choose.

How Hemodialysis Works

Hemodialysis uses a special filter called a dialyzer that functions as an artificial kidney to clean your blood. The dialyzer is a canister connected to the hemodialysis machine.

During treatment, your blood travels through tubes into the dialyzer, which filters out wastes, extra salt, and extra water. Then the cleaned blood flows through another set of tubes back into your body. The hemodialysis machine monitors blood flow and removes wastes from the dialyzer.

Hemodialysis is usually done three times a week. Each treatment lasts from three to five or more hours. During treatment, you can read, write, sleep, talk, or watch TV.

Getting Ready

Several months before your first hemodialysis treatment, an access to your bloodstream will need to be created. You may need to stay overnight in the hospital, but many patients have their access created on an outpatient basis. This access provides an efficient way for blood to be carried from your body to the dialyzer and back without causing discomfort. The two main types of access are a fistula and a graft:

- A surgeon makes a fistula by using your own blood vessels; an artery is connected directly to a vein, usually in your forearm. The increased blood flow makes the vein grow larger and stronger so it can be used for repeated needle insertions. This kind of access is the preferred type. It may take several weeks to be ready for use.

- A graft connects an artery to a vein by using a synthetic tube. It doesn't need to develop as a fistula does, so it can be used sooner after placement. But a graft is more likely to have problems with infection and clotting.

Before dialysis, needles are placed into the access to draw out the blood.

If your kidney disease has progressed quickly, you may not have time to get a permanent vascular access before you start hemodialysis treatments. You may need to use a catheter—a small, soft tube inserted into a vein in your neck, chest, or leg near the groin—as a temporary access. Some people use a catheter for long-term access as well. Catheters that will be needed for more than about three weeks are designed to be placed under the skin to increase comfort and reduce complications.

Who Performs Hemodialysis

Hemodialysis is most often done in a dialysis center by patient care technicians who are supervised by nurses. Medicare pays for three hemodialysis treatments each week. If you choose in-center treatment, you will have a fixed time slot three times per week on Monday-Wednesday-Friday or Tuesday-Thursday-Saturday. If you do not get the time slot you want at first, you can ask to be put on a waiting list for the time slot you prefer. For a special event, you may be able to trade times with someone else. You will want to think about the dialysis schedule if you work or have children to care for. Some centers offer in-center nocturnal dialysis. This treatment is done for a longer period at night, while you sleep at the center. Getting more dialysis means fewer diet and fluid limits, and this treatment leaves your days free for work, child care, hobbies, or other tasks.

You can choose to learn how to do your own hemodialysis treatments at home. When you are the only patient, it is possible to do longer or more frequent dialysis, which comes closer to replacing the steady work healthy kidneys do. Daily home hemodialysis (DHHD) is done five to seven days per week for two to three hours at a time, and you set the schedule. If your health plan will pay for more than three treatments, you might do the short treatments in the mornings or in the evenings. Nocturnal home hemodialysis (NHHD) is done three to six nights per week while you sleep. Either DHHD or NHHD will allow a more normal diet and fluids, with fewer blood pressure and other medications. Most programs want people doing hemodialysis at home to have a trained partner in the home while they do treatments. Learning to do home hemodialysis is like learning to drive a car—it takes a few weeks and is scary at first, but then it becomes routine. The dialysis center provides the machine and training, plus twenty-four-hour support if you have a question or problem. New machines for home dialysis are smaller and easier to use than in-center ones.

You have a choice of dialysis centers, and most towns have more than one center to choose from. You can visit a center to see if it has the treatments you want or the time slot you need. Some centers will let you use a laptop or cell phone or have visitors, and others will not. Medicare has a list of all U.S. centers on its Dialysis Facility Compare website (www.medicare.gov/dialysis) with quality ratings for each. Your health plan may have a list of centers you can use. If you choose in-center treatment, you may want the center to be close to your home to reduce your travel time. If you do a home treatment, once you are trained you need to visit the center only once a month. So, the center can be as far away as you are willing to travel once a month.

Possible Complications

Vascular access problems are the most common reason for hospitalization among people on hemodialysis. Common problems include infection, blockage from clotting, and poor blood flow. These problems can keep your treatments from working. You may need to undergo repeated surgeries in order to get a properly functioning access.

Other problems can be caused by rapid changes in your body's water and chemical balance during treatment. Muscle cramps and hypotension—a sudden drop in blood pressure—are two common side effects. Hypotension can make you feel weak, dizzy, or sick to your stomach.

You'll probably need a few months to adjust to hemodialysis. Side effects can often be treated quickly and easily, so you should always report them to your doctor and dialysis staff. You can avoid many side effects if you follow a proper diet, limit your liquid intake, and take your medicines as directed.

Diet for Hemodialysis

Hemodialysis and a proper diet help reduce the wastes that build up in your blood. A dietitian is available at all dialysis centers to help you plan meals according to your doctor's orders. When choosing foods, remember to do the following things:

- Eat balanced amounts of high-protein foods such as meat, chicken, and fish.

- Control the amount of potassium you eat. Potassium is a mineral found in salt substitutes; some fruits, such as bananas and oranges; vegetables; chocolate; and nuts. Too much potassium can be dangerous to your heart.

- Limit how much you drink. When your kidneys aren't working, water builds up quickly in your body. Too much liquid makes your tissues swell and can lead to high blood pressure, heart trouble, and cramps and low blood pressure during dialysis.

- Avoid salt. Salty foods make you thirsty and make your body hold water.

- Limit foods such as milk, cheese, nuts, dried beans, and dark colas. These foods contain large amounts of the mineral phosphorus. Too much phosphorus in your blood causes calcium to be pulled from your bones, which makes them weak and brittle and can cause arthritis. To prevent bone problems, your doctor may give you special medicines, which you must take with meals every day as directed.

Pros and Cons

Each person responds differently to similar situations. What may be a negative factor for one person may be a positive one for another. See a list of the general advantages and disadvantages of in-center and home hemodialysis below.

Pros and cons of in-center hemodialysis are as follows:

- Pros:
  - Facilities are widely available.
  - Trained professionals are with you at all times.
  - You can get to know other patients.
  - You don't have to have a partner or keep equipment in your home.

- Cons:
  - Treatments are scheduled by the center and are relatively fixed.
  - You must travel to the center for treatment.
  - This treatment has the strictest diet and fluid limits of all.
  - You will need to take—and pay for—more medications.
  - You may have more frequent ups and downs in how you feel from day to day.

- It may take a few hours to feel better after a treatment.

Pros and cons of home hemodialysis are as follows:

- Pros:
  - You can do it at the times you choose—but you still must do it as often as your doctor orders.
  - You don't have to travel to a center.
  - You gain a sense of independence and control over your treatment.
  - Newer machines require less space.
  - You will have fewer ups and downs in how you feel from day to day.
  - Home hemodialysis is more work-friendly than in-center treatment.
  - Your diet and fluids will be much closer to normal.
  - You can take along new, portable machines on car trips, in campers, or on airplanes.
  - You can spend more time with your loved ones.
- Cons:
  - You must have a partner.
  - Helping with treatments may be stressful to your family.
  - You and your partner need training.
  - You need space for storing the machine and supplies at home.
  - You may need to take a leave of absence from work to complete training.
  - You will need to learn to put in the dialysis needles.
  - Daily and nocturnal home hemodialysis are not yet offered in all locations.

Working with Your Healthcare Team

Questions you may want to ask:

- Is hemodialysis the best treatment choice for me? Why?

- If I'm treated at a center, can I go to the center of my choice?

- What should I look for in a dialysis center?

- Will my kidney doctor see me at dialysis?

- What does hemodialysis feel like?

- What is self-care dialysis?

- Is home hemodialysis available in my area? How long does it take to learn? Who will train my partner and me?

- What kind of blood access is best for me?

- As a hemodialysis patient, will I be able to keep working? Can I have treatments at night?

- How much should I exercise?

- Who will be on my healthcare team? How can these people help me?

- With whom can I talk about finances, sexuality, or family concerns?

- How/where can I talk with other people who have faced this decision?

Treatment Choice: Peritoneal Dialysis

Purpose

Peritoneal dialysis is another procedure that removes wastes, chemicals, and extra water from your body. This type of dialysis uses the lining of your abdomen, or belly, to filter your blood. This lining is called the peritoneal membrane and acts as the artificial kidney.

How Peritoneal Dialysis Works

A mixture of minerals and sugar dissolved in water, called dialysis solution, travels through a catheter into your belly. The sugar—called dextrose—draws wastes, chemicals, and extra water from the tiny blood vessels in your peritoneal membrane into the dialysis solution. After several hours, the used solution is drained from your abdomen through the tube, taking the wastes from your blood with it. Then your abdomen is refilled with fresh dialysis solution, and the cycle is repeated. The process of draining and refilling is called an exchange.

Getting Ready

Before your first treatment, a surgeon places a catheter into your abdomen or chest. The catheter tends to work better if there is adequate time—usually from ten days to two or three weeks—for the insertion site to heal. Planning your dialysis access can improve treatment success. This catheter stays there permanently to help transport the dialysis solution to and from your abdomen.

Types of Peritoneal Dialysis

Three types of peritoneal dialysis are available:

- **Continuous ambulatory peritoneal dialysis (CAPD):** CAPD requires no machine and can be done in any clean, well-lit place. With CAPD, your blood is always being cleaned. The dialysis solution passes from a plastic bag through the catheter and into your abdomen, where it stays for several hours with the catheter sealed. The time period that dialysis solution is in your abdomen is called the dwell time. Next, you drain the dialysis solution into an empty bag for disposal. You then refill your abdomen with fresh dialysis solution so the cleaning process can begin again. With CAPD, the dialysis solution stays in your abdomen for a dwell time of four to six hours, or more. The process of draining the used dialysis solution and replacing it with fresh solution takes about thirty to forty minutes. Most people change the dialysis solution at least four times a day and sleep with solution in their abdomens at night. With CAPD, it's not necessary to wake up and perform dialysis tasks during the night.

- **Continuous cycler-assisted peritoneal dialysis (CCPD):** CCPD uses a machine called a cycler to fill and empty your abdomen three to five times during the night while you sleep. In the morning, you begin one exchange with a dwell time that lasts the entire day. You may do an additional exchange in the middle of the afternoon without the cycler to increase the amount of waste removed and to reduce the amount of fluid left behind in your body.

- **Combination of CAPD and CCPD:** If you weigh more than 175 pounds or if your peritoneum filters wastes slowly, you may need a combination of CAPD and CCPD to get the right dialysis dose. For example, some people use a cycler at night but also perform one exchange during the day. Others do four exchanges during the day and use a minicycler to perform one or more exchanges during the night. You'll work with your healthcare team to determine the best schedule for you.

Who Performs Peritoneal Dialysis?

Both types of peritoneal dialysis are usually performed by the patient without help from a partner. CAPD is a form of self-treatment that needs no machine. However, with CCPD, you need a machine to drain and refill your abdomen.

Possible Complications

The most common problem with peritoneal dialysis is peritonitis, a serious abdominal infection. This infection can occur if the opening where the catheter enters your body becomes infected or if contamination occurs as the catheter is connected or disconnected from the bags. Infection is less common in presternal catheters, which are placed in the chest. Peritonitis requires antibiotic treatment by your doctor.

To avoid peritonitis, you must be careful to follow procedures exactly and learn to recognize the early signs of peritonitis, which include fever, unusual color or cloudiness of the used fluid, and redness or pain around the catheter. Report these signs to your doctor or nurse immediately so that peritonitis can be treated quickly to avoid additional problems.

Diet for Peritoneal Dialysis

A peritoneal dialysis diet is slightly different from an in-center hemodialysis diet:

- You'll still need to limit salt and liquids, but you may be able to have more of each, compared with in-center hemodialysis.

- You must eat more protein.

- You may have different restrictions on potassium. You may even need to eat high-potassium foods.

- You may need to cut back on the number of calories you eat because there are calories in the dialysis fluid that may cause you to gain weight.

Your doctor and a dietitian who specializes in helping people with kidney failure will be able to help you plan your meals.

Pros and Cons

Each type of peritoneal dialysis has advantages and disadvantages. Pros and cons of CAPD:

- Pros

  - You can do it alone.

  - You can do it at times you choose as long as you perform the required number of exchanges each day.

  - You can do it in many locations.

  - You don't need a machine.

  - You won't have the ups and downs that many patients on hemodialysis feel.

  - You don't need to travel to a center three times a week.

- Cons

  - It can disrupt your daily schedule.

  - It is a continuous treatment, and all exchanges must be performed seven days a week.

Pros and Cons of CCPD:

- Pros

  - You can do it at night, mainly while you sleep.

  - You are free from performing exchanges during the day.

- Cons

  - You need a machine.

  - Your movement at night is limited by your connection to the cycler.

Working with Your Healthcare Team

Questions you may want to ask:

- Is peritoneal dialysis the best treatment choice for me? Why? If yes, which type is best?

- How long will it take me to learn how to do peritoneal dialysis?

- What does peritoneal dialysis feel like?

- How will peritoneal dialysis affect my blood pressure?
- How will I know if I have peritonitis? How is it treated?
- As a peritoneal dialysis patient, will I be able to continue working?
- How much should I exercise?
- Where do I store supplies?
- How often do I see my doctor?
- Who will be on my healthcare team? How can these people help me?
- Whom do I contact with problems?
- With whom can I talk about finances, sexuality, or family concerns?
- How/where can I talk with other people who have faced this decision?

Dialysis Is Not a Cure

Hemodialysis and peritoneal dialysis are treatments that help replace the work your kidneys did. These treatments help you feel better and live longer, but they don't cure kidney failure. Although patients with kidney failure are now living longer than ever, over the years kidney disease can cause problems such as heart disease, bone disease, arthritis, nerve damage, infertility, and malnutrition. These problems won't go away with dialysis, but doctors now have new and better ways to prevent or treat them. You should discuss these complications and their treatments with your doctor.

Treatment Choice: Kidney Transplantation

Purpose

Kidney transplantation surgically places a healthy kidney from another person into your body. The donated kidney does enough of the work that your two failed kidneys used to do to keep you healthy and symptom free.

How Kidney Transplantation Works

A surgeon places the new kidney inside your lower abdomen and connects the artery and vein of the new kidney to your artery and vein.

Your blood flows through the donated kidney, which makes urine, just like your own kidneys did when they were healthy. The new kidney may start working right away or may take up to a few weeks to make urine. Unless your own kidneys are causing infection or high blood pressure, they are left in place.

Getting Ready

The transplantation process has many steps. First, talk with your doctor because transplantation isn't for everyone. You could have a condition that would make transplantation dangerous or unlikely to succeed.

You may receive a kidney from a deceased donor—a person who has recently died—or from a living donor. A living donor may be related or unrelated—usually a spouse or a friend. If you don't have a living donor, you're placed on a waiting list for a deceased donor kidney. The wait for a deceased donor kidney can be several years.

The transplant team considers three factors in matching kidneys with potential recipients. These factors help predict whether your body's immune system will accept the new kidney or reject it:

- **Blood type:** Your blood type (A, B, AB, or O) must be compatible with the donor's. Blood type is the most important matching factor.

- **Human leukocyte antigens (HLAs):** Your cells carry six important HLAs, three inherited from each parent. Family members are most likely to have a complete match. You may still receive a kidney if the HLAs aren't a complete match as long as your blood type is compatible with the organ donor's and other tests show no problems with matching.

- **Cross-matching antigens:** The last test before implanting an organ is the cross-match. A small sample of your blood will be mixed with a sample of the organ donor's blood in a tube to see if there's a reaction. If no reaction occurs, the result is called a negative cross-match, and the transplant operation can proceed.

The Time Kidney Transplantation Takes

How long you'll have to wait for a kidney varies. Because there aren't enough deceased donors for every person who needs a transplant, you must be placed on a waiting list. However, if a voluntary donor gives you a kidney, the transplant can be scheduled as soon as you're both ready. Avoiding the long wait is a major advantage of living donation.

The surgery takes three to four hours. The usual hospital stay is about a week. After you leave the hospital, you'll have regular follow-up visits.

In a living donation, the donor will probably stay in the hospital about the same amount of time. However, a new technique for removing a kidney for donation uses a smaller incision and may make it possible for the donor to leave the hospital in two to three days.

Between 85 and 90 percent of transplants from deceased donors are working one year after surgery. Transplants from living relatives often work better than transplants from unrelated or deceased donors because they're usually a closer match.

Possible Complications

Transplantation is the closest thing to a cure. But no matter how good the match, your body may reject your new kidney. A common cause of rejection is not taking medication as prescribed.

Your doctor will give you medicines called immunosuppressants to help prevent your body's immune system from attacking the kidney, a process called rejection. You'll need to take immunosuppressants every day for as long as the transplanted kidney is functioning. Sometimes, however, even these medicines can't stop your body from rejecting the new kidney. If this happens, you'll go back to some form of dialysis and possibly wait for another transplant.

Immunosuppressants weaken your immune system, which can lead to infections. Some medicines may also change your appearance. Your face may get fuller; you may gain weight or develop acne or facial hair. Not all patients have these problems, though, and diet and makeup can help.

Immunosuppressants work by diminishing the ability of immune cells to function. In some patients, over long periods of time, this diminished immunity can increase the risk of developing cancer. Some immunosuppressants can cause cataracts, diabetes, extra stomach acid, high blood pressure, and bone disease. When used over time, these drugs may also cause liver or kidney damage in a few patients.

Diet for Kidney Transplantation

Diet for transplant patients is less limited than it is for dialysis patients, although you may still have to cut back on some foods. Your diet will probably change as your medicines, blood values, weight, and blood pressure change:

- You may need to count calories. Your medicine may give you a bigger appetite and cause you to gain weight.

- You may have to eat less salt. Your medications may cause your body to retain sodium, leading to high blood pressure.

Pros and Cons

Kidney transplantation has advantages and disadvantages:

- Pros

  - A transplanted kidney works like a normal kidney.

  - You may feel healthier and "more normal."

  - You have fewer diet restrictions.

  - You won't need dialysis.

  - Patients who successfully go through the selection process have a higher chance of living a longer life.

- Cons

  - It requires major surgery.

  - You may need to wait for a donor.

  - Your body may reject the new kidney, so one transplant may not last a lifetime.

  - You'll need to take immunosuppressants, which may cause complications.

Working with Your Healthcare Team

Questions you may want to ask:

- Is transplantation the best treatment choice for me? Why?

- What are my chances of having a successful transplant?

- How do I find out whether a family member or friend can donate?

- What are the risks to a family member or friend who donates?

- If a family member or friend doesn't donate, how do I get placed on a waiting list for a kidney? How long will I have to wait?

- What symptoms does rejection cause?

- How long does a transplant work?

- What side effects do immunosuppressants cause?

- Who will be on my healthcare team? How can these people help me?

- With whom can I talk about finances, sexuality, or family concerns?

- How or where can I talk with other people who have faced this decision?

Treatment Choice: Refusing or Withdrawing from Treatment

For many people, dialysis and transplantation not only extend life but also improve quality of life. For others who have serious ailments in addition to kidney failure, dialysis may seem a burden that only prolongs suffering. You have the right to refuse or withdraw from dialysis. You may want to speak with your spouse, family, religious counselor, or social worker as you make this decision.

If you withdraw from dialysis treatments or refuse to begin them, you may live for a few days or for several weeks, depending on your health and your remaining kidney function. Your doctor can give you medicines to make you more comfortable during this time. You may start or resume your treatments if you change your mind about refusing dialysis.

Even if you're satisfied with your quality of life on dialysis, you should think about circumstances that might make you want to stop dialysis treatments. At some point in a medical crisis, you might lose the ability to express your wishes to your doctor. An advance directive is a statement or document in which you give instructions either to withhold treatment or to provide it, depending on your wishes and the specific circumstances.

An advance directive may be a living will, a document that details the conditions under which you would want to refuse treatment. You may state that you want your healthcare team to use all available means to sustain your life. Or you may direct that you be withdrawn from dialysis if you become permanently unresponsive or fall into a coma from which you won't awake. In addition to dialysis, other life-sustaining treatments you may choose or refuse include the following:

- Cardiopulmonary resuscitation (CPR)
- Tube feedings
- Mechanical or artificial respiration
- Antibiotics
- Surgery
- Blood transfusions

Another form of advance directive is called a durable power of attorney for healthcare decisions or a healthcare proxy. In this type of advance directive, you assign a person to make healthcare decisions for you if you become unable to make them for yourself. Make sure the person you name understands your values and is willing to follow through on your instructions.

Each state has its own laws governing advance directives. You can obtain a form for an advance medical directive that's valid in your state from the National Hospice and Palliative Care Organization.

Paying for Treatment of Kidney Failure

Treatment for kidney failure is expensive, but Medicare and Medicaid pay much of the cost, usually up to 80 percent. Often, private insurance or state programs pay the rest.

Chapter 44

Diabetes-Related Sexual and Urologic Problems

Troublesome bladder symptoms and changes in sexual function are common health problems as people age. Having diabetes can mean early onset and increased severity of these problems. Sexual and urologic complications of diabetes occur because of the damage diabetes can cause to blood vessels and nerves. Men may have difficulty with erections or ejaculation. Women may have problems with sexual response and vaginal lubrication. Urinary tract infections and bladder problems occur more often in people with diabetes. People who keep their diabetes under control can lower their risk of the early onset of these sexual and urologic problems.

Diabetes and Sexual Problems

Both men and women with diabetes can develop sexual problems because of damage to nerves and small blood vessels. When a person wants to lift an arm or take a step, the brain sends nerve signals to the appropriate muscles. Nerve signals also control internal organs like the heart and bladder, but people do not have the same kind of conscious control over them as they do over their arms and legs. The nerves that control internal organs are called autonomic nerves, which signal the body to digest food and circulate blood without a person

Excerpted from "Sexual and Urologic Problems of Diabetes," National Institute of Diabetes and Digestive and Kidney Diseases, National Institutes of Health, NIH Publication No. 09-5135, December 2008 having to think about it. The body's response to sexual stimuli is also involuntary, governed by autonomic nerve signals that increase blood flow to the genitals and cause smooth muscle tissue to relax. Damage to these autonomic nerves can hinder normal function. Reduced blood flow resulting from damage to blood vessels can also contribute to sexual dysfunction.

What Sexual Problems Can Occur in Men with Diabetes?

Erectile Dysfunction

Erectile dysfunction is a consistent inability to have an erection firm enough for sexual intercourse. The condition includes the total inability to have an erection and the inability to sustain an erection.

Estimates of the prevalence of erectile dysfunction in men with diabetes vary widely, ranging from 20 to 75 percent. Men who have diabetes are two to three times more likely to have erectile dysfunction than men who do not have diabetes. Among men with erectile dysfunction, those with diabetes may experience the problem as much as ten to fifteen years earlier than men without diabetes. Research suggests that erectile dysfunction may be an early marker of diabetes, particularly in men ages forty-five and younger.

In addition to diabetes, other major causes of erectile dysfunction include high blood pressure, kidney disease, alcohol abuse, and blood vessel disease. Erectile dysfunction may also occur because of the side effects of medications, psychological factors, smoking, and hormonal deficiencies.

Men who experience erectile dysfunction should consider talking with a healthcare provider. The healthcare provider may ask about the patient's medical history, the type and frequency of sexual problems, medications, smoking and drinking habits, and other health conditions. A physical exam and laboratory tests may help pinpoint causes of sexual problems. The healthcare provider will check blood glucose control and hormone levels and may ask the patient to do a test at home that checks for erections that occur during sleep. The healthcare provider may also ask whether the patient is depressed or has recently experienced upsetting changes in his life.

Treatments for erectile dysfunction caused by nerve damage, also called neuropathy, vary widely and range from oral pills, a vacuum pump, pellets placed in the urethra, and shots directly into the penis, to surgery. All of these methods have advantages and disadvantages. Psychological counseling to reduce anxiety or address other issues may be necessary. Surgery to implant a device to aid in erection or to repair arteries is usually used as a treatment after all others fail.

Retrograde Ejaculation

Retrograde ejaculation is a condition in which part or all of a man's semen goes into the bladder instead of out the tip of the penis during ejaculation. Retrograde ejaculation occurs when internal muscles, called sphincters, do not function normally. A sphincter automatically opens or closes a passage in the body. With retrograde ejaculation, semen enters the bladder, mixes with urine, and leaves the body during urination without harming the bladder. A man experiencing retrograde ejaculation may notice that little semen is discharged during ejaculation or may become aware of the condition if fertility problems arise. Analysis of a urine sample after ejaculation will reveal the presence of semen.

Poor blood glucose control and the resulting nerve damage can cause retrograde ejaculation. Other causes include prostate surgery and some medications.

Retrograde ejaculation caused by diabetes or surgery may be helped with a medication that strengthens the muscle tone of the sphincter in the bladder. A urologist experienced in infertility treatments may assist with techniques to promote fertility, such as collecting sperm from the urine and then using the sperm for artificial insemination.

What Sexual Problems Can Occur in Women with Diabetes?

Many women with diabetes experience sexual problems. Although research about sexual problems in women with diabetes is limited, one study found 27 percent of women with type 1 diabetes experienced sexual dysfunction. Another study found 18 percent of women with type 1 diabetes and 42 percent of women with type 2 diabetes experienced sexual dysfunction.

Sexual problems may include the following:

• Decreased vaginal lubrication, resulting in vaginal dryness

• Uncomfortable or painful sexual intercourse

• Decreased or no desire for sexual activity

• Decreased or absent sexual response

Decreased or absent sexual response can include the inability to become or remain aroused, reduced or no sensation in the genital area, and the constant or occasional inability to reach orgasm.

Causes of sexual problems in women with diabetes include nerve damage, reduced blood flow to genital and vaginal tissues, and hormonal changes. Other possible causes include some medications, alcohol abuse, smoking, psychological problems such as anxiety or depression, gynecologic infections, other diseases, and conditions relating to pregnancy or menopause.

Women who experience sexual problems or notice a change in sexual response should consider talking with a healthcare provider. The healthcare provider will ask about the patient's medical history, any gynecologic conditions or infections, the type and frequency of sexual problems, medications, smoking and drinking habits, and other health conditions. The healthcare provider may ask whether the patient might be pregnant or has reached menopause and whether she is depressed or has recently experienced upsetting changes in her life. A physical exam and laboratory tests may also help pinpoint causes of sexual problems. The healthcare provider will also talk with the patient about blood glucose control.

Prescription or over-the-counter vaginal lubricants may be useful for women experiencing vaginal dryness. Techniques to treat decreased sexual response include changes in position and stimulation during sexual relations. Psychological counseling may be helpful. Kegel exercises that help strengthen the pelvic muscles may improve sexual response. Studies of drug treatments are under way.

Diabetes and Urologic Problems

Urologic problems that affect men and women with diabetes include bladder problems and urinary tract infections.

Bladder Problems

Many events or conditions can damage nerves that control bladder function, including diabetes and other diseases, injuries, and infections. More than half of men and women with diabetes have bladder dysfunction because of damage to nerves that control bladder function. Bladder dysfunction can have a profound effect on a person's quality of life. Common bladder problems in men and women with diabetes include the following:

- **Overactive bladder:** Damaged nerves may send signals to the bladder at the wrong time, causing its muscles to squeeze without warning. The symptoms of overactive bladder include urinary frequency (urination eight or more times a day or two or more times a night), urinary urgency (the sudden, strong need to urinate immediately), and urge incontinence (leakage of urine that follows a sudden, strong urge to urinate).

- **Poor control of sphincter muscles:** Sphincter muscles surround the urethra—the tube that carries urine from the bladder to the outside of the body—and keep it closed to hold urine in the bladder. If the nerves to the sphincter muscles are damaged, the muscles may become loose and allow leakage or stay tight when a person is trying to release urine.

- **Urine retention:** For some people, nerve damage keeps their bladder muscles from getting the message that it is time to urinate or makes the muscles too weak to completely empty the bladder. If the bladder becomes too full, urine may back up and the increasing pressure may damage the kidneys. If urine remains in the body too long, an infection can develop in the kidneys or bladder. Urine retention may also lead to overflow incontinence—leakage of urine when the bladder is full and does not empty properly.

Diagnosis of bladder problems may involve checking both bladder function and the appearance of the bladder's interior. Tests may include x-rays, urodynamic testing to evaluate bladder function, and cystoscopy, a test that uses a device called a cystoscope to view the inside of the bladder.

Treatment of bladder problems due to nerve damage depends on the specific problem. If the main problem is urine retention, treatment may involve medication to promote better bladder emptying and a practice called timed voiding—urinating on a schedule—to promote more efficient urination. Sometimes people need to periodically insert a thin tube called a catheter through the urethra into the bladder to drain the urine. Learning how to tell when the bladder is full and how to massage the lower abdomen to fully empty the bladder can help as well. If urinary leakage is the main problem, medications, strengthening muscles with Kegel exercises, or surgery can help. Treatment for the urinary urgency and frequency of overactive bladder may involve medications, timed voiding, Kegel exercises, and surgery in some cases.

Urinary Tract Infections

Infections can occur when bacteria, usually from the digestive system, reach the urinary tract. If bacteria are growing in the urethra, the infection is called urethritis. The bacteria may travel up the urinary tract and cause a bladder infection, called cystitis. An untreated infection may go farther into the body and cause pyelonephritis, a kidney infection. Some people have chronic or recurrent urinary tract infections. Symptoms of urinary tract infections can include the following:

- A frequent urge to urinate
- Pain or burning in the bladder or urethra during urination
- Cloudy or reddish urine
- In women, pressure above the pubic bone
- In men, a feeling of fullness in the rectum

If the infection is in the kidneys, a person may have nausea, feel pain in the back or side, and have a fever. Frequent urination can be a sign of high blood glucose, so results from recent blood glucose monitoring should be evaluated.

The healthcare provider will ask for a urine sample, which will be analyzed for bacteria and pus. Additional tests may be done if the patient has frequent urinary tract infections. An ultrasound exam provides images from the echo patterns of sound waves bounced back from internal organs. An intravenous pyelogram uses a special dye to enhance x-ray images of the urinary tract. Cystoscopy might be performed.

Early diagnosis and treatment are important to prevent more serious infections. To clear up a urinary tract infection, the healthcare provider will probably prescribe antibiotic treatment based on the type of bacteria in the urine. Kidney infections are more serious and may require several weeks of antibiotic treatment. Drinking plenty of fluids will help prevent another infection.

Who Is at Risk for Developing Sexual and Urologic Problems of Diabetes?

Risk factors are conditions that increase the chances of getting a particular disease. The more risk factors people have, the greater their chances of developing that disease or condition. Diabetic neuropathy and related sexual and urologic problems appear to be more common in people who:

- have poor blood glucose control;
- have high levels of blood cholesterol;
- have high blood pressure;

- are overweight;

- are older than forty;

- smoke;

- are physically inactive.

Can Diabetes-Related Sexual and Urologic Problems Be Prevented?

People with diabetes can lower their risk of sexual and urologic problems by keeping their blood glucose, blood pressure, and cholesterol levels close to the target numbers their healthcare provider recommends. Being physically active and maintaining a healthy weight can also help prevent the long-term complications of diabetes. For those who smoke, quitting will lower the risk of developing sexual and urologic problems due to nerve damage and also lower the risk for other health problems related to diabetes, including heart attack, stroke, and kidney disease.

Hope through Research

The National Institute of Diabetes and Digestive and Kidney Diseases (NIDDK) was established by Congress in 1950 as one of the National Institutes of Health of the U.S. Department of Health and Human Services. The NIDDK conducts and supports research on diabetes, glucose metabolism, and related conditions. NIDDK-supported research on the sexual and urologic complications of diabetes includes research conducted as part of the Epidemiology of Diabetes Interventions and Complications (EDIC) study. The EDIC is an observational follow-up study of people who originally participated in the Diabetes Control and Complications Trial (DCCT). The DCCT showed that intensive blood glucose control can reduce the risk of complications of type 1 diabetes. EDIC study results suggest that tight glucose control can delay the onset of erectile dysfunction in men with type 1 diabetes.

A recent study focused on urinary incontinence in women at high risk for developing type 2 diabetes who participated in the NIDDK-sponsored Diabetes Prevention Program (DPP). The women had prediabetes, a condition in which blood glucose levels are higher than normal but not high enough for a diagnosis of diabetes. Women who were in the DPP group that used a lifestyle change approach to diabetes prevention and lost 5 to 7 percent of their weight through dietary changes and increased physical activity were compared with those in

391

other DPP groups who received standard education and maintained a stable weight. The women in the lifestyle intervention group had fewer problems with urinary incontinence than women in the other groups. This finding adds to other results of the DPP study that indicate the value of lifestyle changes for preventing or delaying the development of type 2 diabetes.

Chapter 45

Diabetes-Related Tooth and Gum Disease

What are diabetes problems?

Too much glucose in the blood for a long time can cause diabetes problems. This high blood glucose, also called blood sugar, can damage many parts of the body, such as the heart, blood vessels, eyes, and kidneys. Heart and blood vessel disease can lead to heart attacks and strokes. You can do a lot to prevent or slow down diabetes problems.

How can diabetes hurt my teeth and gums?

Tooth and gum problems can happen to anyone. A sticky film full of germs, called plaque, builds up on your teeth. High blood glucose helps germs, also called bacteria, grow. Then you can get red, sore, and swollen gums that bleed when you brush your teeth.

People with diabetes can have tooth and gum problems more often if their blood glucose stays high. High blood glucose can make tooth and gum problems worse. You can even lose your teeth.

Smoking makes it more likely for you to get a bad case of gum disease, especially if you have diabetes and are age forty-five or older.

Red, sore, and bleeding gums are the first sign of gum disease. These problems can lead to periodontitis. Periodontitis is an infection in the

Excerpted from "Prevent Diabetes Problems: Keep Your Teeth and Gums Healthy," National Institute of Diabetes and Digestive and Kidney Diseases, National Institutes of Health, NIH Publication No. 08-4280, April 2008.

gums and the bone that holds the teeth in place. If the infection gets worse, your gums may pull away from your teeth, making your teeth look long.

Call your dentist if you think you have problems with your teeth or gums.

How do I know if I have damage to my teeth and gums?

If you have one or more of these problems, you may have tooth and gum damage from diabetes:

- Red, sore, swollen gums
- Bleeding gums
- Gums pulling away from your teeth so your teeth look long
- Loose or sensitive teeth
- Bad breath
- A bite that feels different
- Dentures—false teeth—that do not fit well

How can I keep my teeth and gums healthy?

- Keep your blood glucose as close to normal as possible.
- Use dental floss at least once a day. Flossing helps prevent the buildup of plaque on your teeth. Plaque can harden and grow under your gums and cause problems. Using a sawing motion, gently bring the floss between the teeth, scraping from bottom to top several times.
- Brush your teeth after each meal and snack. Use a soft tooth-brush. Turn the bristles against the gum line and brush gently. Use small, circular motions. Brush the front, back, and top of each tooth.
- If you wear false teeth, keep them clean.
- Call your dentist right away if you have problems with your teeth and gums.
- Call your dentist if you have red, sore, or bleeding gums; gums that are pulling away from your teeth; a sore tooth that could be infected; or soreness from your dentures.
- Get your teeth cleaned and your gums checked by your dentist twice a year.

- If your dentist tells you about a problem, take care of it right away.

- Be sure your dentist knows that you have diabetes.

- If you smoke, talk with your doctor about ways to quit smoking.

How can my dentist take care of my teeth and gums?

Your dentist can help you take care of your teeth and gums by doing the following things:

- Cleaning and checking your teeth twice a year

- Helping you learn the best way to brush and floss your teeth

- Telling you if you have problems with your teeth or gums and what to do about them

- Making sure your false teeth fit well

Plan ahead. You may be taking a diabetes medicine that can cause low blood glucose, also called hypoglycemia. Talk with your doctor and dentist before the visit about the best way to take care of your blood glucose during the dental work. You may need to bring some diabetes medicine and food with you to the dentist's office.

If your mouth is sore after the dental work, you might not be able to eat or chew for several hours or days. For guidance on how to adjust your normal routine while your mouth is healing, ask your doctor the following things:

- What foods and drinks you should have

- How you should change your diabetes medicines

- How often you should check your blood glucose

Chapter 46

Diabetic Neuropathies

What are diabetic neuropathies?

Diabetic neuropathies are a family of nerve disorders caused by diabetes. People with diabetes can, over time, develop nerve damage throughout the body. Some people with nerve damage have no symptoms. Others may have symptoms such as pain, tingling, or numbness—loss of feeling—in the hands, arms, feet, and legs. Nerve problems can occur in every organ system, including the digestive tract, heart, and sex organs.

About 60 to 70 percent of people with diabetes have some form of neuropathy. People with diabetes can develop nerve problems at any time, but risk rises with age and longer duration of diabetes. The highest rates of neuropathy are among people who have had diabetes for at least twenty-five years. Diabetic neuropathies also appear to be more common in people who have problems controlling their blood glucose, also called blood sugar, as well as those with high levels of blood fat and blood pressure and those who are overweight.

What causes diabetic neuropathies?

The causes are probably different for different types of diabetic neuropathy. Researchers are studying how prolonged exposure to high

Excerpted from "Diabetic Neuropathies: The Nerve Damage of Diabetes," National Institute of Diabetes and Digestive and Kidney Diseases, National Institutes of Health, NIH Publication No. 08-3185, February 2009.

blood glucose causes nerve damage. Nerve damage is likely due to a combination of factors:

- Metabolic factors, such as high blood glucose, long duration of diabetes, abnormal blood fat levels, and possibly low levels of insulin

- Neurovascular factors, leading to damage to the blood vessels that carry oxygen and nutrients to nerves

- Autoimmune factors that cause inflammation in nerves

- Mechanical injury to nerves, such as carpal tunnel syndrome

- Inherited traits that increase susceptibility to nerve disease

- Lifestyle factors, such as smoking or alcohol use

What are the symptoms of diabetic neuropathies?

Symptoms depend on the type of neuropathy and which nerves are affected. Some people with nerve damage have no symptoms at all. For others, the first symptom is often numbness, tingling, or pain in the feet. Symptoms are often minor at first, and because most nerve damage occurs over several years, mild cases may go unnoticed for a long time. Symptoms can involve the sensory, motor, and autonomic—or involuntary—nervous systems. In some people, mainly those with focal neuropathy, the onset of pain may be sudden and severe.

Symptoms of nerve damage may include the following;

- Numbness, tingling, or pain in the toes, feet, legs, hands, arms, and fingers

- Wasting of the muscles of the feet or hands

- Indigestion, nausea, or vomiting

- Diarrhea or constipation

- Dizziness or faintness due to a drop in blood pressure after standing or sitting up

- Problems with urination

- Erectile dysfunction in men or vaginal dryness in women

- Weakness

Symptoms that are not due to neuropathy, but often accompany it, include weight loss and depression.

What are the types of diabetic neuropathy?

Diabetic neuropathy can be classified as peripheral, autonomic, proximal, or focal. Each affects different parts of the body in various ways:

- Peripheral neuropathy, the most common type of diabetic neuropathy, causes pain or loss of feeling in the toes, feet, legs, hands, and arms.

- Autonomic neuropathy causes changes in digestion, bowel and bladder function, sexual response, and perspiration. It can also affect the nerves that serve the heart and control blood pressure, as well as nerves in the lungs and eyes. Autonomic neuropathy can also cause hypoglycemia unawareness, a condition in which people no longer experience the warning symptoms of low blood glucose levels.

- Proximal neuropathy causes pain in the thighs, hips, or buttocks and leads to weakness in the legs.

- Focal neuropathy results in the sudden weakness of one nerve or a group of nerves, causing muscle weakness or pain. Any nerve in the body can be affected.

What is peripheral neuropathy?

Peripheral neuropathy, also called distal symmetric neuropathy or sensorimotor neuropathy, is nerve damage in the arms and legs. Your feet and legs are likely to be affected before your hands and arms. Many people with diabetes have signs of neuropathy that a doctor could note but feel no symptoms themselves. Symptoms of peripheral neuropathy may include the following:

- Numbness or insensitivity to pain or temperature
- A tingling, burning, or prickling sensation
- Sharp pains or cramps
- Extreme sensitivity to touch, even light touch
- Loss of balance and coordination

These symptoms are often worse at night.

Peripheral neuropathy may also cause muscle weakness and loss of reflexes, especially at the ankle, leading to changes in the way a person walks. Foot deformities, such as hammertoes and the collapse of the midfoot, may occur. Blisters and sores may appear on numb areas of the foot because pressure or injury goes unnoticed. If foot injuries are not treated promptly, the infection may spread to the bone, and the foot may then have to be amputated. Some experts estimate that half of all such amputations are preventable if minor problems are caught and treated in time.

What is autonomic neuropathy?

Autonomic neuropathy affects the nerves that control the heart, regulate blood pressure, and control blood glucose levels. Autonomic neuropathy also affects other internal organs, causing problems with digestion, respiratory function, urination, sexual response, and vision. In addition, the system that restores blood glucose levels to normal after a hypoglycemic episode may be affected, resulting in loss of the warning symptoms of hypoglycemia.

Hypoglycemia unawareness. Normally, symptoms such as shakiness, sweating, and palpitations occur when blood glucose levels drop below 70 mg/dL. In people with autonomic neuropathy, symptoms may not occur, making hypoglycemia difficult to recognize. Problems other than neuropathy can also cause hypoglycemia unawareness.

Heart and blood vessels. The heart and blood vessels are part of the cardiovascular system, which controls blood circulation. Damage to nerves in the cardiovascular system interferes with the body's ability to adjust blood pressure and heart rate. As a result, blood pressure may drop sharply after sitting or standing, causing a person to feel light-headed or even to faint. Damage to the nerves that control heart rate can mean that your heart rate stays high, instead of rising and falling in response to normal body functions and physical activity.

Digestive system. Nerve damage to the digestive system most commonly causes constipation. Damage can also cause the stomach to empty too slowly, a condition called gastroparesis. Severe gastroparesis can lead to persistent nausea and vomiting, bloating, and loss of appetite. Gastroparesis can also make blood glucose levels fluctuate widely, due to abnormal food digestion.

Nerve damage to the esophagus may make swallowing difficult, while nerve damage to the bowels can cause constipation alternating with frequent, uncontrolled diarrhea, especially at night. Problems with the digestive system can lead to weight loss.

Urinary tract and sex organs. Autonomic neuropathy often affects the organs that control urination and sexual function. Nerve damage can prevent the bladder from emptying completely, allowing bacteria to grow in the bladder and kidneys and causing urinary tract infections. When the nerves of the bladder are damaged, urinary incontinence may result because a person may not be able to sense when the bladder is full or control the muscles that release urine.

Autonomic neuropathy can also gradually decrease sexual response in men and women, although the sex drive may be unchanged. A man may be unable to have erections or may reach sexual climax without ejaculating normally. A woman may have difficulty with arousal, lubrication, or orgasm.

Sweat glands. Autonomic neuropathy can affect the nerves that control sweating. When nerve damage prevents the sweat glands from working properly, the body cannot regulate its temperature as it should. Nerve damage can also cause profuse sweating at night or while eating.

Eyes. Finally, autonomic neuropathy can affect the pupils of the eyes, making them less responsive to changes in light. As a result, a person may not be able to see well when a light is turned on in a dark room or may have trouble driving at night.

What is proximal neuropathy?

Proximal neuropathy, sometimes called lumbosacral plexus neuropathy, femoral neuropathy, or diabetic amyotrophy, starts with pain in the thighs, hips, buttocks, or legs, usually on one side of the body. This type of neuropathy is more common in those with type 2 diabetes and in older adults with diabetes. Proximal neuropathy causes weakness in the legs and the inability to go from a sitting to a standing position without help. Treatment for weakness or pain is usually needed. The length of the recovery period varies, depending on the type of nerve damage.

What is focal neuropathy?

Focal neuropathy appears suddenly and affects specific nerves, most often in the head, torso, or leg. Focal neuropathy may cause the following:

- Inability to focus the eye
- Double vision

- Aching behind one eye
- Paralysis on one side of the face, called Bell palsy
- Severe pain in the lower back or pelvis
- Pain in the front of a thigh
- Pain in the chest, stomach, or side
- Pain on the outside of the shin or inside of the foot
- Chest or abdominal pain that is sometimes mistaken for heart disease, a heart attack, or appendicitis

Focal neuropathy is painful and unpredictable and occurs most often in older adults with diabetes. However, it tends to improve by itself over weeks or months and does not cause long-term damage.

People with diabetes also tend to develop nerve compressions, also called entrapment syndromes. One of the most common is carpal tunnel syndrome, which causes numbness and tingling of the hand and sometimes muscle weakness or pain. Other nerves susceptible to entrapment may cause pain on the outside of the shin or the inside of the foot.

How can I prevent diabetic neuropathies?

The best way to prevent neuropathy is to keep your blood glucose levels as close to the normal range as possible. Maintaining safe blood glucose levels protects nerves throughout your body.

How are diabetic neuropathies diagnosed?

Doctors diagnose neuropathy on the basis of symptoms and a physical exam. During the exam, your doctor may check blood pressure, heart rate, muscle strength, reflexes, and sensitivity to position changes, vibration, temperature, or light touch.

Foot exams. Experts recommend that people with diabetes have a comprehensive foot exam each year to check for peripheral neuropathy. People diagnosed with peripheral neuropathy need more frequent foot exams. A comprehensive foot exam assesses the skin, muscles, bones, circulation, and sensation of the feet. Your doctor may assess protective sensation or feeling in your feet by touching your foot with a nylon monofilament—similar to a bristle on a hairbrush—attached to a wand or by pricking your foot with a pin. People who cannot sense pressure from a pinprick or monofilament have lost protective sensation and are at risk for developing foot sores that may not heal properly. The doctor may also check temperature perception or use a tuning fork, which is more sensitive than touch pressure, to assess vibration perception.

Other tests. The doctor may perform other tests as part of your diagnosis.

These tests include the following:

- Nerve conduction studies or electromyography are sometimes used to help determine the type and extent of nerve damage. Nerve conduction studies check the transmission of electrical current through a nerve. Electromyography shows how well muscles respond to electrical signals transmitted by nearby nerves. These tests are rarely needed to diagnose neuropathy.

- A check of heart rate variability shows how the heart responds to deep breathing and to changes in blood pressure and posture.

- Ultrasound uses sound waves to produce an image of internal organs. An ultrasound of the bladder and other parts of the urinary tract, for example, can show how these organs preserve a normal structure and whether the bladder empties completely after urination.

How are diabetic neuropathies treated?

The first treatment step is to bring blood glucose levels within the normal range to help prevent further nerve damage. Blood glucose monitoring, meal planning, physical activity, and diabetes medicines or insulin will help control blood glucose levels. Symptoms may get worse when blood glucose is first brought under control, but over time, maintaining lower blood glucose levels helps lessen symptoms. Good blood glucose control may also help prevent or delay the onset of further problems. As scientists learn more about the underlying causes of neuropathy, new treatments may become available to help slow, prevent, or even reverse nerve damage.

Additional treatment depends on the type of nerve problem and symptom. If you have problems with your feet, your doctor may refer you to a foot care specialist.

Pain relief. Doctors usually treat painful diabetic neuropathy with oral medications, although other types of treatments may help some people. People with severe nerve pain may benefit from a combination of medications or treatments. Talk with your healthcare provider about options for treating your neuropathy.

Medications used to help relieve diabetic nerve pain include the following:

- Tricyclic antidepressants, such as amitriptyline, imipramine, and desipramine (Norpramin®, Pertofrane®)

- Other types of antidepressants, such as duloxetine (Cymbalta®), venlafaxine, bupropion (Wellbutrin®), paroxetine (Paxil®), and citalopram (Celexa®)

- Anticonvulsants, such as pregabalin (Lyrica®), gabapentin (Gabarone®, Neurontin®), carbamazepine, and lamotrigine (Lamictal®)

- Opioids and opioid-like drugs, such as controlled-release oxycodone, an opioid, and tramadol (Ultram®), an opioid that also acts as an antidepressant

Duloxetine and pregabalin are approved by the U.S. Food and Drug Administration specifically for treating painful diabetic peripheral neuropathy.

You do not have to be depressed for an antidepressant to help relieve your nerve pain. All medications have side effects, and some are not recommended for use in older adults or those with heart disease. Because over-the-counter pain medicines such as acetaminophen and ibuprofen may not work well for treating most nerve pain and can have serious side effects, some experts recommend avoiding these medications.

Treatments that are applied to the skin—typically to the feet—include capsaicin cream and lidocaine patches (Lidoderm®, Lidopain®). Studies suggest that nitrate sprays or patches for the feet may relieve pain. Studies of alpha-lipoic acid, an antioxidant, and evening primrose oil have shown that they can help relieve symptoms and may improve nerve function.

A device called a bed cradle can keep sheets and blankets from touching sensitive feet and legs. Acupuncture, biofeedback, or physical therapy may help relieve pain in some people. Treatments that involve electrical nerve stimulation, magnetic therapy, and laser or light therapy may be helpful but need further study. Researchers are also studying several new therapies in clinical trials.

Gastrointestinal problems. To relieve mild symptoms of gastroparesis—indigestion, belching, nausea, or vomiting—doctors suggest eating small, frequent meals; avoiding fats; and eating less fiber. When symptoms are severe, doctors may prescribe erythromycin to speed digestion, metoclopramide to speed digestion and help relieve nausea, or other medications to help regulate digestion or reduce stomach acid secretion.

To relieve diarrhea or other bowel problems, doctors may prescribe an antibiotic such as tetracycline, or other medications as appropriate.

Dizziness and weakness. Sitting or standing slowly may help prevent the light-headedness, dizziness, or fainting associated with blood pressure and circulation problems. Raising the head of the bed or wearing elastic stockings may also help. Some people benefit from increased salt in the diet and treatment with salt-retaining hormones. Others benefit from high blood pressure medications. Physical therapy can help when muscle weakness or loss of coordination is a problem.

Urinary and sexual problems. To clear up a urinary tract infection, the doctor will probably prescribe an antibiotic. Drinking plenty of fluids will help prevent another infection. People who have incontinence should try to urinate at regular intervals—every three hours, for example—since they may not be able to tell when the bladder is full.

To treat erectile dysfunction in men, the doctor will first do tests to rule out a hormonal cause. Several methods are available to treat erectile dysfunction caused by neuropathy. Medicines are available to help men have and maintain erections by increasing blood flow to the penis. Some are oral medications and others are injected into the penis or inserted into the urethra at the tip of the penis. Mechanical vacuum devices can also increase blood flow to the penis. Another option is to surgically implant an inflatable or semirigid device in the penis.

Vaginal lubricants may be useful for women when neuropathy causes vaginal dryness. To treat problems with arousal and orgasm, the doctor may refer women to a gynecologist.

Foot care. People with neuropathy need to take special care of their feet. The nerves to the feet are the longest in the body and are the ones most often affected by neuropathy. Loss of sensation in the feet means that sores or injuries may not be noticed and may become ulcerated or infected. Circulation problems also increase the risk of foot ulcers.

More than half of all lower-limb amputations in the United States occur in people with diabetes—eighty-six thousand amputations per year. Doctors estimate that nearly half of the amputations caused by neuropathy and poor circulation could have been prevented by careful foot care.

Follow these steps to take care of your feet:

- Clean your feet daily, using warm—not hot—water and a mild soap. Avoid soaking your feet. Dry them with a soft towel and dry carefully between your toes.

- Inspect your feet and toes every day for cuts, blisters, redness, swelling, calluses, or other problems. Use a mirror—laying a mirror on the floor works well—or get help from someone else if you cannot see the bottoms of your feet. Notify your healthcare provider of any problems.

- Moisturize your feet with lotion, but avoid getting the lotion between your toes.

- After a bath or shower, file corns and calluses gently with a pumice stone.

- Each week or when needed, cut your toenails to the shape of your toes and file the edges with an emery board.

- Always wear shoes or slippers to protect your feet from injuries. Prevent skin irritation by wearing thick, soft, seamless socks.

- Wear shoes that fit well and allow your toes to move. Break in new shoes gradually by first wearing them for only an hour at a time.

- Before putting your shoes on, look them over carefully and feel the insides with your hand to make sure they have no tears, sharp edges, or objects in them that might injure your feet.

- If you need help taking care of your feet, make an appointment to see a foot doctor, also called a podiatrist.

Chapter 47

Gastroparesis

What is gastroparesis?

Gastroparesis, also called delayed gastric emptying, is a disorder in which the stomach takes too long to empty its contents. Normally, the stomach contracts to move food down into the small intestine for digestion. The vagus nerve controls the movement of food from the stomach through the digestive tract. Gastroparesis occurs when the vagus nerve is damaged and the muscles of the stomach and intestines do not work normally. Food then moves slowly or stops moving through the digestive tract.

What causes gastroparesis?

The most common cause of gastroparesis is diabetes. People with diabetes have high blood glucose, also called blood sugar, which in turn causes chemical changes in nerves and damages the blood vessels that carry oxygen and nutrients to the nerves. Over time, high blood glucose can damage the vagus nerve.

Some other causes of gastroparesis are as follows:

- Surgery on the stomach or vagus nerve

- Viral infections

Excerpted from "Gastroparesis," National Institute of Diabetes and Digestive and Kidney Diseases, National Institutes of Health, NIH Publication No. 07-4348, July 2007.

- Anorexia nervosa or bulimia

- Medications—anticholinergics and narcotics—that slow contractions in the intestine

- Gastroesophageal reflux disease

- Smooth muscle disorders, such as amyloidosis and scleroderma

- Nervous system diseases, including abdominal migraine and Parkinson disease

- Metabolic disorders, including hypothyroidism

Many people have what is called idiopathic gastroparesis, meaning the cause is unknown and cannot be found even after medical tests.

What are the symptoms of gastroparesis?

Signs and symptoms of gastroparesis are as follows:

- Heartburn

- Pain in the upper abdomen

- Nausea

- Vomiting of undigested food—sometimes several hours after a meal

- Early feeling of fullness after only a few bites of food

- Weight loss due to poor absorption of nutrients or low calorie intake

- Abdominal bloating

- High and low blood glucose levels

- Lack of appetite

- Gastroesophageal reflux

- Spasms in the stomach area

Eating solid foods, high-fiber foods such as raw fruits and vegetables, fatty foods, or drinks high in fat or carbonation may contribute to these symptoms.

The symptoms of gastroparesis may be mild or severe, depending on the person. Symptoms can happen frequently in some people and less often in others. Many people with gastroparesis experience a wide range of symptoms, and sometimes the disorder is difficult for the physician to diagnose.

What are the complications of gastroparesis?

If food lingers too long in the stomach, it can cause bacterial overgrowth from the fermentation of food. Also, the food can harden into solid masses called bezoars that may cause nausea, vomiting, and obstruction in the stomach. Bezoars can be dangerous if they block the passage of food into the small intestine.

Gastroparesis can make diabetes worse by making blood glucose control more difficult. When food that has been delayed in the stomach finally enters the small intestine and is absorbed, blood glucose levels rise. Since gastroparesis makes stomach emptying unpredictable, a person's blood glucose levels can be erratic and difficult to control.

How is gastroparesis diagnosed?

After performing a full physical exam and taking your medical history, your doctor may order several blood tests to check blood counts and chemical and electrolyte levels. To rule out an obstruction or other conditions, the doctor may perform the following tests:

- **Upper endoscopy:** After giving you a sedative to help you become drowsy, the doctor passes a long, thin tube called an endoscope through your mouth and gently guides it down the throat, also called the esophagus, into the stomach. Through the endoscope, the doctor can look at the lining of the stomach to check for any abnormalities.

- **Ultrasound:** To rule out gallbladder disease and pancreatitis as sources of the problem, you may have an ultrasound test, which uses harmless sound waves to outline and define the shape of the gallbladder and pancreas.

- **Barium x-ray:** After fasting for twelve hours, you will drink a thick liquid called barium, which coats the stomach, making it show up on the x-ray. If you have diabetes, your doctor may have special instructions about fasting. Normally, the stomach will be empty of all food after twelve hours of fasting. Gastroparesis is likely if the x-ray shows food in the stomach. Because a person with gastroparesis can sometimes have normal emptying, the doctor may repeat the test another day if gastroparesis is suspected.

Once other causes have been ruled out, the doctor will perform one of the following gastric emptying tests to confirm a diagnosis of gastroparesis:

- **Gastric emptying scintigraphy:** This test involves eating a bland meal, such as eggs or egg substitute, that contains a small amount of a radioactive substance, called radioisotope, that shows up on scans. The dose of radiation from the radioisotope is not dangerous. The scan measures the rate of gastric emptying at one, two, three, and four hours. When more than 10 percent of the meal is still in the stomach at four hours, the diagnosis of gastroparesis is confirmed.

- **Breath test:** After ingestion of a meal containing a small amount of isotope, breath samples are taken to measure the presence of the isotope in carbon dioxide, which is expelled when a person exhales. The results reveal how fast the stomach is emptying.

- **SmartPill:** Approved by the U.S. Food and Drug Administration (FDA) in 2006, the SmartPill is a small device in capsule form that can be swallowed. The device then moves through the digestive tract and collects information about its progress that is sent to a cell phone–sized receiver worn around your waist or neck. When the capsule is passed from the body with the stool in a couple of days, you take the receiver back to the doctor, who enters the information into a computer.

How is gastroparesis treated?

Treatment of gastroparesis depends on the severity of the symptoms. In most cases, treatment does not cure gastroparesis—it is usually a chronic condition. Treatment helps you manage the condition so you can be as healthy and comfortable as possible.

Medication. Several medications are used to treat gastroparesis. Your doctor may try different medications or combinations to find the most effective treatment. Discussing the risk of side effects of any medication with your doctor is important.

Medications used include the following:

- **Metoclopramide (Reglan):** This drug stimulates stomach muscle contractions to help emptying. Metoclopramide also helps reduce nausea and vomiting. Metoclopramide is taken twenty to thirty minutes before meals and at bedtime. Side effects of this drug include fatigue, sleepiness, depression, anxiety, and problems with physical movement.

- **Erythromycin:** This antibiotic also improves stomach emptying. It works by increasing the contractions that move food through the stomach. Side effects include nausea, vomiting, and abdominal cramps.

- **Domperidone:** This drug works like metoclopramide to improve stomach emptying and decrease nausea and vomiting. The FDA is reviewing domperidone, which has been used elsewhere in the world to treat gastroparesis. Use of the drug is restricted in the United States.

- **Other medications:** Other medications may be used to treat symptoms and problems related to gastroparesis. For example, an antiemetic can help with nausea and vomiting. Antibiotics will clear up a bacterial infection. If you have a bezoar in the stomach, the doctor may use an endoscope to inject medication into it to dissolve it.

Dietary changes. Changing your eating habits can help control gastroparesis. Your doctor or dietitian may prescribe six small meals a day instead of three large ones. If less food enters the stomach each time you eat, it may not become overly full. In more severe cases, a liquid or pureed diet may be prescribed.

The doctor may recommend that you avoid high-fat and high-fiber foods. Fat naturally slows digestion—a problem you do not need if you have gastroparesis—and fiber is difficult to digest. Some high-fiber foods like oranges and broccoli contain material that cannot be digested. Avoid these foods because the indigestible part will remain in the stomach too long and possibly form bezoars.

Feeding tube. If a liquid or pureed diet does not work, you may need surgery to insert a feeding tube. The tube, called a jejunostomy, is inserted through the skin on your abdomen into the small intestine. The feeding tube bypasses the stomach and places nutrients and medication directly into the small intestine. These products are then digested and delivered to your bloodstream quickly. You will receive special liquid food to use with the tube. The jejunostomy is used only when gastroparesis is severe or the tube is necessary to stabilize blood glucose levels in people with diabetes.

Parenteral nutrition. Parenteral nutrition refers to delivering nutrients directly into the bloodstream, bypassing the digestive system. The doctor places a thin tube called a catheter in a chest vein, leaving an opening to it outside the skin. For feeding, you attach a bag containing liquid nutrients or medication to the catheter. The fluid enters your bloodstream through the vein. Your doctor will tell you what type of liquid nutrition to use.

This approach is an alternative to the jejunostomy tube and is usually a temporary method to get you through a difficult period with gastroparesis. Parenteral nutrition is used only when gastroparesis is severe and is not helped by other methods.

Gastric electrical stimulation. A gastric neurostimulator is a surgically implanted battery-operated device that releases mild electrical pulses to help control nausea and vomiting associated with gastroparesis. This option is available to people whose nausea and vomiting do not improve with medications. Further studies will help determine who will benefit most from this procedure, which is available in a few centers across the United States.

Botulinum toxin. The use of botulinum toxin has been associated with improvement in symptoms of gastroparesis in some patients; however, further research on this form of therapy is needed.

What if I have diabetes and gastroparesis?

The primary treatment goals for gastroparesis related to diabetes are to improve stomach emptying and regain control of blood glucose levels. Treatment includes dietary changes, insulin, oral medications, and, in severe cases, a feeding tube and parenteral nutrition.

Dietary changes. The doctor will suggest dietary changes such as six smaller meals to help restore your blood glucose to more normal levels before testing you for gastroparesis. In some cases, the doctor or dietitian may suggest you try eating several liquid or pureed meals a day until your blood glucose levels are stable and the symptoms improve. Liquid meals provide all the nutrients found in solid foods, but can pass through the stomach more easily and quickly.

Insulin for blood glucose control. If you have gastroparesis, food is being absorbed more slowly and at unpredictable times. To control blood glucose, you may need to take insulin more often or change the type of insulin you take; take your insulin after you eat instead of before; or check your blood glucose levels frequently after you eat and administer insulin whenever necessary.

Your doctor will give you specific instructions for taking insulin based on your particular needs.

Chapter 48

Hyperglycemic Hyperosmolar Syndrome

Diabetic hyperglycemic hyperosmolar syndrome (HHS) is a complication of type 2 diabetes that involves extremely high blood sugar (glucose) levels without the presence of ketones. Ketones are byproducts of fat breakdown.

Causes

Diabetic hyperglycemic hyperosmolar syndrome is a condition of:

- extremely high blood sugar (glucose) levels;
- extreme lack of water (dehydration);
- decreased consciousness.

The buildup of ketones in the body (ketoacidosis) may also occur.

This condition is usually seen in people with type 2 diabetes. It may occur in those who have not been diagnosed with diabetes, or in people who have not been able to control their diabetes. The condition may be brought on by:

- infection;
- other illness;
- medications that lower glucose tolerance or increase fluid loss (in people who are losing or not getting enough fluid).

Normally, the kidneys try to make up for high glucose levels in the blood by allowing the extra glucose to leave the body in the urine. If you do not drink enough fluids, or you drink fluids that contain sugar, the kidneys can no longer get rid of the extra glucose. Glucose levels in the blood can become very high as a result. The blood then becomes much more concentrated than normal (hyperosmolarity).

Hyperosmolarity is a condition in which the blood has a high concentration of salt (sodium), glucose, and other substances that normally cause water to move into the bloodstream. This draws the water out of the body's other organs, including the brain. Hyperosmolarity creates a cycle of increasing blood glucose levels and dehydration.

Risk factors include:

- a stressful event such as infection, heart attack, stroke, or recent surgery;

- congestive heart failure;

- impaired thirst;

- limited access to water (especially in patients with dementia or who are bed-bound);

- older age;

- poor kidney function;

- poor management of diabetes—not following the treatment plan as directed;

- stopping insulin or other medications that lower glucose levels.

Symptoms

- Coma

- Confusion

- Convulsions

- Increased thirst

- Increased urination (at the beginning of the syndrome)

- Lethargy

- Nausea

- Weakness

- Weight loss

Symptoms may get worse over a period of days or weeks. Other symptoms that may occur with this disease:

- Dysfunctional movement

- Loss of feeling or function of muscles

- Speech impairment

Exams and Tests

Signs may include:

- extreme dehydration;

- high temperature—higher than 38 degrees Centigrade (100.4 degrees Fahrenheit);

- increased heart rate;

- low systolic blood pressure.

Test results include:

- high serum osmolarity (concentration);

- higher than normal blood urea nitrogen (BUN) and creatinine;

- higher than normal serum sodium;

- mild ketone buildup (ketosis);

- very high blood glucose.

Evaluation for possible causes may include:

- blood cultures;

- chest x-ray;

- electrocardiogram (ECG);

- urinalysis.

Treatment

The goal of treatment is to correct the dehydration. This will improve the blood pressure, urine output, and circulation.

Fluids and potassium will be given through a vein (intravenously). High glucose levels are treated with intravenous insulin.

Outlook (Prognosis)

Patients who develop this syndrome are often already ill. The death rate with this condition is as high as 40 percent.

Possible Complications

- Acute circulatory collapse (shock)
- Blood clot formation
- Brain swelling (cerebral edema)
- Increased blood acid levels (lactic acidosis)

When to Contact a Medical Professional

This condition is a medical emergency. Go to the emergency room or call the local emergency number (such as 911) if you develop symptoms of diabetic hyperglycemic hyperosmolar syndrome.

Prevention

Controlling type 2 diabetes and recognizing the early signs of dehydration and infection can help prevent this condition.

Alternative Names

Hyperglycemic hyperosmolar coma; nonketotic hyperglycemic hyperosmolar coma (NKHHC); hyperosmolar nonketotic coma (HONK)

References

Kitabchi AE, Umpierrez GE, Murphy MB, Kreisberg RA. Hyperglycemic crises in adult patients with diabetes: a consensus statement from the American Diabetes Association. *Diabetes Care*. 2006;29:2739–48.

Cydulka RK, Maloney Jr. GE. Diabetes mellitus and disorders of glucose homeostasis. In: Marx J, Hockberger R, Walls R, eds. *Rosen's Emergency Medicine*. *7th ed*. Philadelphia, Pa: Saunders Elsevier; 2009.

Chapter 49

Hypoglycemia

What Is Hypoglycemia?

Hypoglycemia, also called low blood glucose or low blood sugar, occurs when blood glucose drops below normal levels. Glucose, an important source of energy for the body, comes from food. Carbohydrates are the main dietary source of glucose. Rice, potatoes, bread, tortillas, cereal, milk, fruit, and sweets are all carbohydrate-rich foods.

After a meal, glucose is absorbed into the bloodstream and carried to the body's cells. Insulin, a hormone made by the pancreas, helps the cells use glucose for energy. If a person takes in more glucose than the body needs at the time, the body stores the extra glucose in the liver and muscles in a form called glycogen. The body can use glycogen for energy between meals. Extra glucose can also be changed to fat and stored in fat cells. Fat can also be used for energy.

When blood glucose begins to fall, glucagon—another hormone made by the pancreas—signals the liver to break down glycogen and release glucose into the bloodstream. Blood glucose will then rise toward a normal level. In some people with diabetes, this glucagon response to hypoglycemia is impaired and other hormones such as epinephrine, also called adrenaline, may raise the blood glucose level. But with diabetes treated with insulin or pills that increase insulin production, glucose levels can't easily return to the normal range.

Excerpted from "Hypoglycemia," National Institute of Diabetes and Digestive and Kidney Diseases, National Institutes of Health, NIH Publication No.: 09-3926, October 2008.

Hypoglycemia can happen suddenly. It is usually mild and can be treated quickly and easily by eating or drinking a small amount of glucose-rich food. If left untreated, hypoglycemia can get worse and cause confusion, clumsiness, or fainting. Severe hypoglycemia can lead to seizures, coma, and even death.

In adults and children older than ten years, hypoglycemia is uncommon except as a side effect of diabetes treatment. Hypoglycemia can also result, however, from other medications or diseases, hormone or enzyme deficiencies, or tumors.

What Are the Symptoms of Hypoglycemia?

Hypoglycemia causes symptoms such as the following:

- Hunger
- Shakiness
- Nervousness
- Sweating
- Dizziness or light-headedness
- Sleepiness
- Confusion
- Difficulty speaking
- Anxiety
- Weakness

Hypoglycemia can also happen during sleep. Some signs of hypoglycemia during sleep include the following:

- Crying out or having nightmares
- Finding pajamas or sheets damp from perspiration
- Feeling tired, irritable, or confused after waking up

What Causes Hypoglycemia in People with Diabetes?

Diabetes Medications

Hypoglycemia can occur as a side effect of some diabetes medications, including insulin and oral diabetes medications—pills—that increase insulin production, such as the following:

- Chlorpropamide (Diabinese®)
- Glimepiride (Amaryl®)
- Glipizide (Glucotrol®, Glucotrol XL®)
- Glyburide (DiaBeta®, Glynase®, Micronase®)
- Nateglinide (Starlix®)
- Repaglinide (Prandin®)
- Sitagliptin (Januvia®)
- Tolazamide
- Tolbutamide

Certain combination pills can also cause hypoglycemia, including the following:

- Glipizide + metformin (Metaglip®)
- Glyburide + metformin (Glucovance®)
- Pioglitazone + glimepiride (Duetact®)
- Rosiglitazone + glimepiride (Avandaryl®)
- Sitagliptin + metformin (Janumet®)

Other types of diabetes pills, when taken alone, do not cause hypoglycemia. Examples of these medications are as follows:

- Acarbose (Precose®)
- Metformin (Glucophage®)
- Miglitol (Glyset®)
- Pioglitazone (Actos®)
- Rosiglitazone (Avandia®)

However, taking these pills along with other diabetes medications—insulin, pills that increase insulin production, or both—increases the risk of hypoglycemia.

In addition, use of the following injectable medications can cause hypoglycemia:

- Pramlintide (Symlin®), which is used along with insulin
- Exenatide (Byetta®), which can cause hypoglycemia when used in combination with chlorpropamide, glimepiride, glipizide, glyburide, tolazamide, and tolbutamide

Other Causes of Hypoglycemia

In people on insulin or pills that increase insulin production, low blood glucose can be due to the following causes:

- Meals or snacks that are too small, delayed, or skipped

- Increased physical activity

- alcoholic beverages

How Can Hypoglycemia Be Prevented?

Diabetes treatment plans are designed to match the dose and timing of medication to a person's usual schedule of meals and activities. Mismatches could result in hypoglycemia. For example, taking a dose of insulin—or other medication that increases insulin levels—but then skipping a meal could result in hypoglycemia.

To help prevent hypoglycemia, people with diabetes should always consider the following:

- **Their diabetes medications:** A healthcare provider can explain which diabetes medications can cause hypoglycemia and explain how and when to take medications. For good diabetes management, people with diabetes should take diabetes medications in the recommended doses at the recommended times. In some cases, healthcare providers may suggest that patients learn how to adjust medications to match changes in their schedule or routine.

- **Their meal plan:** A registered dietitian can help design a meal plan that fits one's personal preferences and lifestyle. Following one's meal plan is important for managing diabetes. People with diabetes should eat regular meals, have enough food at each meal, and try not to skip meals or snacks. Snacks are particularly important for some people before going to sleep or exercising. Some snacks may be more effective than others in preventing hypoglycemia overnight. The dietitian can make recommendations for snacks.

- **Their daily activity:** To help prevent hypoglycemia caused by physical activity, healthcare providers may advise the following:

  - Checking blood glucose before sports, exercise, or other physical activity and having a snack if the level is below 100 milligrams per deciliter (mg/dL)

- Adjusting medication before physical activity

- Checking blood glucose at regular intervals during extended periods of physical activity and having snacks as needed

- Checking blood glucose periodically after physical activity

- **Their use of alcoholic beverages:** Drinking alcoholic beverages, especially on an empty stomach, can cause hypoglycemia, even a day or two later. Heavy drinking can be particularly dangerous for people taking insulin or medications that increase insulin production. Alcoholic beverages should always be consumed with a snack or meal at the same time. A healthcare provider can suggest how to safely include alcohol in a meal plan.

- **Their diabetes management plan:** Intensive diabetes management—keeping blood glucose as close to the normal range as possible to prevent long-term complications—can increase the risk of hypoglycemia. Those whose goal is tight control should talk with a healthcare provider about ways to prevent hypoglycemia and how best to treat it if it occurs.

How Is Hypoglycemia Treated?

Signs and symptoms of hypoglycemia vary from person to person. People with diabetes should get to know their signs and symptoms and describe them to their friends and family so they can help if needed. School staff should be told how to recognize a child's signs and symptoms of hypoglycemia and how to treat it.

People who experience hypoglycemia several times in a week should call their healthcare provider. They may need a change in their treatment plan: less medication or a different medication, a new schedule for insulin or medication, a different meal plan, or a new physical activity plan.

Prompt Treatment for Hypoglycemia

When people think their blood glucose is too low, they should check the blood glucose level of a blood sample using a meter. If the level is below 70 mg/dL, one of these quick-fix foods should be consumed right away to raise blood glucose:

- Three or four glucose tablets

- One serving of glucose gel—the amount equal to fifteen grams of carbohydrate

- One-half cup, or four ounces, of any fruit juice

- One-half cup, or four ounces, of a regular—not diet—soft drink

- One cup, or eight ounces, of milk

- Five or six pieces of hard candy

- One tablespoon of sugar or honey

Recommended amounts may be less for small children. The child's doctor can advise about the right amount to give a child.

The next step is to recheck blood glucose in fifteen minutes to make sure it is 70 mg/dL or above. If it's still too low, another serving of a quick-fix food should be eaten. These steps should be repeated until the blood glucose level is 70 mg/dL or above. If the next meal is an hour or more away, a snack should be eaten once the quick-fix foods have raised the blood glucose level to 70 mg/dL or above.

For People Who Take Acarbose (Precose®) or Miglitol (Glyset®)

People who take either of these diabetes medications should know that only pure glucose, also called dextrose—available in tablet or gel form—will raise their blood glucose level during a low blood glucose episode. Other quick-fix foods and drinks won't raise the level quickly enough because acarbose and miglitol slow the digestion of other forms of carbohydrate.

Help from Others for Severe Hypoglycemia

Severe hypoglycemia—very low blood glucose—can cause a person to pass out and can even be life threatening. Severe hypoglycemia is more likely to occur in people with type 1 diabetes. People should ask a health-care provider what to do about severe hypoglycemia. Another person can help someone who has passed out by giving an injection of glucagon. Glucagon will rapidly bring the blood glucose level back to normal and help the person regain consciousness. A healthcare provider can prescribe a glucagon emergency kit. Family, friends, or co-workers—the people who will be around the person at risk of hypoglycemia—can learn how to give a glucagon injection and when to call 911 or get medical help.

Physical Activity and Blood Glucose Levels

Physical activity has many benefits for people with diabetes, including lowering blood glucose levels. However, physical activity can make levels too low and can cause hypoglycemia up to twenty-four hours afterward. A healthcare provider can advise about checking the blood glucose level before exercise. For those who take insulin or one of the oral medications that increase insulin production, the healthcare provider may suggest having a snack if the glucose level is below 100 mg/dL or adjusting medication doses before physical activity to help avoid hypoglycemia. A snack can prevent hypoglycemia. The healthcare provider may suggest extra blood glucose checks, especially after strenuous exercise.

Hypoglycemia When Driving

Hypoglycemia is particularly dangerous if it happens to someone who is driving. People with hypoglycemia may have trouble concentrating or seeing clearly behind the wheel and may not be able to react quickly to road hazards or to the actions of other drivers. To prevent problems, people at risk for hypoglycemia should check their blood glucose level before driving. During longer trips, they should check their blood glucose level frequently and eat snacks as needed to keep the level at 70 mg/dL or above. If necessary, they should stop for treatment and then make sure their blood glucose level is 70 mg/dL or above before starting to drive again.

Hypoglycemia Unawareness

Some people with diabetes do not have early warning signs of low blood glucose, a condition called hypoglycemia unawareness. This condition occurs most often in people with type 1 diabetes, but it can also occur in people with type 2 diabetes. People with hypoglycemia unawareness may need to check their blood glucose level more often so they know when hypoglycemia is about to occur. They also may need a change in their medications, meal plan, or physical activity routine.

Hypoglycemia unawareness develops when frequent episodes of hypoglycemia lead to changes in how the body reacts to low blood glucose levels. The body stops releasing the hormone epinephrine and other stress hormones when blood glucose drops too low. The loss of the body's ability to release stress hormones after repeated episodes of hypoglycemia is called hypoglycemia-associated autonomic failure, or HAAF.

Epinephrine causes early warning symptoms of hypoglycemia such as shakiness, sweating, anxiety, and hunger. Without the release of epinephrine and the symptoms it causes, a person may not realize that hypoglycemia is occurring and may not take action to treat it. A vicious cycle can occur in which frequent hypoglycemia leads to hypoglycemia unawareness and HAAF, which in turn leads to even more severe and dangerous hypoglycemia. Studies have shown that preventing hypoglycemia for a period as short as several weeks can sometimes break this cycle and restore awareness of symptoms. Healthcare providers may therefore advise people who have had severe hypoglycemia to aim for higher-than-usual blood glucose targets for short-term periods.

Being Prepared for Hypoglycemia

People who use insulin or take an oral diabetes medication that can cause low blood glucose should always be prepared to prevent and treat low blood glucose by doing the following:

- Learning what can trigger low blood glucose levels

- Having their blood glucose meter available to test glucose levels; frequent testing may be critical for those with hypoglycemia unawareness, particularly before driving a car or engaging in any hazardous activity

- Always having several servings of quick-fix foods or drinks handy

- Wearing a medical identification bracelet or necklace

- Planning what to do if they develop severe hypoglycemia

- Telling their family, friends, and co-workers about the symptoms of hypoglycemia and how they can help if needed

For people with diabetes, a blood glucose level below 70 mg/dL is considered hypoglycemia.

Table 49.1. Normal and Target Blood Glucose Ranges

Normal Blood Glucose Levels in People Who Do Not Have Diabetes	
Upon waking—fasting	70 to 99 mg/dL
After meals	70 to 140 mg/dL
Target Blood Glucose Levels in People Who Have Diabetes	
Before meals	70 to 130 mg/dL
One to two hours after the start of a meal	below 180 mg/dL

Source: American Diabetes Association. Standards of Medical Care in Diabetes—2008. *Diabetes Care.* 2008;31:S12–S54.

Hypoglycemia in People Who Do Not Have Diabetes

Two types of hypoglycemia can occur in people who do not have diabetes:

* Reactive hypoglycemia, also called postprandial hypoglycemia, occurs within four hours after meals.

* Fasting hypoglycemia, also called postabsorptive hypoglycemia, is often related to an underlying disease.

Symptoms of both reactive and fasting hypoglycemia are similar to diabetes-related hypoglycemia. Symptoms may include hunger, sweating, shakiness, dizziness, light-headedness, sleepiness, confusion, difficulty speaking, anxiety, and weakness.

To find the cause of a patient's hypoglycemia, the doctor will use laboratory tests to measure blood glucose, insulin, and other chemicals that play a part in the body's use of energy.

Reactive Hypoglycemia

Diagnosis. To diagnose reactive hypoglycemia, the doctor may ask about signs and symptoms; test blood glucose while the patient is having symptoms by taking a blood sample from the arm and sending it to a laboratory for analysis; and check to see whether the symptoms ease after the patient's blood glucose returns to 70 mg/dL or above after eating or drinking

A blood glucose level below 70 mg/dL at the time of symptoms and relief after eating will confirm the diagnosis. The oral glucose tolerance test is no longer used to diagnose reactive hypoglycemia because experts now know the test can actually trigger hypoglycemic symptoms.

Causes and treatment. The causes of most cases of reactive hypoglycemia are still open to debate. Some researchers suggest that certain people may be more sensitive to the body's normal release of the hormone epinephrine, which causes many of the symptoms of hypoglycemia. Others believe deficiencies in glucagon secretion might lead to reactive hypoglycemia.

A few causes of reactive hypoglycemia are certain, but they are uncommon. Gastric—or stomach—surgery can cause reactive hypoglycemia because of the rapid passage of food into the small intestine. Rare enzyme deficiencies diagnosed early in life, such as hereditary fructose intolerance, also may cause reactive hypoglycemia.

To relieve reactive hypoglycemia, some health professionals recommend the following:

- Eating small meals and snacks about every three hours

- Being physically active

- Eating a variety of foods, including meat, poultry, fish, or non-meat sources of protein; starchy foods such as whole-grain bread, rice, and potatoes; fruits; vegetables; and dairy products

- Eating foods high in fiber

- Avoiding or limiting foods high in sugar, especially on an empty stomach

The doctor can refer patients to a registered dietitian for personalized meal planning advice. Although some health professionals recommend a diet high in protein and low in carbohydrates, studies have not proven the effectiveness of this kind of diet to treat reactive hypoglycemia.

Fasting Hypoglycemia

Diagnosis. Fasting hypoglycemia is diagnosed from a blood sample that shows a blood glucose level below 50 mg/dL after an overnight fast, between meals, or after physical activity.

Causes and treatment. Causes of fasting hypoglycemia include certain medications, alcoholic beverages, critical illnesses, hormonal deficiencies, some kinds of tumors, and certain conditions occurring in infancy and childhood.

Medications, including some used to treat diabetes, are the most common cause of hypoglycemia. Other medications that can cause hypoglycemia include the following:

- Salicylates, including aspirin, when taken in large doses

- Sulfa medications, which are used to treat bacterial infections

- Pentamidine, which treats a serious kind of pneumonia

- Quinine, which is used to treat malaria

If using any of these medications causes a person's blood glucose level to fall, the doctor may advise stopping the medication or changing the dose.

Drinking alcoholic beverages, especially binge drinking, can cause hypoglycemia. The body's breakdown of alcohol interferes with the liver's efforts to raise blood glucose. Hypoglycemia caused by excessive drinking can be serious and even fatal.

Some illnesses that affect the liver, heart, or kidneys can cause hypoglycemia. Sepsis, which is an overwhelming infection, and starvation are other causes of hypoglycemia. In these cases, treating the illness or other underlying cause will correct the hypoglycemia.

Hormonal deficiencies may cause hypoglycemia in very young children, but rarely in adults. Shortages of cortisol, growth hormone, glucagon, or epinephrine can lead to fasting hypoglycemia. Laboratory tests for hormone levels will determine a diagnosis and treatment. Hormone replacement therapy may be advised.

Insulinomas are insulin-producing tumors in the pancreas. Insulinomas can cause hypoglycemia by raising insulin levels too high in relation to the blood glucose level. These tumors are rare and do not normally spread to other parts of the body. Laboratory tests can pinpoint the exact cause. Treatment involves both short-term steps to correct the hypoglycemia and medical or surgical measures to remove the tumor.

Children rarely develop hypoglycemia. If they do, causes may include the following:

- Brief intolerance to fasting, often during an illness that disturbs regular eating patterns. Children usually outgrow this tendency by age ten.

- Hyperinsulinism, which is the overproduction of insulin. This condition can result in temporary hypoglycemia in newborns, which is common in infants of mothers with diabetes. Persistent hyperinsulinism in infants or children is a complex disorder that requires prompt evaluation and treatment by a specialist.

- Enzyme deficiencies that affect carbohydrate metabolism. These deficiencies can interfere with the body's ability to process natural sugars, such as fructose and galactose, glycogen, or other metabolites.

- Hormonal deficiencies such as lack of pituitary or adrenal hormones.

Chapter 50

Ketoacidosis

Diabetic ketoacidosis is a complication of diabetes that occurs when the body cannot use sugar (glucose) as a fuel source because the body has no insulin or not enough insulin, and fat is used instead. Byproducts of fat breakdown, called ketones, build up in the body.

Causes

People with type 1 diabetes lack enough insulin, a hormone the body uses to process glucose (blood sugar) for energy. When glucose is not available, body fat is broken down instead.

As fats are broken down, acids called ketones build up in the blood and urine. In high levels, ketones are poisonous. This condition is known as ketoacidosis

Blood glucose levels rise (usually higher than 300 mg/dL) because the liver produces glucose to try to combat the problem. However the cells cannot pull in that glucose without insulin.

Diabetic ketoacidosis may lead to a diagnosis of type 1 diabetes, because it is often the first symptom that causes a person to see a doctor. It can also be the result of increased insulin needs in someone already diagnosed with type 1 diabetes. Infection, trauma, heart attack, or surgery can lead to diabetic ketoacidosis in such cases. Missing doses of insulin can also lead to ketoacidosis in people with diabetes.

People with type 2 diabetes can develop ketoacidosis, but it is rare. It is usually triggered by a severe illness. People of Hispanic and African-American ethnicity seem to be more likely to have ketoacidosis as a complication of type 2 diabetes.

Symptoms

The warning signs that you are becoming very sick might include:

- deep, rapid breathing;
- dry skin and mouth;
- flushed face;
- fruity breath (breath odor);
- nausea and vomiting;
- stomach pain.

Other symptoms that can occur include:

- fatigue;
- frequent urination or thirst for a day or more;
- mental stupor that may progress to coma;
- muscle stiffness or aching;
- shortness of breath;
- abdominal pain;
- breathing difficulty while lying down;
- decreased appetite;
- decreased consciousness;
- headache.

Exams and Tests

Ketone testing may be used in type 1 diabetes to screen for early ketoacidosis. The ketones test is done using a urine sample. Ketone testing is usually done at the following times:

- When the blood sugar is higher than 240 mg/dL

- During an illness such as pneumonia, heart attack, or stroke
- When nausea or vomiting occur
- During pregnancy

Other tests that may be done to diagnose ketoacidosis include:

- arterial blood gas;
- blood glucose test;
- blood pressure measurement;
- amylase blood test;
- potassium blood test.

This disease may also affect the results of the following tests:

- Carbon dioxide ($CO_{2)}$
- Cerebrospinal fluid (CSF) collection
- Potassium urine test
- Magnesium blood test
- Phosphorus blood test
- Sodium blood test
- Sodium urine test
- Urine pH

Treatment

The goal of treatment is to correct the high blood glucose level by giving more insulin. Another goal is to replace fluids lost through excessive urination and vomiting. You may be able to recognize the early warning signs and make appropriate corrections at home before the condition gets worse.

Most of the time, you will need to go to the hospital. The following will be done at the hospital:

- Insulin replacement will be given.
- Fluids and electrolytes will be replaced.

- The cause of the condition (such as infection) will be found and treated.

Outlook (Prognosis)

Acidosis can lead to severe illness or death. Improved therapy for young people with diabetes has decreased the death rate from this condition. However, it remains a significant risk in the elderly, and in people who fall into a coma when treatment has been delayed.

Possible Complications

- Fluid buildup in the brain (cerebral edema)

- Heart attack and death of bowel tissue due to low blood pressure

- Renal failure

When to Contact a Medical Professional

This condition can become a medical emergency. Call your healthcare provider if you notice early symptoms of diabetic ketoacidosis.

Go to the emergency room or call the local emergency number (such as 911) if you experience:

- decreased consciousness;

- difficulty breathing;

- fruity breath;

- mental stupor;

- nausea;

- vomiting.

Prevention

People with diabetes should learn to recognize the early warning signs and symptoms of ketoacidosis. In people with infections or who are on insulin pump therapy, measuring urine ketones can give more information than glucose measurements alone.

Insulin pump users need to check often to see that insulin is still flowing through the tubing, and that there are no blockages, kinks, or disconnections.

Alternative Names

DKA; ketoacidosis

References

Eisenbarth GS, Polonsky KS, Buse JB. Type 1 Diabetes Mellitus. In: Kronenberg HM, Melmed S, Polonsky KS, Larsen PR. Kronenberg: *Williams Textbook of Endocrinology. 11th ed.* Philadelphia, Pa: Saunders Elsevier; 2008: chap 31.

Chapter 51

Osteoporosis and Diabetes

What Is Diabetes?

Diabetes is a disorder of metabolism, a term that describes the way our bodies chemically change the foods we eat into growth and energy. After we digest food, glucose (sugar) enters the bloodstream, where it is used by the cells for energy. For glucose to get into the cells, insulin must be present.

Insulin is a hormone produced by the pancreas, an organ located behind the stomach. It is responsible for moving glucose from the bloodstream into the cells to provide energy needed for daily life. In people with diabetes, the body produces too little or no insulin or it does not respond properly to the insulin that is produced. As a result, glucose builds up in the blood and may overflow into the urine where it is excreted from the body. Therefore, the cells lose their main source of energy.

More than twenty million Americans have diabetes. Of these, approximately 5 to 10 percent have type 1 diabetes and 90 to 95 percent have type 2 diabetes:

- In type 1 diabetes, the body produces little or no insulin. This form of the disease typically appears in children and young adults, but it can develop at any age.

Excerpted from "What People with Diabetes Need to Know about Osteoporosis," National Instituted of Arthritis and Musculoskeletal and Skin Diseases, National Institutes of Health, May 2009.

- In type 2 diabetes, the body produces insulin but not enough, and the body does not respond properly to the insulin that is produced. This form of the disease is more common in people who are older, overweight, and inactive.

What Is Osteoporosis?

Osteoporosis is a condition in which the bones become less dense and more likely to fracture. Fractures from osteoporosis can result in pain and disability. Osteoporosis is a major health threat for an estimated forty-four million Americans, 68 percent of whom are women.

Risk factors for developing osteoporosis include the following:

- Being thin or having a small frame

- Having a family history of the disease

- For women, being postmenopausal, having an early menopause, or not having menstrual periods (amenorrhea)

- Using certain medications, such as glucocorticoids

- Not getting enough calcium

- Not getting enough physical activity

- Smoking

- Drinking too much alcohol

Osteoporosis is a disease that often can be prevented. If undetected, it can progress for many years without symptoms until a fracture occurs.

The Diabetes-Osteoporosis Link

Type 1 diabetes is linked to low bone density, although researchers don't know exactly why. Insulin, which is deficient in type 1 diabetes, may promote bone growth and strength. The onset of type 1 diabetes typically occurs at a young age when bone mass is still increasing. It is possible that people with type 1 diabetes achieve lower peak bone mass, the maximum strength and density that bones reach. People usually reach their peak bone mass by age thirty. Low peak bone mass increases one's risk of developing osteoporosis later in life. Some people with type 1 diabetes also have celiac disease, which is associated with reduced bone mass. It is also possible that cytokines, substances produced by various cells in the body, play a role in the development of both type 1 diabetes and osteoporosis.

Recent research also suggests that women with type 1 diabetes may have an increased fracture risk, since vision problems and nerve damage associated with the disease have been linked to an increased risk of falls and related fractures. Hypoglycemia, or low blood sugar reactions, may also contribute to falls.

Increased body weight can reduce one's risk of developing osteoporosis. Since excessive weight is common in people with type 2 diabetes, affected people were long believed to be protected against osteoporosis. However, although bone density is increased in people with type 2 diabetes, fractures are increased. As with type 1 diabetes, this may be due to increased falls because of vision problems and nerve damage. Moreover, the sedentary lifestyle common in many people with type 2 diabetes also interferes with bone health.

Managing Osteoporosis

Strategies to prevent and treat osteoporosis in people with diabetes are the same as for those without diabetes:

- **Nutrition:** A diet rich in calcium and vitamin D is important for healthy bones. Good sources of calcium include low-fat dairy products; dark green, leafy vegetables; and calcium-fortified foods and beverages. Many low-fat and low-sugar sources of calcium are available. Also, supplements can help you meet the daily requirements of calcium and other important nutrients. Vitamin D plays an important role in calcium absorption and bone health. It is synthesized in the skin through exposure to sunlight. Although many people are able to obtain enough vitamin D naturally, older individuals are often deficient in this vitamin due, in part, to limited time spent outdoors. They may require vitamin D supplements to ensure an adequate daily intake.

- **Exercise:** Like muscle, bone is living tissue that responds to exercise by becoming stronger. The best exercise for your bones is weight-bearing exercise that forces you to work against gravity. Some examples include walking, stair climbing, and dancing. Regular exercise can help prevent bone loss and, by enhancing balance and flexibility, reduce the likelihood of falling and breaking a bone. Exercise is especially important for people with diabetes since exercise helps insulin lower blood glucose levels.

- **Healthy lifestyle:** Smoking is bad for bones as well as for the heart and lungs. Women who smoke tend to go through menopause earlier, triggering earlier bone loss. In addition, smokers may absorb less calcium from their diets. Alcohol can also negatively affect bone health. Heavy drinkers are more prone to bone loss and fracture because of poor nutrition as well as an increased risk of falling. Avoiding smoking and alcohol can also help with managing diabetes.

- **Bone density test:** Specialized tests known as bone mineral density (BMD) tests measure bone density in various parts of the body. These tests can detect osteoporosis before a bone fracture occurs and predict one's chances of fracturing in the future. The most widely recognized bone mineral density test is called a dual-energy x-ray absorptiometry or DXA test. It is painless: a bit like having an x-ray, but with much less exposure to radiation. It can measure bone density at your hip and spine. People with diabetes should talk to their doctors about whether they might be candidates for a bone density test.

- **Medication:** Like diabetes, there is no cure for osteoporosis. However, several medications are approved by the Food and Drug Administration for the prevention and treatment of osteoporosis in postmenopausal women and men. Medications are also approved for use in both women and men with glucocorticoid-induced osteoporosis.

Chapter 52

Polycystic Ovary Syndrome and Diabetes

What is polycystic ovary syndrome (PCOS)?

Polycystic ovary syndrome (PCOS) is a health problem that can affect a woman's:

- menstrual cycle;
- hormones;
- blood vessels;
- ability to have children;
- heart;
- appearance.

With PCOS, women typically have the following:

- High levels of androgens (these are sometimes called male hormones, though females also make them.)
- Missed or irregular periods (monthly bleeding)
- Many small cysts (fluid-filled sacs) in their ovaries

How many women have PCOS?

Between one in ten and one in twenty women of childbearing age has PCOS. As many as five million women in the United States may be affected. It can occur in girls as young as eleven years old.

Reprinted from "Polycystic Ovary Syndrome: Frequently Asked Questions," National Women's Health Information Center, March 17, 2010.

What causes PCOS?

The cause of PCOS is unknown. But most experts think that several factors, including genetics, could play a role. Women with PCOS are more likely to have a mother or sister with PCOS.

A main underlying problem with PCOS is a hormonal imbalance. In women with PCOS, the ovaries make more androgens than normal. Androgens are male hormones that females also make. High levels of these hormones affect the development and release of eggs during ovulation.

Researchers also think insulin may be linked to PCOS. Insulin is a hormone that controls the change of sugar, starches, and other food into energy for the body to use or store. Many women with PCOS have too much insulin in their bodies because they have problems using it. Excess insulin appears to increase production of androgen. High androgen levels can lead to the following:

- Acne

- Excessive hair growth

- Weight gain

- Problems with ovulation

What are the symptoms of PCOS?

The symptoms of PCOS can vary from woman to woman. Some of the symptoms of PCOS include the following:

- Infertility (not able to get pregnant) because of not ovulating. In fact, PCOS is the most common cause of female infertility.

- Infrequent, absent, and/or irregular menstrual periods.

- Hirsutism—increased hair growth on the face, chest, stomach, back, thumbs, or toes.

- Cysts on the ovaries.

- Acne, oily skin, or dandruff.

- Weight gain or obesity, usually with extra weight around the waist.

- Male-pattern baldness or thinning hair.

- Patches of skin on the neck, arms, breasts, or thighs that are thick and dark brown or black.

- Skin tags—excess flaps of skin in the armpits or neck area.

- Pelvic pain.

- Anxiety or depression.

- Sleep apnea—when breathing stops for short periods of time while asleep.

Why do women with PCOS have trouble with their menstrual cycle and fertility?

The ovaries, where a woman's eggs are produced, have tiny fluid-filled sacs called follicles or cysts. As the egg grows, the follicle builds up fluid. When the egg matures, the follicle breaks open, the egg is released, and the egg travels through the fallopian tube to the uterus (womb) for fertilization. This is called ovulation.

In women with PCOS, the ovary doesn't make all of the hormones it needs for an egg to fully mature. The follicles may start to grow and build up fluid but ovulation does not occur. Instead, some follicles may remain as cysts. For these reasons, ovulation does not occur and the hormone progesterone is not made. Without progesterone, a woman's menstrual cycle is irregular or absent. Plus, the ovaries make male hormones, which also prevent ovulation.

Does PCOS change at menopause?

Yes and no. PCOS affects many systems in the body. So, many symptoms may persist even though ovarian function and hormone levels change as a woman nears menopause. For instance, excessive hair growth continues, and male-pattern baldness or thinning hair gets worse after menopause. Also, the risks of complications (health problems) from PCOS, such as heart attack, stroke, and diabetes, increase as a woman gets older.

How do I know if I have PCOS?

There is no single test to diagnose PCOS. Your doctor will take the following steps to find out if you have PCOS or if something else is causing your symptoms.

Medical history. Your doctor will ask about your menstrual periods, weight changes, and other symptoms.

Physical exam. Your doctor will want to measure your blood pressure, body mass index (BMI), and waist size. He or she also will check the areas of increased hair growth. You should try to allow the natural hair to grow for a few days before the visit.

Pelvic exam. Your doctor might want to check to see if your ovaries are enlarged or swollen by the increased number of small cysts.

Blood tests. Your doctor may check the androgen hormone and glucose (sugar) levels in your blood.

Vaginal ultrasound (sonogram). Your doctor may perform a test that uses sound waves to take pictures of the pelvic area. It might be used to examine your ovaries for cysts and check the endometrium (lining of the womb). This lining may become thicker if your periods are not regular.

How is PCOS treated?

Because there is no cure for PCOS, it needs to be managed to prevent problems. Treatment goals are based on your symptoms, whether or not you want to become pregnant, and lowering your chances of getting heart disease and diabetes. Many women will need a combination of treatments to meet these goals. Some treatments for PCOS include the following.

Lifestyle modification. Many women with PCOS are overweight or obese, which can cause health problems. You can help manage your PCOS by eating healthy and exercising to keep your weight at a healthy level. Healthy eating tips include the following:

- Limiting processed foods and foods with added sugars

- Adding more whole-grain products, fruits, vegetables, and lean meats to your diet

This helps to lower blood glucose (sugar) levels, improve the body's use of insulin, and normalize hormone levels in your body. Even a 10 percent loss in body weight can restore a normal period and make your cycle more regular.

Birth control pills. For women who don't want to get pregnant, birth control pills can do the following:

- Control menstrual cycles

- Reduce male hormone levels

- Help to clear acne

Keep in mind that the menstrual cycle will become abnormal again if the pill is stopped. Women may also think about taking a pill that only has progesterone, like Provera®, to control the menstrual cycle and reduce the risk of endometrial cancer. But, progesterone alone does not help reduce acne and hair growth.

Diabetes medications. The medicine metformin (Glucophage®) is used to treat type 2 diabetes. It has also been found to help with PCOS symptoms, though it isn't approved by the U.S Food and Drug Administration (FDA) for this use. Metformin affects the way insulin controls blood glucose (sugar) and lowers testosterone production. It slows the growth of abnormal hair and, after a few months of use, may help ovulation to return. Recent research has shown metformin to have other positive effects, such as decreased body mass and improved cholesterol levels. Metformin will not cause a person to become diabetic.

Fertility medications. Lack of ovulation is usually the reason for fertility problems in women with PCOS. Several medications that stimulate ovulation can help women with PCOS become pregnant. Even so, other reasons for infertility in both the woman and man should be ruled out before fertility medications are used. Also, some fertility medications increase the risk for multiple births (twins, triplets). Treatment options include the following:

- Clomiphene (Clomid®, Serophene®)—the first choice therapy to stimulate ovulation for most patients.

- Metformin taken with clomiphene—may be tried if clomiphene alone fails. The combination may help women with PCOS ovulate on lower doses of medication.

- Gonadotropins—given as shots, but are more expensive and raise the risk of multiple births compared to clomiphene.

Another option is in vitro fertilization (IVF). IVF offers the best chance of becoming pregnant in any given cycle. It also gives doctors better control over the chance of multiple births. But, IVF is very costly.

Surgery. "Ovarian drilling" is a surgery that may increase the chance of ovulation. It's sometimes used when a woman does not respond to fertility medicines. The doctor makes a very small cut above or below the navel (belly button) and inserts a small tool that acts like a telescope into the abdomen (stomach). This is called laparoscopy. The doctor then punctures the ovary with a small needle carrying an electric current to destroy a small portion of the ovary.

This procedure carries a risk of developing scar tissue on the ovary. This surgery can lower male hormone levels and help with ovulation. But, these effects may last only a few months. This treatment doesn't help with loss of scalp hair or increased hair growth on other parts of the body.

Medicine for increased hair growth or extra male hormones. Medicines called anti-androgens may reduce hair growth and clear acne. Spironolactone (Aldactone®), first used to treat high blood pressure, has been shown to reduce the impact of male hormones on hair growth in women. Finasteride (Propecia®), a medicine taken by men for hair loss, has the same effect. Anti-androgens are often combined with birth control pills. These medications should not be taken if you are trying to become pregnant.

Before taking Aldactone, tell your doctor if you are pregnant or plan to become pregnant. Do not breastfeed while taking this medicine. Women who may become pregnant should not handle Propecia.

Other options include the following:

- Vaniqa® cream to reduce facial hair

- Laser hair removal or electrolysis to remove hair

- Hormonal treatment to keep new hair from growing

Other treatments. Some research has shown that bariatric (weight loss) surgery may be effective in resolving PCOS in morbidly obese women. Morbid obesity means having a BMI of more than 40, or a BMI of 35 to 40 with an obesity-related disease. The drug troglitazone was shown to help women with PCOS. But, it was taken off the market because it caused liver problems. Similar drugs without the same side effect are being tested in small trials.

Researchers continue to search for new ways to treat PCOS. Talk to your doctor about whether taking part in a clinical trial might be right for you.

How does PCOS affect a woman while pregnant?

Women with PCOS appear to have higher rates of the following:

- Miscarriage

- Gestational diabetes

- Pregnancy-induced high blood pressure (preeclampsia)

- Premature delivery

Babies born to women with PCOS have a higher risk of spending time in a neonatal intensive care unit or of dying before, during, or shortly after birth. Most of the time, these problems occur in multiple-birth babies (twins, triplets).

Researchers are studying whether the diabetes medicine metformin can prevent or reduce the chances of having problems while pregnant. Metformin also lowers male hormone levels and limits weight gain in women who are obese when they get pregnant.

Metformin is an FDA pregnancy category B drug. It does not appear to cause major birth defects or other problems in pregnant women. But, there have only been a few studies of metformin use in pregnant women to confirm its safety. Talk to your doctor about taking metformin if you are pregnant or are trying to become pregnant. Also, metformin is passed through breast milk. Talk with your doctor about metformin use if you are a nursing mother.

Does PCOS put women at risk for other health problems?

Women with PCOS have greater chances of developing several serious health conditions, including life-threatening diseases. Recent studies found that:

- more than 50 percent of women with PCOS will have diabetes or pre-diabetes (impaired glucose tolerance) before the age of forty;

- the risk of heart attack is four to seven times higher in women with PCOS than women of the same age without PCOS;

- women with PCOS are at greater risk of having high blood pressure;

- women with PCOS have high levels of low-density lipoprotein (LDL, or bad) cholesterol and low levels of high-density lipoprotein (HDL, or good) cholesterol;

- women with PCOS can develop sleep apnea—when breathing stops for short periods of time during sleep.

Women with PCOS may also develop anxiety and depression. It is important to talk to your doctor about treatment for these mental health conditions.

Women with PCOS are also at risk for endometrial cancer. Irregular menstrual periods and the lack of ovulation cause women to produce the hormone estrogen, but not the hormone progesterone. Progesterone causes the endometrium (lining of the womb) to shed each month as a menstrual period. Without progesterone, the endometrium becomes thick, which can cause heavy or irregular bleeding. Over time, this can lead to endometrial hyperplasia, when the lining grows too much, and cancer.

I have PCOS. What can I do to prevent complications?

If you have PCOS, get your symptoms under control at an earlier age to help reduce your chances of having complications like diabetes and heart disease. Talk to your doctor about treating all your symptoms, rather than focusing on just one aspect of your PCOS, such as problems getting pregnant. Also, talk to your doctor about getting tested for diabetes regularly. Other steps you can take to lower your chances of health problems include the following:

- Eating right
- Exercising
- Not smoking

How can I cope with the emotional effects of PCOS?

Having PCOS can be difficult. You may feel:

- embarrassed by your appearance;
- worried about being able to get pregnant;
- depressed.

Getting treatment for PCOS can help with these concerns and help boost your self-esteem. You may also want to look for support groups in your area or online to help you deal with the emotional effects of PCOS. You are not alone and there are resources available for women with PCOS.

Part Six

Diabetes in
Specific Populations

Chapter 53

Diabetes in Children

Chapter Contents

Section 53.1

Dealing with Your Child's Diagnosis of Diabetes

Discovering that your young child has type 1 or type 2 diabetes can give rise to many emotions. You may feel angry, sad, upset, guilty, helpless, or anxious, and you may worry whether you will be able to cope with the level of care your child will need every day.

Because your child is so young, you will have the responsibility for looking after his or her diabetes, which can make your job as a parent even more demanding. You are not alone, however. Many services are available to help you and your child learn more about diabetes and what you, and others who care for your child, need to do to manage the disease.

Here are some suggestions to help you and your family adjust to a diagnosis of diabetes in your child:

- Accept your child's diagnosis without guilt. While no one really knows what causes type 1 diabetes, we do know it is not caused by eating too much sugar and there is nothing you could have done to prevent the disease, even if you had taken your child to see the doctor sooner.

- Learn as much as you can about diabetes. The more you learn, the less fear you will have and the more comfortable you will be in caring for your child. Your knowledge and confidence will help your child feel more secure.

- Take your child to see his or her diabetes healthcare professional on a regular basis to discuss your child's growth, development, and diabetes management.

- If you haven't been introduced to the pediatric diabetes team, ask for a referral. You and your child will benefit tremendously from the wisdom and experience of a nurse, dietitian, social worker, and physician with expertise in pediatric diabetes.

- Make family communication a priority. Your child's diagnosis affects everyone in the family, but not everyone will respond in the same way. Talking to each other about these feelings—whether fear, sadness, anger, even jealousy—will help your family come to terms with your new life with diabetes. Don't forget to share your own emotions with someone who understands, such as another parent of a child with diabetes or your healthcare professional.

- Be prepared to answer other people's questions about your child's diabetes. You might want to research some stock answers to common questions such as "What's diabetes?" "How did he get it?" or "Will she grow out of it?" If people try to give you advice, you could answer, "Thank you, I'll think about that," or "I've been told diabetes is very individual." You may sometimes receive conflicting advice from other people. Talk this through with your diabetes health professional to see how it relates specifically to your child.

- Take time for family fun. While diabetes is now part of your life, it is not your—or your child's—entire life.

Section 53.2

Managing Diabetes from Childhood through the Teen Years

Children and Type 1 Diabetes

Parenting is a tough job under the best of circumstances. When your child is diagnosed with type 1 diabetes, you suddenly have to take on a whole new list of responsibilities and concerns. Although family life and daily routines may be more complicated, especially in the beginning, over time and with the help and support of your diabetes team you will discover that your child can have a healthy, full life in which diabetes plays an important but not all-encompassing role.

Parent's Role

As the parent of a child with type 1 diabetes, you will need to test your child's blood glucose level, inject insulin, make sure that she eats regular meals and snacks, and ensure that her medication, food intake, and activities are balanced for optimum diabetes management. If your child is very young, she may not be able to recognize or express how she feels, so you will also need to be alert to the signs of low blood glucose (hypoglycemia).

The idea of testing blood, injecting insulin, and learning about diabetes care may seem frightening to you right now. As you work with your diabetes team (physician, diabetes educator, nurse, dietitian, and/ or pharmacist), you will gain knowledge and confidence. It is important that you become at ease with your child's diabetes care so that you can instill this confidence in your child.

Talking to Your Child about Diabetes

The way you talk to your child about his diabetes will have a tremendous impact on how he perceives the disease, his body, and himself.

452

Avoid judgmental terms when describing food or blood glucose levels, For example, no single food should be described as "bad" or "junk"; rather, talk to your child about how food fits into a healthy lifestyle. Similarly, blood glucose levels are best described as "high, low, or normal" rather than "good or bad." Young children, especially, may attach to themselves the negative terms you use to describe their diabetes. By being positive and supportive, you help boost your child's self-esteem at a time that it may be most threatened.

Talking to Caregivers

You need to make sure that anyone who looks after your child with diabetes has enough information in order to keep her safe. In particular, they need to know your child's eating and drinking requirements; what treatments and blood glucose tests she needs and when; what symptoms suggest high blood glucose (hyperglycemia) and low blood glucose (hypoglycemia) and what to do if your child has low blood glucose levels. You will also need to advise those caring for your child of situations when you must be contacted and how you can be reached at all times. In some situations, parents will need to make sure that caregivers are competent with either testing blood glucose and giving insulin or supervising these routines. Members of your diabetes team can help you make sure that your child's caregivers are adequately educated.

As Your Child Grows

As with any other parenting issue, your role regarding your child's diabetes will change as he matures. Encourage your child to be involved in his diabetes management right from the beginning. Even a very young child can pick which finger is to be tested and read the numbers on the meter. As he grows and becomes more independent, he can learn to test his blood, interpret the results, and perform injections.

The toughest job for many parents is to learn to let go of controlling their child's care and to trust her to take responsibility for her health. This should be a gradual process for both of you. Don't expect your child to assume complete responsibility for testing and injections at a young age. Diabetes care will always be shared to some extent. With your support and guidance, your child will learn to incorporate diabetes care into her daily routine and become the manager of her diabetes.

Children and Type 2 Diabetes

Type 2 diabetes was once a disease that occurred primarily, if not exclusively, in adults. Today, however, the disease is increasingly appearing in adolescents and even in children. Recent research offers these alarming statistics:

- There has been a ten- to thirty-fold increase in American children with type 2 diabetes in the past ten to fifteen years. Most of these children are from ethnic groups at high risk for type 2 diabetes, i.e. African, Hispanic, and Asian descent. Given that 77 percent of new Canadians are from these populations, the rate of type 2 diabetes in Canada is expected to skyrocket in coming years.

- One in every three American children born in 2000 will likely be diagnosed with diabetes in their lifetime; similar rates are anticipated for Canadian children.

- Type 2 diabetes is being diagnosed in children as young as eight years of age, and the incidence appears to be increasing rapidly.

- In the next fifteen years, it is anticipated that the global incidence of type 2 diabetes in children will increase by up to 50 percent.

Who Is at Risk?

The development of type 2 diabetes is closely related to obesity; about 95 percent of children with type 2 diabetes are overweight at diagnosis. Given that the proportion of children who are overweight has tripled in the last thirty years, it is not surprising that incidence of type 2 diabetes among youth is rising.

In addition to obesity, factors that increase a child's risk for developing type 2 diabetes include:

- being a member of a high-risk ethnic group;

- having a family history of the disease (especially being born to a mother whose pregnancy was complicated by diabetes);

- having dark, velvety patches in skin folds (a skin condition known as acanthosis nigricans);

- having high levels of fat in the blood (dyslipidemia);

- having high blood pressure (hypertension); and

- having polycystic ovarian syndrome (a disorder in females that is marked by lack of menstrual periods, unusual hair growth, and excess weight).

About half of all children with type 2 diabetes do not have any symptoms and are diagnosed only when screened for other disorders related to obesity. The Canadian Diabetes Association recommends screening for type 2 diabetes in obese children ten years of age and older (or when puberty starts, if earlier than age ten) who have at least two of the risk factors noted above.

Prevention

A healthy lifestyle can significantly reduce the risk of developing type 2 diabetes. In fact, studies in adults suggest that moderate weight loss and regular physical activity can reduce the risk of type 2 diabetes by more than 50 percent.

Try these simple lifestyle changes that can make a big difference in the health of your family:

- Switch from regular pop to sugar-free pop or water.

- Switch to lower-fat dairy products, such as 1 percent or skim milk.

- Offer children healthy snack choices, such as fresh fruits and cut-up veggies.

- Model healthy eating and activity habits for your children.

- Leave the car at home; walk or bike whenever possible.

- Gradually reduce screen time (television computers, etc.) and replace it with active play time. Try a family walk after dinner.

Teens and Diabetes

When children are diagnosed with diabetes, parents need to be very involved in learning about the condition, participating in the routines at an appropriate level, and sharing management decisions. While it is critical that older school-age children and teens learn the details of the condition and how to care for themselves, parents must understand diabetes and its management. This parental competence promotes a safe, supportive home environment for the newly diagnosed teen and reduces stress in both parents and the child.

Learning to Let Go

As a child matures, the challenge for many families is finding the balance between parental monitoring and teen independence. On the one hand, careful diabetes management is vitally important to the immediate and long-term health of your child. On the other hand, you can't be with your child 24/7. Even if you could take total control of your child's diabetes (which you can't), teens are more likely to rebel against tight restrictions. Rather, you may want to strive for a supporting rather than controlling role in your teen's diabetes care. Here are some suggestions:

- Recognize how devastating diabetes can be to a teen. She wants to be carefree and independent, just like her friends. Instead, she feels burdened with a lifelong condition and restricted by tests and injections. Help her figure out ways to fit diabetes into her schedule; share the load where you can (e.g., help her record her blood glucose results or offer to give one of her injections each day). Look for support from your diabetes team, including the social worker. Find out if your teen is interested in joining a peer support group and where this might be available.

- Be positive and nonjudgmental about your teen's diabetes management. Avoid using terms such as "good" or "bad" when referring to blood glucose levels. Instead, focus on helping him evaluate his blood glucose levels and determining a course of action. For example, ask, "Your blood glucose is higher than your target, so what do you need to do?"

- Understand, and help your teen understand, that adolescents with diabetes require more insulin as they grow and go through puberty. This is normal. It is not a sign of worsening diabetes.

- Encourage your teen to participate in sports and other activities, which are great for building self-esteem. Help her to figure out how to prevent low blood glucose (hypoglycemia), which often accompanies increased activity, by testing frequently and either reducing insulin or increasing food intake.

- Ensure that your teen understands the potentially devastating consequences that smoking, alcohol, and drugs can have for people with diabetes. If you are not comfortable talking with your teen about these issues, be sure to ask your diabetes professional to raise the subject with him.

- Avoid focusing on weight and body shape in your teen. Rather, focus on promoting a healthy lifestyle for all members of the family. Some teens discover that when they are getting inadequate amounts of insulin they lose weight. Although the discovery may be accidental, some teens (particularly girls) are tempted to reduce or skip their insulin repeatedly in order to lose weight. This risky behavior leads to poor glucose management, a risk of diabetes ketoacidosis (a life-threatening condition that arises from a serious insulin shortage), and a high risk for long-term complications. Parents who suspect this behavior in their teen should take steps to supervise each insulin injection while they seek the advice from their diabetes team.

- Be flexible and willing to help or step back as your teen needs. Watch for signs that your teen is struggling with his diabetes management: signs of high blood glucose levels (frequent urination, extreme thirst), low blood glucose episodes (hypoglycemia), poor school attendance, depression, or a significant change in behavior. If your child shows any of these signs, re-involve yourself in your teen's diabetes and talk to his diabetes professional for further advice.

- Keep the lines of communication open. Instead of nagging or criticizing, use open-ended questions that encourage conversation. For example, ask: "How do you feel you are coping with your diabetes?" "What are you finding most difficult about it?" or "What would help you now?"

- With patience and a positive attitude, you can help your teen become a responsible, independent, and healthy young adult.

Section 53.3

School and Diabetes: Advice for Teens

You probably spend about six hours or more at school each day— more than one-third of your waking hours. If you have diabetes, chances are you'll need to check your blood sugar levels or give yourself an insulin injection during that time. So how do you deal with diabetes at school?

Talking to Teachers and School Staff about Diabetes

Maybe you just found out you have diabetes. Perhaps you've been living with it for a while but switched to a new school. Your first step is to let school staff know.

Set up a meeting with your school principal's office. Your mom or dad should be there, and you may want to suggest the school nurse join you.

Give your school nurse, teacher, and principal's office a copy of your diabetes management plan. This plan talks about what you will need to do during the school day, like test your blood sugar, give yourself injections, or eat lunch at a certain time each day. Your diabetes management plan also contains contact info for your doctors and diabetes healthcare team, so the school will know how to get in touch if you're sick.

Some schools might work with you to create a special plan for managing your diabetes at school. This may mean letting you eat lunch a little early or having a school nurse help with insulin injections if you need it.

Tell your teachers. When your teachers know what needs to be done, they can schedule time for you to do stuff like test your blood glucose levels or get shots. Some teachers don't allow you to eat in class, which is why it's good to let your teacher know what's going on.

Ask to meet your teacher before or after class to talk about what you might need to do. If teachers know you have diabetes, they can watch for symptoms of diabetes problems and can call for medical help if you need it.

Teachers are busy. You might need to remind them once in a while about what you have to do to take care of your diabetes. If you have a substitute teacher, let him or her know that you have diabetes and may need to do things like go to the bathroom or get a snack.

If you feel uncomfortable talking to teachers or school staff about your diabetes, write a note or letter that goes over what you'll need to do to take care of your diabetes.

Get to know your school nurse. At many schools, students with diabetes need to get their diabetes medicines or test blood sugar levels in the nurse's office. Most schools won't let students carry needles or medications with them. Don't let that worry you, though. Even in an emergency, the extra time needed to get to the school nurse won't cause a problem.

Taking Care of Diabetes at School

Keep a stock of medications, testing equipment, and other supplies at school. You'll need the same supplies and equipment that you use at home. You'll probably need to keep these in the school nurse's office, but your school may want you to store them somewhere else. Ask the principal's office what your school's policy is.

Keep a copy of your diabetes management plan with you. Even if your school has your plan, it's good to keep one in your purse, backpack, locker, or car as well. If you run into any diabetes problems at school or start having symptoms of hypoglycemia or hyperglycemia, do what your plan tells you to do. That may mean having a snack, checking your blood glucose levels, or heading to the nurse's office — whatever your plan says.

Prepare to handle different situations. What if the school nurse isn't in? Is there someone else who can help? Who do you call if something unexpected happens—your doctor or your parent? Which kinds of problems can wait until after school and which ones should you handle right away?

Ask your doctor what you need to know about managing diabetes in school and how to handle special situations. Write down what you should do and who you should go to and keep this information with your management plan. Knowing what to do can help you feel more confident if you do have a problem at school.

Talking to Friends and Classmates about Diabetes

It's your call whether you tell friends and classmates about your diabetes. If they know, it can mean less worry for you about what they think when they see you doing things like leaving class to go to the nurse's office for a blood sugar level check.

But what about teasing? Some kids will tease anyone who seems the slightest bit different from anyone else. If this happens to you, you're definitely not alone: About one in three kids and teens with problems like diabetes have had to deal with bullying.

What can you do when people tease you? Get your friends' help to remind people that diabetes is no big deal. Ignoring a bully is a good strategy too. Bullies thrive on the reaction they get, and if you walk away, you're telling the bully that you just don't care. Sooner or later the bully will probably get bored with trying to bother you.

It may also help to talk to a guidance counselor, teacher, or friend—anyone who can give you the support you need. Talking can be a good outlet for the fears and frustrations that can build when you're being bullied.

Whatever happens, though, don't try to hide your condition by skipping treatments or eating foods that aren't on your meal plan—it'll just make you feel worse and risk getting sick at school.

Section 53.4

Celebrating Special Occasions

Having diabetes shouldn't prevent a child from having fun during special occasions. A little planning and a question or two allows kids with diabetes to participate in just about everything.

On special occasions, such as sporting events, pizza days at school, or birthday parties, contact the organizer to find out what food will be served and when, and what physical activities are planned. How the food "fits in" depends on when it's being served. Meals or snacks can be split as needed to allow your child to eat with the other children. Your diabetes educator can give you some good ideas about how to handle this.

For holidays and celebrations, it's important to keep as many traditions as possible, but you may need to modify those that involve food. Consider creating new traditions that put the focus on fun and activity, not food.

Halloween

Emphasize the non-food-related aspects of Halloween, such as costume preparation and decoration.

After trick-or-treating, sort through your child's sack of loot, allowing her to set aside the candies she loves best. Ration these out to ensure she enjoys them at the right times—after supper for dessert, for instance, or after her lunch at school.

Remember that there aren't good or bad choices when it comes to candy. A gram of carbohydrate, whether it comes from a chocolate bar or a lollipop, affects blood glucose levels in the same way. However, a Halloween-size candy, which contains between eight and fifteen grams of carbohydrates, is a better choice than a big bag of chips, which is chock full of fat and calories.

Leftover treats can be traded with brothers or sisters, given to less fortunate kids, or "sold" to parents in exchange for non-food-related treats, such as a new toy or book.

Consider tucking one or two of your child's least-favorite candies in his schoolbag to treat hypoglycemia (low blood glucose levels). Don't give a child a candy he really likes for this, since he may find it hard to resist and won't save it for a low.

Christmas

Moderation and balance are the keys to a healthy holiday. Be sure to include fun physical activities, such as skating, tobogganing, or a winter walk.

Spread treats, such as gingerbread and candy canes, over the holiday season rather than offering them all at once.

Make sure nutritious snacks are always available.

Have Santa stuff stockings with non-food items, such as hair clips, stickers, coloring books, movie tickets, etc.

Activity

Encourage your child to get involved in physical activities. Taking part in activities can help a child to make friends, feel good, and achieve and maintain a healthy body weight.

Activity can have an impact on a child's blood glucose levels, especially if she is taking insulin, so she will need to have her blood glucose tested before, during, and after activities. She may need to adjust her insulin dose or eat an extra snack to prevent low blood glucose. Talk to your healthcare provider for guidance.

If your child takes insulin, exercise—especially activity that lasts more than thirty minutes—can cause blood glucose to drop too low (below 4mmol/L). Make sure your child always has a fast-acting carbohydrate, such as six LifeSavers® or a juice box, on hand.

Be aware that blood glucose levels can drop long after the activity is finished. Check your child's blood glucose levels to see if he needs an extra bedtime snack if he has been very active during the day.

Whatever the occasion, kids with diabetes should be encouraged to be involved. By determining the details in advance, you and your child will be prepared to participate and have fun.

Section 53.5

Surviving Children's Sick Days

"Managing Your Child's Diabetes on Sick Days," August 2010, reprinted with permission from www.kidshealth.org. Copyright © 2010 The Nemours Foundation. This information was provided by KidsHealth, one of the largest resources online for medically reviewed health information written for parents, kids, and teens. For more articles like this one, visit www.KidsHealth.org, or www.TeensHealth.org.

How Illness Affects Blood Sugar Levels

Kids with diabetes get sick once in a while, just like other kids. However, because the effects of illness on the body can raise or lower blood sugar levels in people with diabetes, a few extra precautions are needed to keep blood sugar levels under control.

With proper planning and some advice from your doctor, you'll be prepared to handle sick days with confidence.

When your child gets sick—whether it's a minor illness like a sore throat or cold or a bigger problem like dehydration or surgery—the body perceives the illness as stress. To relieve the stress, the body fights the illness. This process requires more energy than the body normally uses.

On one hand, this is good because it helps supply the extra fuel the body needs. On the other hand, in a person with diabetes, this can lead to high blood sugar levels. While stress tends to make blood sugar rise in people with diabetes, some illnesses cause loss of appetite, nausea, or vomiting. The poor intake of food in such cases can result in low blood sugar levels in someone taking the usual doses of insulin.

In a nutshell: Blood sugar levels can be very unpredictable on sick days. Because you can't be sure exactly how the illness will affect your child's diabetes control, it's important to check your child's blood sugar levels often on sick days and adjust insulin doses as needed.

Advance Preparation

Your child's diabetes healthcare team will include sick-day instructions in the diabetes management plan, which might include:

- how to monitor both blood sugar levels and ketones when your child is sick;

- which over-the-counter and prescription medicines are ok to give your child;

- what adjustments you should make to your child's food and drink and medications;

- when to call the doctor or another member of the diabetes healthcare team.

In addition, kids with diabetes should get the pneumococcal conjugate vaccine (PCV), which protects against some serious infections, including certain types of pneumonia, blood infections, and bacterial meningitis. Kids with diabetes should also get a flu shot every year. These vaccines may help cut down on sick days.

When Your Child Is Sick

While your doctor will give you specific advice about what to do when your child is sick, here are some general guidelines:

- **Stay on track:** Unless the doctor tells you to make changes, be sure your child keeps taking the same diabetes medications. It's important for your child to keep taking insulin during illness, even though food intake may be reduced. The liver produces glucose and releases stored glucose into the blood, so even if your child is not eating very much, the body still needs insulin to process the glucose. In fact, some people need more insulin than usual on sick days—and some with type 2 diabetes who don't take insulin might need some. Without insulin, the body starts to burn fat, ketones build up in the blood, and diabetic ketoacidosis can occur.

- **Keep a close eye on blood sugar and ketone levels:** Blood sugar levels should be checked frequently—your doctor will advise you on how often. Urine tests for ketones are often positive during illness (even in kids without diabetes) when a child's intake is poor and the body has shifted to using stored fat for energy. But for kids with diabetes, testing can provide an early warning sign that levels in the blood may be building up enough to cause diabetic ketoacidosis. The diabetes treatment plan should guide you as to when and how often to check ketones.

- **Pay special attention to nausea and vomiting:** Kids with diabetes occasionally catch a bug that causes nausea, vomiting, or abdominal pain. But because these can also be symptoms of diabetic ketoacidosis, it's important to closely monitor blood glucose and ketone levels and seek medical help according to the guidelines in the diabetes treatment plan.

- **Prevent dehydration:** Have your child drink plenty of fluids. Offer beverages that your child likes that won't worsen symptoms like nausea. Your doctor can advise you about what to give to help manage the illness and maintain control of the diabetes.

- **Use medications wisely:** Although doctors' opinions vary as to whether they're really helpful, over-the-counter (OTC) medications are often given to kids to control symptoms of illnesses like a cold or the flu. These may contain ingredients that raise or lower blood sugar or that imitate symptoms of high or low blood sugar levels. Check with your doctor before giving an OTC medication to your child. Guidelines for using common medications are often included in the diabetes management plan, including what to check on the labels. If OTC medications are given at the right dose, they generally won't have a significant effect on diabetes control. But prescription drugs such as glucocorticoids (like those given for a severe asthma flare-up) can significantly raise blood sugar. Make sure you know the possible effects on your child's diabetes of any prescribed drugs. Contact your doctor if you think adjustments to the diabetes treatment plan might be needed.

- **Take notes:** When you talk to your doctor, keep information handy about the illness, your child's symptoms, medications and doses taken, what food and drink was consumed, and whether your child kept it down. Also, note any weight loss or fever and record blood sugar and ketone level test results.

- **Help your child rest:** Kids need rest when they're sick, so encourage sleeping and resting as much as possible. Kids who usually manage diabetes on their own might need help doing so for a day or two.

When to Call the Doctor

Your child's diabetes management plan will include specific guidelines to help you recognize when medical help is required and recommend what actions to take and whom to call.

Generally, though, call your doctor if your child is sick and:

- has a lack of appetite or inability to eat or drink;

- has persistent vomiting or diarrhea;

- has low blood sugar because of poor food intake—but remember to try to bring it back up (such as by injecting glucagon, if necessary) before calling the doctor or rushing to the emergency department;

- has blood sugar levels that are high for several checks or don't decrease with extra insulin;

- has moderate or large amounts of ketones in the urine;

- might be having symptoms of diabetic ketoacidosis;

- his or her food or fluids will be restricted for things like diagnostic tests, surgery, or a dental procedure.

Whenever you have questions or concerns, check in with your doctor. Together, you can make sure that your child feels well again soon.

Section 53.6

Weight and Diabetes in Children

"Obese Children Twice as Likely to Have Diabetes," January 30, 2006. Reprinted with permission of the University of Michigan Health System. © 2006 Regents of the University of Michigan. All rights reserved. This article refers to the following study: "An Epidemiologic Profile of Children With Diabetes in the U.S.," by Joyce Lee, MD, MPH, et al. *Diabetes Care*, February 2006, pp. 420–21. Reviewed by David A. Cooke, M.D., FACP, February 2011.

Childhood obesity can carry with it some heavy health risks that often last well into adulthood—heart disease, high blood pressure, and depression, to name a few.

Obese children also are twice as likely to have diabetes than children who are of normal weight, according to a new study from the University of Michigan Health System.

The study, published in the February 2006 issue of *Diabetes Care*, is the most recent national study to estimate the prevalence of children with diabetes. It found that more than 229,000 children—approximately 3.2 cases for every 1,000 American children under the age of eighteen— currently have diabetes. And one-third of those children are obese.

The study, was conducted by researchers with the Child Health Evaluation Research (CHEAR) Unit in the Division of General Pediatrics at the U-M C.S. Mott Children's Hospital. It is based on data from the National Survey of Children's Health (NSCH), a population-based household telephone survey sponsored by the Maternal and Child Health Bureau, the National Center for Health Statistics, and the Centers for Disease Control and Prevention.

As children's waistlines have continued to grow so has concern that obesity will lead to even more children developing diabetes before they've graduated from high school. And caring for the combination of these children's diabetes and obesity may place more strain on the healthcare system, says study lead author Joyce Lee, M.D., with the Division of Pediatric Endocrinology and CHEAR Unit at U-M.

"Among school-aged children, obese children have a greater than twofold chance of having diabetes, compared with children of normal weight," says Lee.

"The large number of children with diabetes in the U.S., and the potential for increasing numbers of children developing diabetes with the obesity epidemic, has serious implications for how these children will receive appropriate healthcare now and as they grow into adulthood."

For their study, Lee and her colleagues used a subset of information gathered from NSCH interviews with the parents and guardians of 102,353 children from January 2003 through July 2004.

As part of the interviews, the parents and guardians were asked if their child's healthcare professional had ever told them that their child has diabetes.

The children were grouped into three categories based on their body mass index, or BMI: not overweight, overweight, and obese. BMI was calculated using the height and weight of the child reported by his parent or guardian.

Children with a BMI above the eighty-fifth percentile for their age and sex are classified as overweight, while those with a BMI above the ninety-fifth percentile are considered obese. For example, a ten-year-old boy of average height would be defined as obese if he weighed approximately 101 pounds or greater, says Lee.

These data provided researchers with evidence of an association between childhood obesity and diabetes. The study found that children ages six to eleven and ages twelve to seventeen who were obese were more than twice as likely to have diabetes than children of the same age who were of normal weight.

The study estimates that nationally, 229,240 children have diabetes. Prevalence of diabetes was higher among older children, and the disease was more common among non-Hispanic white children than non-Hispanic black or Hispanic children.

While one form of diabetes, type 2, is usually associated with obesity, data used for this study did not distinguish between the two types.

Still, results point to a greater need for public health strategies to curb childhood obesity and reduce the number of children with diabetes, says Lee.

"These data create cause for concern, especially with a nationwide shortage of specialists who care for children with diabetes," notes Lee. "From a clinical, public health and health resources perspective, we need to address childhood obesity head-on to help reduce the future burden of diabetes in the U.S."

In addition to Lee, Melissa L. McPheeters, Ph.D., MPH; and James G. Gurney, Ph.D., with the CHEAR team in the U-M Division of General Pediatrics; and William H. Herman, M.D., MPH, with the

Department of Internal Medicine at the U-M Medical School and the Department of Epidemiology at the U-M School of Public Health, co-authored the study.

The study was funded by a National Institutes of Health Pediatric Health Services Research Grant.

Chapter 54

Diabetes and Pregnancy

Introduction

You have type 1 or type 2 diabetes and you are pregnant or hoping to get pregnant soon. You can learn what to do to have a healthy baby. You can also learn how to take care of yourself and your diabetes before, during, and after your pregnancy.

Pregnancy and new motherhood are times of great excitement, worry, and change for any woman. If you have diabetes and are pregnant, your pregnancy is automatically considered a high-risk pregnancy. Women carrying twins—or more—or who are beyond a certain age are also considered to have high-risk pregnancies. High risk doesn't mean you'll have problems. Instead, high risk means you need to pay special attention to your health and you may need to see specialized doctors. Millions of high-risk pregnancies produce perfectly healthy babies without the mom's health being affected. Special care and attention are the keys.

Taking Care of Your Baby and Yourself

Keeping your blood glucose as close to normal as possible before you get pregnant and during your pregnancy is the most important thing you can do to stay healthy and have a healthy baby. Your healthcare

Reprinted from "For Women with Diabetes: Your Guide to Pregnancy," National Institute of Diabetes and Digestive and Kidney Diseases, National Institutes of Health, NIH Publication No. 08-5491, February 2008.

team can help you learn how to use meal planning, physical activity, and medications to reach your blood glucose goals. Together, you'll create a plan for taking care of yourself and your diabetes.

Pregnancy causes a number of changes in your body, so you might need to make changes in the ways you manage your diabetes. Even if you've had diabetes for years, you may need changes in your meal plan, physical activity routine, and medications. In addition, your needs might change as you get closer to your delivery date.

How Diabetes Can Affect You and Your Baby

High blood glucose levels before and during pregnancy can do the following things:

- Worsen your long-term diabetes complications, such as vision problems, heart disease, and kidney disease

- Increase the chance of problems for your baby, such as being born too early, weighing too much or too little, and having low blood glucose or other health problems at birth

- Increase the risk of your baby having birth defects

- increase the risk of losing your baby through miscarriage or stillbirth

However, research has shown that when women with diabetes keep blood glucose levels under control before and during pregnancy, the risk of birth defects is about the same as in babies born to women who don't have diabetes.

Glucose in a pregnant woman's blood passes through to the baby. If your blood glucose level is too high during pregnancy, so is your baby's glucose level before birth.

Your Diabetes, Before and during Your Pregnancy

As you know, in diabetes, blood glucose levels are above normal. Whether you have type 1 or type 2 diabetes, you can manage your blood glucose levels and lower the risk of health problems.

A baby's brain, heart, kidneys, and lungs form during the first eight weeks of pregnancy. High blood glucose levels are especially harmful during this early part of pregnancy. Yet many women don't realize they're pregnant until five or six weeks after conception. Ideally, you will work with your health care provider to get your blood glucose under control before you get pregnant.

If you're already pregnant, see your healthcare provider as soon as possible to make a plan for taking care of yourself and your baby. Even if you learn you're pregnant later in your pregnancy, you can still do a lot for your baby's health and your own.

The checklist below can help you make a plan for a safe and healthy pregnancy. More information on each topic then follows. Your healthcare team can help you with tasks that are difficult for you. Tackle one thing at a time to keep from being overwhelmed.

My Diabetes Care Plan for Pregnancy

Things I can do to get ready for a healthy pregnancy and continue to do during my pregnancy,

Planning ahead:

- I'll get my diabetes under control three to six months before I try to get pregnant.
- If I'm already pregnant, I'll see my healthcare provider right away.

My healthcare team:

- I'll make sure I have the right team of healthcare providers.
- I'll meet with members of my team.

My blood glucose levels:

- I'll set goals with my healthcare team for my daily blood glucose levels.
- I'll set a goal with my healthcare team for my A1C test result.
- I'll learn how and when to check my blood glucose on my own.
- I'll learn what to do if my blood glucose is too low.
- I'll make sure my family or friends know how to give me glucagon for low blood glucose.
- I'll learn what to do if my blood glucose is too high.

My ketone levels:

- I'll learn how and when to check my urine or blood for ketones.
- I'll learn what to do if I have ketones in my urine or blood.

My checkups:

- I'll get the recommended checkups and laboratory tests for

- blood pressure;
- eye disease;
- heart and blood vessel disease;
- nervous system disease;
- kidney function;
- thyroid disease;
- average blood glucose level—the A1C test.

Smoking:

- If I smoke, I'll quit.

My meal plan:

- I'll see a dietitian or diabetes educator about what, when, and how much to eat.
- I'll ask whether I need vitamin and mineral supplements and will take them as directed.
- I'll skip alcoholic beverages.

My physical activity routine:

- I'll talk with my healthcare team about what physical activities are safe for me.
- I'll make a plan with my healthcare team for regular physical activity.

My medications:

- I'll talk with my healthcare team about my diabetes medications—what kinds, how much, how to take them, and when to take them.
- I'll talk with my healthcare team about my other medications—what to keep taking and what to stop taking.

Changes in my daily routine:

- I'll make a plan for taking care of myself when I'm ill—what to do about food, insulin, blood glucose testing, and ketone testing.
- I'll make a plan for what I need to have with me when I'm away from home—for several hours or for a longer trip.

Planning Ahead

Before you get pregnant, talk with your healthcare team about your wish to have a baby. Your team can work with you to make sure your blood glucose levels are on target. If you have questions or worries, bring them up. If you're already pregnant, see your doctor right away.

My Healthcare Team

Regular visits with healthcare providers who are experts in diabetes and pregnancy will ensure you get the very best care. Your team may include the following:

- A medical doctor who specializes in diabetes care, such as an endocrinologist or a diabetologist. You will continue to need monitoring and advice on glucose control throughout your pregnancy and after.

- An obstetrician-gynecologist, or "OB/GYN," who has managed pregnancies of women with diabetes. Ask for a referral if your current gynecologist does not also deliver babies, as not all gynecologists do. When calling around to find an OB/GYN, ask about experience with women with diabetes. Maternal-fetal medicine specialists, also called perinatologists, have special training to take care of women with high-risk pregnancies. You will see your OB/GYN regularly throughout your pregnancy.

- A nurse educator or nurse practitioner, who provides prenatal care and advice on managing diabetes.

- A registered dietitian to help with meal planning. A good diet—for glucose control and nutrition—has never been more important than now. The phrase "You're eating for two" is not about quantity as much as food choices.

- Specialists who diagnose and treat diabetes-related complications, such as ophthalmologists and optometrists for vision problems, nephrologists for kidney disease, and cardiologists for heart disease. If you are already experiencing complications from diabetes, you'll need those conditions monitored throughout your pregnancy as well.

- A social worker or psychologist to help you cope with stress, worry, and the extra demands of pregnancy. You may already have this kind of support, or you may suddenly need it. If anxiety mounts, do not hesitate to mention your uneasiness to your OB/

GYN. Ask for a referral if you need more help working through issues.

- A pediatrician—a doctor who cares for children. You might want to ask friends, family, or your healthcare team for recommendations. Many pediatricians visit their newest patients at the hospital soon after their arrival.

- A neonatologist—a doctor who cares for newborn babies. The hospital will assign a neonatologist if urgent care for your baby is needed at the hospital.

You are the most important member of the team. Your healthcare providers can give you expert advice. But you'll be responsible for the day-to-day actions needed to keep your diabetes under control.

My Blood Glucose Levels

Daily blood glucose levels. You'll check your blood glucose levels using a blood glucose meter several times a day. Most healthcare providers recommend testing at least four times a day. Ask your healthcare provider when you should check your blood glucose levels.

I should check my blood glucose levels at the following times:

- Fasting—when I wake up, before I eat or drink anything
- Before each meal
- One hour after the start of a meal
- Two hours after the start of a meal
- Before bedtime
- In the middle of the night—for example, at 2 or 3 a.m.

The daily goals recommended by the American Diabetes Association for most pregnant women are shown in Table 54.1.

Table 54.1. American Diabetes Association Daily Goals for Blood Glucose Levels

When	Plasma Blood Glucose (mg/dL)
Before meals and when you wake up	80 to 110
Two hours after the start of a meal	Below 155

Source: American Diabetes Association. Preconception care of women with diabetes. *Diabetes Care.* 2004;27(Supplement 1):S76–78.

See Table 54.2 for goals recommended by the American College of Obstetricians and Gynecologists.

Table 54.2. American College of Obstetricians and Gynecologists Daily Goals for Blood Glucose Levels

When	Plasma Blood Glucose (mg/dL)
Fasting	105 or less
Before meals	110 or less
One hour after the start of a meal	155 or less
Two hours after the start of a meal	135 or less
During the night	Not less than 65

Source: American College of Obstetricians and Gynecologists (ACOG) Committee on Practice Bulletins. ACOG Practice Bulletin Number 60: Pregestational diabetes mellitus. *Obstetrics and Gynecology.* 2005;105(3):675–85.

The A1C test. Another way to see whether you're meeting your goals is to have an A1C blood test.

Results of the A1C test show your average blood glucose levels during the past two to three months.

Table 54.3. Goals for the A1C Test

Source of Recommendation	Target Number
American Diabetes Association	4 to 6 percent—normal, or less than 1 percent above the upper limits of normal
American College of Obstetricians and Gynecologists	No higher than 6 percent

Low blood glucose. When you're pregnant, you're at increased risk of having low blood glucose, also called hypoglycemia. When blood glucose levels are too low, your body can't get the energy it needs. Usually hypoglycemia is mild and can easily be treated by eating or drinking something with carbohydrate. But left untreated, hypoglycemia can make you pass out.

Although hypoglycemia can happen suddenly, it can usually be treated quickly, bringing your blood glucose level back to normal. Low blood glucose can be caused by the following things:

- Meals or snacks that are too small, delayed, or skipped
- Doses of insulin that are too high
- Increased activity or exercise

Low blood glucose also can be caused by drinking too much alcohol. However, women who are trying to get pregnant or who are already pregnant should avoid all alcoholic beverages.

Using glucagon for severe low blood glucose. If you have severe low blood glucose and pass out, you'll need help to bring your blood glucose level back to normal. Your healthcare team can teach your family members and friends how to give you an injection of glucagon, a hormone that raises blood glucose levels right away.

High blood glucose. High blood glucose, also called hyperglycemia, can happen when you don't have enough insulin or when your body isn't able to use insulin correctly. High blood glucose can result from the following things:

- A mismatch between food and medication
- Eating more food than usual
- Being less active than usual
- Illness
- Stress

In addition, if your blood glucose level is already high, physical activity can make it go even higher. Symptoms of high blood glucose include the following:

- Frequent urination
- Thirst
- Weight loss

Talk with your healthcare provider about what to do when your blood glucose is too high—whether it happens once in a while or at the same time every day for several days in a row. Your provider might suggest a change in your insulin, meal plan, or physical activity routine.

My Ketone Levels

When your blood glucose is too high or if you're not eating enough, your body might make chemicals called ketones. Ketones are produced when your body doesn't have enough insulin and glucose can't be used for energy. Then the body uses fat instead of glucose for energy. Burning fat instead of glucose can be harmful to your health and your baby's health. Harmful ketones can pass from you to your baby. Your healthcare provider can teach you how and when to test your urine or blood for ketones.

If ketones build up in your body, you can develop a condition called ketosis. Ketosis can quickly turn into diabetic ketoacidosis, which can be very dangerous. Symptoms of ketoacidosis are as follows:

- Stomach pain
- Frequent urination or frequent thirst, for a day or more
- Fatigue
- Nausea and vomiting
- Muscle stiffness or aching
- Feeling dazed or in shock
- Rapid deep breathing
- Breath that smells fruity

Checking your urine or blood ketone levels. Your healthcare provider might recommend you test your urine or blood daily for ketones and also when your blood glucose is high, such as higher than 200 mg/dL.

You can prevent serious health problems by checking for ketones as recommended. Ask your healthcare team about when to check for ketones and what to do if you have them.

If you use an insulin infusion pump, your healthcare provider might also recommend that you test for ketones when your blood glucose level is unexpectedly high.

Your healthcare provider might teach you how to make changes in the amount of insulin you take or when you take it. Or your provider may prefer that you call for advice when you have ketones.

My Checkups

Pregnancy can make some diabetes-related health problems worse. Your healthcare provider can talk with you about how pregnancy might affect any problems you have had since before pregnancy. If you plan your pregnancy enough in advance, you may want to work with your healthcare provider to arrange for treatments, such as laser treatment for eye problems, before you get pregnant. Your diabetes-related health conditions can also affect your pregnancy.

Have a complete checkup before you get pregnant or at the start of your pregnancy. Your doctor should check for the following things:

- High blood pressure, also called hypertension

- Eye disease, also called diabetic retinopathy

- Heart and blood vessel disease, also called cardiovascular disease

- Nerve damage, also called diabetic neuropathy

- Kidney disease, also called diabetic nephropathy

- Thyroid disease

You'll also get regular checkups throughout your pregnancy to check your blood pressure and average blood glucose levels and to monitor the protein in your urine.

Smoking

Smoking can increase your chance of having a stillborn or premature baby. Smoking is also especially harmful for people with diabetes. If you smoke, talk with your healthcare provider about how to quit.

My Meal Plan

If you don't already see a dietitian, now would be an excellent time to start. Your dietitian can help you learn what to eat, how much to eat, and when to eat. Together, you'll create a meal plan tailored to your needs, usual schedule, food preferences, medical conditions, medications, and physical fitness routine.

Many women need changes in their diet, such as extra calories and protein, during pregnancy. You might need to see your dietitian every few months during pregnancy as your needs change. Eating a well-balanced diet helps ensure that you and your baby are healthy.

How much to eat. Talk with your dietitian about how many servings to have at each meal and snack. Your dietitian can also provide advice about portion sizes. Your meal plan will be based on how many calories you need for pregnancy and your goals for weight gain during the pregnancy. For most women whose weight is in the normal range before pregnancy, gaining twenty-five to thirty-five pounds is recommended. If you're underweight or overweight at the start of your pregnancy, your weight goal may differ. For overweight women, the recommended weight gain is no more than fifteen pounds.

Vitamin and mineral supplements. Your healthcare team will tell you whether you need to take a vitamin and mineral supplement before and during pregnancy. Many pregnant women need supplements because their diets don't supply enough of the following important vitamins and minerals:

- *Iron:* To help make extra blood for pregnancy and for the baby's supply of iron

- *Folic acid:* To prevent birth defects in the brain and spinal cord

- *Calcium:* To build strong bones

Alcoholic beverages. You should avoid alcoholic beverages while you're trying to get pregnant and throughout pregnancy. When you drink, the alcohol also goes to your baby. Alcohol can lead to serious, lifelong problems for your baby.

Artificial sweeteners. Artificial sweeteners can be used in moderate amounts. If you choose to use sweeteners, talk with your dietitian about how much to have.

My Physical Activity Routine

Daily physical activity can help you reach your target blood glucose levels. It can also help you reach your blood pressure and cholesterol target levels, relieve stress, improve muscle tone, strengthen your heart and bones, and keep your joints flexible. Talk with your healthcare team about moderate physical activity, such as walking or swimming. Consider whether you have any health problems and which exercises would be best for you. Your healthcare team may advise you to avoid exercises that increase your risk of falling, such as downhill skiing.

A sensible goal for most women is to aim for thirty minutes or more of activity, most days of the week. If you've been active before pregnancy, you may be able to continue with a more moderate version of your usual exercise routine. But if you haven't been active, start with an activity such as walking. Vigorous physical activity, such as walking briskly, can lead to low blood glucose. Pregnant women sometimes do not have the typical signs of low blood glucose.

My Medications

Medications for diabetes. During pregnancy, the safest diabetes medication is insulin. Your healthcare team will work with you to make a personalized plan for your insulin routine. If you've been taking diabetes pills to control your blood glucose levels, you'll need to stop taking them. Researchers have not yet determined whether diabetes pills are safe for use throughout pregnancy. Instead, your healthcare team will show you how to take insulin.

If you're already taking insulin, you might need a change in the kind, the amount, and how or when you take it. The amount of insulin you take is likely to increase as you go through pregnancy because your body becomes less able to respond to the action of insulin, a condition called insulin resistance. Your insulin needs may double or even triple as you get closer to your delivery date. Insulin can be taken in several ways. Your healthcare team can help you decide which way is best for you.

Other medications. Some medications are not safe during pregnancy and should be discontinued before you get pregnant. Tell your healthcare provider about all the medications you currently take, such as those for high cholesterol and high blood pressure. Your provider can tell you which medications to stop taking.

Changes in My Daily Routine

Sick days. When you're ill, your blood glucose levels can rise rapidly. Diabetic ketoacidosis, a dangerous condition for you and your baby, can occur. Talk with your healthcare team about what you should do if you get sick. Be sure you know the following:

- What to do if you're nauseated or vomiting

- How often you should check your blood glucose

- How often you should check your urine or blood for ketones

- When you should call your healthcare provider

Being away from home. When you're away from home—for several hours or for a longer trip—you'll want to be prepared for problems. Make sure you always have the following with you:

- A snack or a meal

- Food or drinks to treat low blood glucose

- Your diabetes medicines and supplies
- Your blood glucose meter and supplies
- Your glucagon kit
- Your healthcare team's phone numbers for emergencies

Checking Your Baby's Health during Pregnancy

You are likely to have tests all through your pregnancy to check your baby's health. Your healthcare team can tell you which of the following tests you'll have and when you might have them. Your healthcare provider might also suggest other tests. If certain diseases or conditions run in your family, you might meet with a genetic counselor. The counselor may recommend tests based on your family history and can explain the risk of certain conditions for your baby.

Maternal Blood Screening Test

The maternal blood screening test is also called the multiple marker screen test, the triple screen, or quad screen. It measures several substances in your blood. Results can tell you whether your baby is at risk for spinal cord and brain problems, Down syndrome, and other birth defects. If the results show an increased risk for problems, additional tests such as ultrasound or amniocentesis can provide more information.

Ultrasound

Ultrasound uses sound waves to provide a picture of areas inside the body. The picture produced by ultrasound is called a sonogram. Ultrasound can show the baby's size, position, structures, and sex. It can also help estimate age, evaluate growth, and show some types of birth defects.

Fetal Echocardiogram

The fetal echocardiogram uses ultrasound to check for problems in the structures of the baby's heart.

Amniocentesis

Amniocentesis uses a thin needle inserted through the abdomen into the uterus to obtain a small amount of the fluid that surrounds the baby. Cells from the fluid are grown in a lab and then analyzed. Amniocentesis can help tell whether your baby has health problems and if your baby's lungs have finished developing. Developed lungs are needed for the baby to breathe without help after delivery.

Chorionic Villus Sampling (CVS)

CVS involves a thin needle inserted into the placenta to obtain cells. Cells then are analyzed to look for health problems. Ultrasound is used to guide the needle into the placenta, either through the vagina and cervix or through the abdomen and uterus. The placenta is composed of tissue and blood vessels that develop to attach the baby to the mother's uterus so the developing baby can get nutrition from mom.

Kick Counts (Fetal Movement Counting)

Counting kicks is an easy way to keep track of your baby's activity. You'll count how many times the baby moves during a certain period of time.

Nonstress Test

A fetal monitor checks whether your baby's heart rate increases as it should when the baby is active.

Biophysical Profile

Ultrasound checks your baby's muscle tone, breathing, and movement to obtain a biophysical profile. Ultrasound also estimates the amount of amniotic fluid surrounding the baby.

Contraction Stress Test

This test measures the baby's heart rate during contractions using a fetal monitor. The results can help your doctor decide whether the baby needs to be delivered early.

About Labor and Delivery

Timing of Delivery

Your healthcare team will consider your health, your baby's health, and the state of your pregnancy in deciding how and when delivery should occur. Some doctors prefer to deliver babies of women with diabetes one or two weeks before their due dates to lower the risk of problems. Your doctor may recommend inducing labor before your due date or delivering the baby surgically using a cesarean section, also called a c-section. However, most women with diabetes have the option of delivering vaginally. You'll want to talk with your healthcare team about your options well ahead of time.

The factors your healthcare team will consider in deciding what type of delivery is best for you and your baby may include the following:

- Your baby's size and position
- Your baby's lung maturity
- Your baby's movements
- Your baby's heart rate
- The amount of amniotic fluid
- Your blood glucose and blood pressure levels
- Your general health

Blood Glucose Control during Labor and Delivery

Keeping your blood glucose levels under control helps ensure your baby won't have low blood glucose after birth. Because you'll be physically active when you're in labor, you may not need much insulin. Hospital staff will check your blood glucose levels frequently. Some women take both insulin and glucose, as well as fluids, through an intravenous (IV) line during labor. Infusing insulin and glucose directly into your bloodstream through a vein provides good control of blood glucose levels. If you are using an insulin pump, you might continue to use it throughout labor.

If you are having a c-section, your blood glucose levels may increase because of the stress of surgery. Your healthcare team will closely monitor your blood glucose levels and will likely use an IV for insulin and glucose to keep your levels under control.

After Your Baby Arrives

About Breastfeeding

Breastfeeding is highly recommended for the babies of women with diabetes. Breastfeeding provides the best nutrition and helps your baby stay healthy.

Your Meal Plan

If you're breastfeeding, you might need more calories each day than you needed during your pregnancy. Your dietitian can provide personalized recommendations and answer any questions you have about what, when, and how much to eat.

Your Medications

After you've given birth, you might need less insulin than usual for several days. Breastfeeding can also lower the amount of insulin you need. Diabetes pills are not recommended during breastfeeding.

Low Blood Glucose

You'll be at increased risk for low blood glucose, especially if you're breastfeeding. You might need to have a snack before or after you breastfeed your baby. Your healthcare team may suggest that you check your blood glucose more often than usual.

Chapter 55

Diabetes in the Elderly

Chapter Contents

Section 55.1

Diabetes in Seniors: An Overview

"Diabetes in Seniors," reprinted with permission from
www.mydr.com.au © 2009 CMPMedica Australia.

What is diabetes?

Diabetes (also called diabetes mellitus) is a chronic (ongoing) condition characterized by high blood glucose (blood sugar) levels due to the body's inability to produce or respond to insulin, a hormone that allows blood glucose to enter the cells of the body and be used for energy.

Why are seniors at risk of diabetes?

Of course, seniors (those over sixty-five) are not the only people to be affected by diabetes: type 1 diabetes (previously known as insulin-dependent diabetes or juvenile-onset diabetes) is usually diagnosed during childhood, while type 2 diabetes (previously known as non-insulin-dependent diabetes or adult-onset diabetes), the most common type, is usually diagnosed in adults over the age of forty-five, although a growing number of young people are developing type 2 diabetes. Gestational diabetes is a type of diabetes that occurs only during pregnancy.

Type 2 diabetes is linked to an unhealthy lifestyle. Major risk factors for diabetes include age, being overweight, genetic predisposition to diabetes, and a reduction in activity levels. The rates of type 2 diabetes steadily increase with age.

Type 2 diabetes is most likely to occur if you:

- are over forty-five years old and have high blood pressure;

- are over forty-five years old and are overweight;

- are over forty-five and have (or have had) one or more family members with diabetes;

- are over fifty-five years of age;

- have had a heart attack in the past;

- have heart disease;

- have or have had a blood sugar test that is borderline-high;

- have or have had high blood sugar levels during pregnancy (a condition called gestational diabetes);

- have polycystic ovary syndrome and are overweight;

- are an Aboriginal Australian or Torres Strait Islander and are over thirty-five years old (or younger if overweight); or

- are a Pacific Islander, are from a Chinese cultural background or are from the Indian subcontinent and are over thirty-five years old.

What are the effects of diabetes on seniors?

A key issue for seniors with diabetes is that, sometimes, the symptoms may not be very obvious.

The well-known symptoms of diabetes, such as urinating excessively and feeling thirsty all the time, are not as obvious in the elderly as in young people.

In addition, symptoms of type 2 diabetes, such as feeling tired and lethargic, can often be misinterpreted as just part of the normal aging process.

As a result, older people with diabetes may be relatively free of symptoms and may remain undiagnosed until damage has been done.

If left unchecked, the accumulation of glucose in the blood can cause enormous damage to nearly every major organ in the body, including kidney damage; artery damage, which increases the risk of stroke and heart attack; eye damage, leading to vision loss; erectile dysfunction (impotence) in men; and nerve damage, which can lead to traumatic injury and infection, possibly leading to limb amputation.

It's unlikely you'll be able to mend the damage that has already been done, but you and your doctor can work together to control your blood sugar and help minimize the impact of diabetes in the future.

With many people now living to the age of eighty-plus years, preventing long-term complications of diabetes from further damaging your health is vital. For example, your doctor might recommend that you take a small dose of aspirin every day to help reduce your chances of having a heart attack or stroke, especially if you have vascular (blood vessel) problems.

How do other conditions affect my diabetes?

Many older people also have other conditions as well as diabetes, and this can complicate diabetes management.

For example, high blood pressure or high levels of certain fats in the blood can speed up the progression of common complications of diabetes, such as kidney problems, eye problems, foot problems, and heart and blood vessel problems.

People with diabetes whose blood glucose levels are high are more prone to infections than people with normal blood glucose levels, so, as well as keeping your blood glucose levels in check, you should also take precautionary measures against additional infection, for example, by having regular vaccinations against flu and pneumonia.

Some medications, herbs, and supplements can also have an impact on your blood glucose levels, so make sure you tell each doctor, pharmacist, and complementary healthcare practitioner who treats you that you have diabetes so they can recommend the appropriate treatment for you.

What can my doctor do to help me manage my condition?

Your doctor can:

- run blood tests regularly to check that your diabetes is under control;

- check your eyes regularly to keep track of possible eye disease (diabetic retinopathy);

- monitor your weight and help you lose weight if you need to;

- measure your blood pressure regularly and provide treatment for high blood pressure, if present;

- check the health of your feet for any signs of foot ulcers or infections and recommend a specialist or podiatrist to help manage any diabetic foot problems, if necessary;

- monitor your levels of cholesterol and triglycerides (types of fat found in the bloodstream) regularly, and provide treatment if your levels are outside the normal range;

- conduct regular urine tests to check for any kidney problems (diabetic nephropathy);

- keep vaccinations against flu and pneumococcal disease up-to-date to help prevent additional illness; and

- prescribe tablets known as oral hypoglycemic agents (or insulin, if necessary), if adopting a healthier lifestyle hasn't helped you to control your diabetes.

What can I do to help manage my condition?

You can:

- work with your doctor and any other healthcare professionals, such as diabetes educators, to learn how to keep control of your diabetes;

- keep in regular contact with your doctor;

- see a podiatrist for regular check-ups;

- wear proper footwear and examine your feet every night to check for problems;

- tell all the health professionals with whom you come in contact that you have diabetes;

- conduct regular blood glucose monitoring to keep track of your condition;

- watch your diet and make healthy choices such as eating less fat and more healthy, carbohydrate-containing foods such as fruit, vegetables, bread, and legumes;

- quit smoking, if you smoke;

- lose weight if you need to;

- do some form of physical activity, under the guidance of your doctor;

- keep any recommended vaccinations up-to-date; and

- ensure you take your medication according to your doctor's instructions.

Remember, while untreated diabetes puts you at significant risk of a range of serious health problems, this risk can be vastly improved by appropriate medical and lifestyle treatment.

Section 55.2

Particular Diabetes Management Challenges for Seniors

According to the American Diabetes Association, approximately 18.3 percent (8.6 million) of Americans age sixty and older have diabetes. The prevalence of the disease increases with age; an estimated 50 percent of all diabetes happens in those aged fifty-five and older. The risk of developing type 2 diabetes also increases with age.

Seniors face unique diabetes management challenges. For those with type 2 diabetes, age causes a decline in insulin production and an increase in glucose intolerance. Older Americans are also more likely to have complicating conditions such as retinopathy, hypertension, and kidney problems.

Other environmental and physical issues that may impact diabetes care for older Americans include:

- **Economic barriers:** Seniors on a fixed income may skimp on appropriate diabetes care, medications, and proper nutrition.

- **Transportation:** Seniors who can no longer drive may have difficulty getting to medical appointments and keeping up with appropriate diabetes preventative care.

- **Mobility:** Conditions such as arthritis that are more prevalent with age can keep older adults from regular exercise. By age seventy-five, approximately one in three men and half of all women are physically inactive.

- **Isolation:** Seniors may lack an adequate peer or family network for emotional and social support. They may be more apt to suffer from depression.

There are solutions. For those who don't have access to public transportation due to location or physical limitations, community-sponsored senior transportation may be available at little to no charge; check with your municipality to find out more. Your local senior center may also provide transportation, as well as meal service.

Part Seven

New Research
in Diabetes Care

Chapter 56

Diabetes Yesterday, Today, and Tomorrow

Type 1 Diabetes

Yesterday

In the 1950s about one in five people died within twenty years after a diagnosis of type 1 diabetes. One in three people died within twenty-five years of diagnosis.

About one in four people developed kidney failure within twenty-five years of a type 1 diabetes diagnosis. Doctors could not detect early kidney disease and had no tools for slowing its progression to kidney failure. Survival after kidney failure was poor, with one of ten patients dying each year.

About 90 percent of people with type 1 diabetes developed diabetic retinopathy within twenty-five years of diagnosis. Blindness from diabetic retinopathy was responsible for about 12 percent of new cases of blindness between the ages of forty-five and seventy-four.

Studies had not proven the value of laser surgery in reducing blindness.

Major birth defects in the offspring of mothers with type 1 diabetes were three times higher than in the general population.

Patients relied on injections of animal-derived insulin. The insulin pump would soon be introduced but would not become widely used for years.

Reprinted from "Type 1 Diabetes Fact Sheet," January 2010, and "Type 2 Diabetes Fact Sheet," June 2008, National Institutes of Health.

Studies had not yet shown the need for intensive glucose control to delay or prevent the debilitating eye, nerve, kidney, heart, and blood vessel complications of diabetes. Also, the importance of blood pressure control in preventing complications had not been established yet.

Patients monitored their glucose levels with urine tests, which recognized high but not dangerously low glucose levels and reflected past, not current, glucose levels. More reliable methods for testing glucose levels in the blood had not been developed yet.

Researchers had just discovered autoimmunity as the underlying cause of type 1 diabetes. However, they couldn't assess an individual's level of risk for developing type 1 diabetes, and they didn't know enough to even consider ways to prevent type 1 diabetes.

Today

The long-term survival of those with type 1 diabetes has dramatically improved in the last thirty years. For people born between 1975 and 1980, about 3.5 percent die within twenty years of diagnosis, and 7 percent die within twenty-five years of diagnosis. These death rates are much lower than those of patients born in the 1950s, but are still significantly increased compared to the general population.

After twenty years of annual increases from 5 to 10 percent, rates for new kidney failure cases have leveled off. The most encouraging trend is in diabetes, where rates for new cases in whites under age forty are the lowest in twenty years. Improved control of glucose and blood pressure and the use of specific antihypertensive drugs called angiotensin-converting enzyme (ACE) inhibitors and angiotensin receptor blockers (ARBs) prevent or delay the progression of kidney disease to kidney failure. With good care, fewer than 10 percent of people with diabetes develop kidney failure.

Annual eye exams are recommended because, with timely laser surgery and appropriate follow-up care, people with advanced diabetic retinopathy can reduce their risk of blindness by 90 percent.

For expectant mothers with type 1 diabetes, tight control of glucose that begins before conception lowers the risk of birth defects, miscarriage, and newborn death to a range that is close to that of the general population.

Patients use genetically engineered human insulin in a variety of formulations, e.g., rapid-acting, intermediate-acting, and long-acting insulin, to control their blood glucose. Insulin pumps are widely used, and inhaled insulin is available. Components of an artificial pancreas are being tested in clinical studies.

A major clinical trial, the Diabetes Control and Complications Trial (DCCT), showed that intensive glucose control dramatically delays or prevents the eye, nerve, and kidney complications of type 1 diabetes. A paradigm shift in the way type 1 diabetes is controlled was based on this finding. As researchers continued to follow study participants, they found that tight glucose control also prevents or delays the cardiovascular complications of type 1 diabetes, such as heart attack and stroke.

The DCCT and its follow-up study also showed that recurrent episodes of low blood sugar (hypoglycemia) do not affect patients' long-term cognitive function and do not result in long-term damage to patients' brains.

Patients can regularly monitor their blood glucose with precise, less painful methods, including a continuous glucose monitor. The widely used hemoglobin A1c test (HbA1c) shows average blood glucose over the past three months. The HbA1c Standardization Program has enabled the translation of tight blood glucose control into common practice.

In addition to identifying a key gene region that contributes nearly half the increased risk of developing type 1 diabetes, scientists have identified other genes associated with susceptibility to developing the disease. With new technologies and biosample collections, we are poised to discover additional genes and gene regions associated with type 1 diabetes.

Researchers have learned a great deal about the underlying biology of autoimmune diabetes and can now predict who is at high, moderate, and low risk for developing type 1 diabetes. This knowledge and recent advances in immunology have enabled researchers to design studies that seek to prevent type 1 diabetes and to preserve insulin production in newly diagnosed patients. This new understanding has prevented life-threatening complications in clinical trial participants at risk for developing diabetes.

Many people who received islet transplants for poorly controlled type 1 diabetes are free of the need for insulin administration a year later, and episodes of dangerously low blood glucose are greatly reduced for as long as five years after transplant, according to studies at nineteen medical centers in the United States and Canada. However, the function of transplanted islets is lost over time, and patients have side effects from immunosuppressive drugs.

The SEARCH for Diabetes in Youth Study has provided the first national data on prevalence of diabetes in youth: 1 of every 523 youth had physician-diagnosed diabetes in 2001 (this number included both type 1 and type 2 diabetes). SEARCH has also provided the first data on the rate of development of new cases of childhood diabetes and will continue to monitor trends in the future.

Tomorrow

The National Institutes of Health (NIH) are poised to make major discoveries in the prediction of who will develop type 1 diabetes and its complications, to personalize individual treatments, and to use this information to preempt disease onset and development of complications. This knowledge will have a major impact on reducing the human and economic toll of type 1 diabetes.

By finding all the genes and environmental factors (e.g., viruses, toxins, dietary factors) that contribute to type 1 diabetes, researchers will develop ways to safely prevent or reverse the autoimmune destruction of insulin-producing cells.

New therapies will preempt the vascular changes in the eye that are currently treated with laser therapy.

Methods for safely imaging the insulin-producing beta cells will help scientists better understand the disease process and assess the benefits of treatments and preventions that are under study.

Knowledge about biological pathways regulating development and growth of insulin-producing beta cells will help scientists generate beta cells in the lab. This progress may relieve the shortage of beta cells for transplantation and lead to ways to promote beta cell regeneration in people with type 1 diabetes.

Toxic suppression of the immune system to prevent rejection of transplanted organs and tissues will be replaced with safer, more targeted methods of immune modulation.

New technologies, such as a closed loop system that automatically senses blood glucose and adjusts insulin dosage precisely, will become available—allowing patients to more easily control their blood glucose levels and develop fewer complications.

As the molecular pathways by which blood glucose causes cell injury are better understood, scientists will develop medicines that prevent and repair the damage.

Some of the most important progress in type 1 diabetes has been gained from clinical studies in patients with diabetes and those at risk for the disease. To maintain the rapid pace of discovery, it is critical for individuals to take part in well-designed clinical studies. As one leading researcher put it, "The patient is the most important member of the research team."

Type 2 Diabetes

Thirty Years Ago

No proven disease prevention strategies existed.

The only ways to treat diabetes were the now obsolete forms of insulin from cows and pigs, and drugs that stimulate insulin release from the beta cells of the pancreas (sulfonylureas). Both of these therapies cause dangerous low blood sugar reactions and weight gain.

No proven strategies existed to prevent disease complications, such as blindness, kidney disease, nerve damage, and heart disease.

No proven tests were available for assessing patient control of their blood sugar levels.

While scientists knew that genes played a role (i.e., the disease often runs in families), they had not identified any specific culprit genes.

National efforts were not being made to combat obesity—a serious risk factor for the disease. Fewer people developed type 2 diabetes compared to today because overweight, obesity, and physical inactivity were not pervasive.

Patients were almost exclusively adults—the reason that the disease was formerly called "adult-onset diabetes." It was rare in children or young adults.

Today

Type 2 diabetes can be prevented or delayed! The National Institutes of Health (NIH)-funded Diabetes Prevention Program (DPP) clinical trial studied over three thousand adults at high risk for developing type 2 diabetes due to elevated blood sugar levels and overweight. The lifestyle intervention reduced by 58 percent the risk of getting type 2 diabetes. This dramatic result was achieved through modest weight loss (5 to 7 percent of body weight) and thirty minutes of exercise five times weekly. In another arm of the study, the drug metformin reduced development of diabetes by 31 percent. Both Caucasian and minority populations benefited from the interventions.

Based on the DPP findings, the NIH developed the education campaign, Small Steps, Big Rewards, Prevent Type 2 Diabetes, to help people at high risk take the necessary steps to prevent the disease. The Centers for Disease Control and Prevention (CDC) and over two hundred private partners have joined this effort. Moreover, the NIH has launched translation research initiatives to determine the best ways to promote adoption of the DPP prevention-oriented findings in real-world settings.

Vigorous research continues to combat type 2 diabetes, which—even with proven prevention strategies—is escalating in the United States. The escalation appears linked to the rising rate of obesity. Approximately 23.6 million Americans have type 2 diabetes, which represents 7.8 percent of the U.S. population and about one quarter of them don't even know it. In addition, we now know that at least another 57 million Americans have "pre-diabetes." Diabetes is conservatively estimated to be the seventh leading cause of death in the United States.

Minority populations are disproportionately affected (African Americans, Hispanics, American Indians, Alaska Natives, Asian Americans, and Pacific Islanders). For example, African Americans are 1.8 times more likely to develop type 2 diabetes compared to non-Hispanic whites.

Increased diagnosis of type 2 diabetes in children is also associated with rising rates of obesity. This trend is especially alarming because, as younger people develop the disease, the complications, morbidity, and mortality associated with diabetes are all likely to occur earlier. Furthermore, offspring of women with type 2 diabetes are more likely to develop the disease. Therefore, the burgeoning of diabetes in younger populations could lead to a vicious cycle of ever-growing rates of diabetes.

The SEARCH for Diabetes in Youth Study has provided the first national data on prevalence of diabetes in youth: 1 of every 523 youth had physician-diagnosed diabetes in 2001(this number included both type 1 and type 2 diabetes.) SEARCH has also provided the first data on the rate of development of new cases of childhood diabetes and will continue to monitor trends in the future.

The NIH launched a major clinical trial, called HEALTHY, which is examining whether an intervention given to middle-schoolers will prevent development of type 2 diabetes risk factors. For youngsters who already have the disease, the TODAY clinical trial is determining the best treatment strategies.

Research has vastly expanded understanding of the molecular underpinnings leading to diabetes and its complications and has laid the foundation for improvements in the survival and quality of life for people with the disease.

Studies have dramatically increased knowledge about the complex genetic underpinnings of type 2 diabetes. Recent studies have boosted to sixteen the total number of gene regions associated with increased risk of type 2 diabetes.

New drug development has been aided by NIH-supported clinical trials that validated a marker, called hemoglobin A1c (HbA1c). This marker reflects average blood sugar control over a three-month period.

Thus, a simple lab test can tell patients whether they are achieving good control of blood sugar levels.

Tight control of blood sugar has become a standard of treatment based on results from NIH clinical trials demonstrating that tight control (i.e., HbA1c less than 7) can prevent or delay the development of devastating complications. Unfortunately, few patients currently achieve the close control needed for preventing complications. Researchers are urgently seeking improved methods of achieving tight control.

New and more effective treatments have become available through research. New oral agents targeting the specific metabolic abnormalities of type 2 diabetes are available. Patients are benefiting from improved forms of insulin, a range of oral medications to control blood sugar and reduce the need for insulin, and new drugs that may not only control blood sugar, but also strengthen the activity of patients' own insulin-producing cells.

New technologies are emerging, such as the recently approved continuous glucose monitors. These devices have the potential to dramatically improve patients' ability to control their sugar levels—key for preventing complications—and to improve their quality of life by eliminating the need for invasive finger sticks.

Kidney disease can be detected earlier by standardized blood tests to estimate renal function and monitor urine protein excretion. Therefore, patients can be treated earlier to slow the rate of kidney damage. Improved control of glucose and blood pressure and the use of antihypertensive drugs called angiotensin-converting enzyme (ACE) inhibitors and angiotensin receptor blockers (ARBs) prevent or delay the progression of kidney disease to kidney failure. With good care, fewer than 10 percent of patients develop kidney failure.

Clinical trials have shown that blood pressure and lipid control reduce diabetes complications by up to 50 percent. Physicians are now much better equipped to control hypertension and unhealthy blood fats, which often accompany diabetes and raise the risk of heart disease, the leading cause of death of people with diabetes.

Results from a large clinical trial showed that patients with type 2 diabetes at high risk of heart disease do not benefit from intensive blood glucose control below current recommendations. Although these findings are important, they will not change therapy for most patients with type 2 diabetes because they are not treated to blood sugar levels as low as those tested in this trial.

With timely laser surgery and appropriate follow-up care, people with advanced diabetic retinopathy can reduce their risk of blindness by 90 percent.

The NIH spends $1.037 billion on diabetes research. In 2007, total costs attributable to diabetes for Americans was estimated at $174 billion—an increase of 32 percent since 2002.

Tomorrow

The NIH is poised to make major discoveries in the prediction of who will develop type 2 diabetes and its complications, to personalize individual treatments, and to use this information to preempt disease onset and development of complications. This knowledge will have a major impact on reducing the human and economic toll that type 2 diabetes places on the United States.

Researchers are pursuing earlier and more aggressive treatment approaches that will help to preempt diabetes complications.

New understanding of the molecular links between obesity and insulin resistance will inform the development of new therapeutic targets for preventing and treating type 2 diabetes.

Identification of susceptibility genes for diabetes and its complications will enable earlier implementation of prevention measures targeted to those at highest risk.

Preempting diabetes will eliminate the life-threatening complications, which will mean that people will live longer, healthier lives without fear—such as the fear of going blind or losing a lower limb.

Research on the effect of maternal diabetes on offspring will help to break the vicious intergenerational cycle.

Continued research on the mechanisms underlying the development and progression of disease complications will result in the ability to predict who is likely to develop them. Personalized treatments could then be developed to preempt complications. This strategy would dramatically improve the health and wellbeing of patients.

Results from NIH clinical trials will help to identify strategies to preempt type 2 diabetes in children, thereby stemming the alarming trend of increased rates of this disease in youth.

Chapter 57

Diabetes Control and Prevention Studies

Chapter Contents

Section 57.1

Diabetes Control and Complications Trial and Follow-up Study

Reprinted from "DCCT and EDIC: The Diabetes Control and Complications Trial and Follow-up Study," National Institute of Diabetes and Digestive and Kidney Diseases, National Institutes of Health, NIH Publication No. 08-3874, May 2008.

What Is the DCCT?

The Diabetes Control and Complications Trial (DCCT) was a major clinical study conducted from 1983 to 1993 and funded by the National Institute of Diabetes and Digestive and Kidney Diseases. The study showed that keeping blood glucose levels as close to normal as possible slows the onset and progression of the eye, kidney, and nerve damage caused by diabetes. In fact, it demonstrated that any sustained lowering of blood glucose, also called blood sugar, helps, even if the person has a history of poor control.

The DCCT involved 1,441 volunteers, ages thirteen to thirty-nine, with type 1 diabetes and twenty-nine medical centers in the United States and Canada. Volunteers had to have had diabetes for at least one year but no longer than fifteen years. They also were required to have no, or only early signs of, diabetic eye disease.

The study compared the effects of standard control of blood glucose versus intensive control on the complications of diabetes. Intensive control meant keeping hemoglobin A1C levels as close as possible to the normal value of 6 percent or less. The A1C blood test reflects a person's average blood glucose over the last two to three months. Volunteers were randomly assigned to each treatment group.

What Is the EDIC?

When the DCCT ended in 1993, researchers continued to study more than 90 percent of participants. The follow-up study, called Epidemiology of Diabetes Interventions and Complications (EDIC), is assessing the incidence and predictors of cardiovascular disease events such as heart attack, stroke, or needed heart surgery, as well as diabetic complications related to the eye, kidney, and nerves. The EDIC study is also examining the impact of intensive control versus standard control on quality of life. Another objective is to look at the cost-effectiveness of intensive control.

DCCT Study Findings

Intensive blood glucose control reduces risk of the following things:

- Eye disease: 76 percent reduced risk
- Kidney disease: 50 percent reduced risk
- Nerve disease: 60 percent reduced risk

EDIC Study Findings

Intensive blood glucose control reduces risk of the following things:

- Any cardiovascular disease event: 42 percent reduced risk
- Nonfatal heart attack, stroke, or death from cardiovascular causes: 57 percent reduced risk

How Did Intensive Treatment Affect Diabetic Eye Disease?

All DCCT participants were monitored for diabetic retinopathy, an eye disease that affects the retina. Study results showed that intensive therapy reduced the risk for developing retinopathy by 76 percent. In participants who had some eye damage at the beginning of the study, intensive management slowed the progression of the disease by 54 percent.

The retina is the light-sensing tissue at the back of the eye. According to the National Eye Institute, one of the National Institutes of Health, as many as twenty-four thousand people with diabetes lose their sight each year. In the United States, diabetic retinopathy is the leading cause of blindness in adults less than sixty-five years of age.

How Did Intensive Treatment Affect Diabetic Kidney Disease?

Participants in the DCCT were tested to assess the development of diabetic kidney disease, or nephropathy. Findings showed that intensive treatment prevented the development and slowed the progression of diabetic kidney disease by 50 percent.

Diabetic kidney disease is the most common cause of kidney failure in the United States. After having diabetes for fifteen years, one-third of people with type 1 diabetes develop kidney disease. Diabetes damages the small blood vessels in the kidneys, impairing their ability to filter impurities from blood for excretion in the urine. People with kidney failure must have a kidney transplant or rely on dialysis to cleanse their blood.

How Did Intensive Treatment Affect Diabetic Nerve Disease?

Participants in the DCCT were examined to detect the development of nerve damage, or diabetic neuropathy. Study results showed the risk of nerve damage was reduced by 60 percent in people on intensive treatment.

Diabetic nerve disease can cause pain and loss of feeling in the feet, legs, and fingertips. It can also affect the parts of the nervous system that control blood pressure, heart rate, digestion, and sexual function. Neuropathy is a major contributing factor in foot and leg amputations among people with diabetes.

Elements of Intensive Management in the DCCT

- Testing blood glucose levels four or more times a day
- Injecting insulin at least three times daily or using an insulin pump
- Adjusting insulin doses according to food intake and exercise
- Following a diet and exercise plan
- Making monthly visits to a healthcare team composed of a physician, nurse educator, dietitian, and behavioral therapist

How Did Intensive Treatment Affect Diabetes-Related Cardiovascular Disease?

People with type 1 diabetes have a tenfold greater risk of heart disease compared with nondiabetic patients because high blood glucose can damage the heart and blood vessels. That damage can lead to heart attacks and strokes, the leading causes of death for people with diabetes.

Another condition related to heart disease and common in people with diabetes is peripheral arterial disease (PAD), also called peripheral vascular disease (PVD). With this condition, the blood vessels in the legs are narrowed or blocked by fatty deposits, decreasing blood flow to the legs and feet. PAD is a sign of widespread atherosclerosis, and people with PAD are at increased risk of heart attack or stroke. Poor circulation in the legs and feet also raises the risk of amputation.

When the initial findings of the DCCT were announced in 1993, it was too early to detect the effects of the therapies on cardiovascular disease because patients were young. In 2005, however, EDIC researchers reported that the risk of any heart disease was reduced by 42 percent in people who had been in the intensive treatment group. Volunteers in the intensive treatment group also cut their risk of nonfatal heart attack, stroke, or death from cardiovascular causes by 57 percent.

Patients received the intensive therapy for an average of 6.5 years in the DCCT. More than 10 years after the DCCT ended, when both groups began receiving similar care, the benefits to the heart of the earlier treatment emerged. Moreover, the EDIC study found the benefits of tight glucose control on eye, kidney, and nerve problems persisted long after the DCCT ended. Researchers call the long-lasting benefit of tight control "metabolic memory." Following the DCCT, blood glucose levels in the intensive treatment group rose, and those of the conventional treatment group declined, so that blood glucose levels are now nearly the same between treatment groups.

What Are the Risks of Intensive Treatment?

In the DCCT, the most significant side effect of intensive treatment was an increase in the risk for hypoglycemia, also called low blood glucose, including episodes severe enough to require assistance from another person.

When blood glucose falls too low, a person can become confused, behave irrationally, have seizures, lose consciousness, or even die. The good news is that such episodes, while dangerous at the time, do not lead to a long-term loss of cognitive function—the ability to perceive, reason, and remember—as scientists originally feared. Researchers recently reported this finding after examining 1,144 of the original DCCT participants a mean of eighteen years after enrollment in the DCCT.

The DCCT did not study intensive therapy in young children or in patients with severe complications, frequent hypoglycemia, or those with a limited life expectancy. While most patients benefit from keeping their blood glucose levels as close to normal as possible, less stringent goals may be appropriate for some patients.

DCCT researchers estimate that intensive management doubles the cost of managing diabetes because of increased visits to a healthcare professional and the need for more frequent blood testing at home. However, this cost is offset by the reduction in medical expenses related to long-term complications and by the improved quality of life of people with diabetes.

What Do the Results of the DCCT and EDIC Studies Mean for People with Type 2 Diabetes?

Results of the DCCT and EDIC studies have important implications for preventing diabetes complications in people with type 2 diabetes because the microvascular disease development process is likely to be similar for both type 1 and type 2 diabetes. One study of people with type 2 diabetes, the United Kingdom Prospective Diabetes Study, demonstrated that controlling blood glucose levels reduced the risk of diabetic eye disease and kidney disease.

Other studies of the role of blood glucose control in people with type 2 diabetes are still under way. For example, the Action to Control Cardiovascular Risk in Diabetes (ACCORD) trial, a multi-center, randomized trial, is studying approaches to preventing major cardiovascular events in individuals with type 2 diabetes. ACCORD is designed to compare current practice guidelines with more intensive glycemic control in ten thousand individuals with type 2 diabetes, including those at especially high risk for cardiovascular disease (CVD) events because of age, evidence of subclinical atherosclerosis, or existing clinical CVD. More intensive control of blood pressure than is called for in current guidelines and a medication to reduce triglyceride levels and raise HDL cholesterol levels will also be studied in subgroups of these ten thousand volunteers. Each treatment strategy will be accompanied by standard advice regarding lifestyle choices, including diet, physical activity, and smoking cessation, appropriate for individuals with diabetes.

The primary outcome to be measured is the first occurrence of a major CVD event, specifically heart attack, stroke, or cardiovascular death. In addition, the study will investigate the impact of the treatment strategies on other cardiovascular outcomes; total mortality;

limb amputation; eye, kidney, or nerve disease; health-related quality of life; and cost-effectiveness.

In February 2008, the National Heart, Lung, and Blood Institute decided to stop one part of the study—the intensive glycemic control treatment—before the end of the entire trial because of safety concerns. However, the trial continued with the other treatments until the planned end in 2009.

What Are the Most Important Factors in Preventing Diabetes Complications?

Research studies have shown that control of blood glucose, blood pressure, and blood lipid levels helps prevent complications in people with type 1 or type 2 diabetes.

- Results of the DCCT are reported in the *New England Journal of Medicine*, 329(14), September 30, 1993.

- Results of the EDIC are reported in the *New England Journal of Medicine*, 353(25), December 22, 2005.

Section 57.2

Diabetes Prevention Program

Excerpted from "Diabetes Prevention Program," National Institute of Diabetes and Digestive and Kidney Diseases, National Institutes of Health, NIH Publication No. 09-5099, October 2008.

The Diabetes Prevention Program (DPP) was a major multicenter clinical research study aimed at discovering whether modest weight loss through dietary changes and increased physical activity or treatment with the oral diabetes drug metformin (Glucophage®) could prevent or delay the onset of type 2 diabetes in study participants. At the beginning of the DPP, participants were all overweight and had blood glucose, also called blood sugar, levels higher than normal but not high enough for a diagnosis of diabetes—a condition called pre-diabetes.

The DPP found that participants who lost a modest amount of weight through dietary changes and increased physical activity sharply reduced their chances of developing diabetes. Taking metformin also reduced risk, although less dramatically. The DPP resolved its research questions earlier than projected and, following the recommendation of an external monitoring board, the study was halted a year early. The researchers published their findings in the February 7, 2002, issue of the *New England Journal of Medicine*.

DPP Study Design and Goals

In the DPP, participants from twenty-seven clinical centers around the United States were randomly divided into different treatment groups. The first group, called the lifestyle intervention group, received intensive training in diet, physical activity, and behavior modification. By eating less fat and fewer calories and exercising for a total of 150 minutes a week, they aimed to lose 7 percent of their body weight and maintain that loss.

The second group took 850 mg of metformin twice a day. The third group received placebo pills instead of metformin. The metformin and placebo groups also received information about diet and exercise but no intensive motivational counseling. A fourth group was treated with the drug troglitazone (Rezulin®), but this part of the study was discontinued after researchers discovered that troglitazone can cause serious liver damage. The participants in this group were followed but not included as one of the intervention groups.

All 3,234 study participants were overweight and had pre-diabetes, which are well-known risk factors for the development of type 2 diabetes. In addition, 45 percent of the participants were from minority groups—African American, Alaska Native, American Indian, Asian American, Hispanic/Latino, or Pacific Islander—at increased risk of developing diabetes.

Type 2 Diabetes and Pre-Diabetes

Type 2 diabetes is a disorder that affects the way the body uses digested food for growth and energy. Normally, the food one eats is broken down into glucose, a form of sugar. The glucose then passes into the bloodstream, where it is used by the cells for growth and energy. For glucose to reach the cells, however, insulin must be present. Insulin is a hormone produced by the pancreas, a fist-sized gland behind the stomach.

Most people with type 2 diabetes have two problems: insulin resistance—a condition in which muscle, liver, and fat cells do not use insulin properly—and reduced insulin production by the pancreas. As a result, glucose builds up in the blood, overflows into the urine, and passes out of the body, never fulfilling its role as the body's main source of fuel.

About 23.6 million people in the United States have diabetes. Of those, 17.9 million are diagnosed and 5.7 million are undiagnosed. Between 90 and 95 percent of people with diabetes have type 2 diabetes. Diabetes is the main cause of kidney failure, limb amputation, and new-onset blindness in American adults. People with diabetes are more likely than people without diabetes to develop and die from diseases of the heart and blood vessels, called cardiovascular disease. Adults with diabetes have heart disease death rates about two to four times higher than adults without diabetes, and the risk for stroke is two to four times higher among people with diabetes.

Pre-diabetes is a condition in which blood glucose levels are higher than normal but not high enough for a diagnosis of diabetes. Pre-diabetes is also called impaired glucose tolerance (IGT) or impaired fasting glucose (IFG), depending on the test used to measure blood glucose levels. Having pre-diabetes puts one at higher risk for developing type 2 diabetes. People with pre-diabetes are also at increased risk for developing cardiovascular disease.

Pre-diabetes is becoming more common in the United States. The U.S. Department of Health and Human Services estimates that about one in four U.S. adults aged twenty years or older—or fifty-seven million people—had pre-diabetes in 2007. Those with pre-diabetes are likely to develop type 2 diabetes within ten years, unless they take steps to prevent or delay diabetes.

Who Should Be Tested for Pre-Diabetes and Diabetes?

The American Diabetes Association recommends that testing to detect pre-diabetes and type 2 diabetes be considered in adults without symptoms who are overweight or obese and have one or more additional risk factors for diabetes. In those without these risk factors, testing should begin at age forty-five.

Risk factors for pre-diabetes and diabetes—in addition to being overweight or obese or being age forty-five or older—include the following:

- Being physically inactive

- Having a parent, brother, or sister with diabetes

- Having a family background that is African American, Alaska Native, American Indian, Asian American, Hispanic/Latino, or Pacific Islander

- Giving birth to a baby weighing more than nine pounds or being diagnosed with gestational diabetes—diabetes first found during pregnancy

- Having high blood pressure—140/90 mmHg or above—or being treated for high blood pressure

- having high-density lipoprotein (HDL), or "good," cholesterol below 35 mg/dL, or a triglyceride level above 250 mg/dL

- Having polycystic ovary syndrome, also called PCOS

- Having impaired fasting glucose (IFG) or impaired glucose tolerance (IGT) on previous testing

- Having other conditions associated with insulin resistance, such as severe obesity or a condition called acanthosis nigricans, characterized by a dark, velvety rash around the neck or armpits

- Having a history of cardiovascular disease

If results of testing are normal, testing should be repeated at least every three years. Doctors may recommend more frequent testing depending on initial results and risk status.

DPP Results

The DPP's results indicate that millions of high-risk people can delay or avoid developing type 2 diabetes by losing weight through regular physical activity and a diet low in fat and calories. Weight loss and physical activity lower the risk of diabetes by improving the body's ability to use insulin and process glucose. The DPP also suggests that metformin can help delay the onset of diabetes.

Participants in the lifestyle intervention group—those receiving intensive individual counseling and motivational support on effective diet, exercise, and behavior modification—reduced their risk of developing diabetes by 58 percent. This finding was true across all participating ethnic groups and for both men and women. Lifestyle changes worked particularly well for participants aged sixty and older, reducing their risk by 71 percent. About 5 percent of the lifestyle intervention group developed diabetes each year during the study period, compared with 11 percent of those in the placebo group.

Participants taking metformin reduced their risk of developing diabetes by 31 percent. Metformin was effective for both men and women, but it was least effective in people aged forty-five and older. Metformin was most effective in people twenty-five to forty-four years old and in those with a body mass index of 35 or higher, meaning they were at least sixty pounds overweight. About 7.8 percent of the metformin group developed diabetes each year during the study, compared with 11 percent of the group receiving the placebo.

Further Analyses of DPP Data

In the years since the DPP was completed, further analyses of DPP data continue to yield important insights into the value of lifestyle changes in helping people prevent type 2 diabetes and associated conditions. For example, one analysis confirmed that DPP participants carrying two copies of a gene variant, or mutation, that significantly increased their risk of developing diabetes benefited from lifestyle changes as much as or more than those without the gene variant. Another analysis found that weight loss was the main predictor of reduced risk for developing diabetes in DPP lifestyle intervention group participants. The authors concluded that diabetes risk reduction efforts should focus on weight loss, which is helped by increased exercise.

Analyses of DPP data have added to the evidence that changes in diet and physical activity leading to weight loss are especially effective in helping reduce risk factors associated with both diabetes and cardiovascular disease, including high blood pressure and metabolic syndrome. A person with metabolic syndrome has several of a specific group of risk factors for developing diabetes and heart disease, such as having excess fat deposited around the waist, high triglyceride levels, and high fasting blood glucose levels. One analysis found that DPP participants in the lifestyle intervention group who did not have metabolic syndrome at the beginning of the study—about half of the participants—were less likely to develop it than those in the other groups. Another analysis of DPP data found that the presence of high blood pressure in DPP participants decreased in the lifestyle intervention group but increased in the metformin and placebo groups over time. Measures of triglyceride and HDL cholesterol levels also improved in the lifestyle intervention group. A third analysis found that levels of C-reactive protein and fibrinogen—risk factors for heart disease—were lower in the metformin and lifestyle intervention groups, with a larger reduction in the lifestyle group.

In addition, one study focused on urinary incontinence in women who participated in the DPP. Women in the lifestyle intervention group who lost 5 to 7 percent of their body weight through dietary changes and exercise had fewer problems with urinary incontinence than women in the other study groups.

Hope through Research

The DPP contributed to a better understanding of how diabetes develops in people at risk and how they can prevent or delay the development of diabetes by making behavioral changes leading to weight loss. These findings are reflected in recommendations from the American Diabetes Association for the prevention or delay of type 2 diabetes, which stress the importance of lifestyle changes and weight loss. The DPP's impact continues as new research, building on the study's results, seeks the most effective ways to prevent, delay, or even reverse diabetes.

DPP researchers continue to examine the roles of lifestyle and metformin and other diabetes medications in preventing type 2 diabetes. They also continue to monitor participants to learn more about the study's long-term effects through the Diabetes Prevention Program Outcomes Study (DPPOS), a follow-up to the DPP. DPPOS is examining the impact of long-term risk reduction on diabetes-related health problems, such as nerve damage and heart, kidney, and eye disease.

Chapter 58

Genetic Risk for Type 2 Diabetes: Recent Research Advances

Researchers Identify New Genetic Risk Factors for Type 2 Diabetes

In the most comprehensive look at genetic risk factors for type 2 diabetes to date, a U.S.-Finnish team, working in close collaboration with two other groups, has identified at least four new genetic variants associated with increased risk of diabetes and confirmed existence of another six. The findings of the three groups, published simultaneously in the April 26, 2007, online edition of the journal *Science*, boost to at least ten the number of genetic variants confidently associated with increased susceptibility to type 2 diabetes—a disease that affects more than two hundred million people worldwide.

"This achievement represents a major milestone in our battle against diabetes. It will accelerate efforts to understand the genetic risk factors for this disease, as well as explore how these genetic factors interact with each other and with lifestyle factors," said National Institutes of Health (NIH) director Elias A. Zerhouni, M.D. "Such research is opening the door to the era of personalized medicine. Our current one-size-fits-all approach will soon give way to more individualized strategies based on each person's unique genetic make-up."

Reprinted from "Researchers Identify New Genetic Risk Factors for Type 2 Diabetes," *NIH News*, February 6, 2010; "Major Collaboration Uncovers Surprising New Genetic Clues to Diabetes," *NIH News*, April 24, 2010; and "Newly Identified Genes Influence Insulin and Glucose Regulation," *NIH News*, June 29, 2010.

Led by Michael Boehnke, Ph.D., of the University of Michigan's School of Public Health, Ann Arbor; Francis Collins, M.D., Ph.D., of the National Human Genome Research Institute (NHGRI); Richard Bergman, Ph.D., of the University of Southern California, Los Angeles; Karen Mohlke, Ph.D. of the University of North Carolina, Chapel Hill; and Jaakko Tuomilehto, M.D., Ph.D. of the University of Helsinki and National Public Health Institute in Finland; the U.S.-Finnish team received major support from the National Institute of Diabetes and Digestive and Kidney Diseases (NIDDK) and NHGRI's Division of Intramural Research, both part of the NIH. The laboratory analysis of genetic variants in the first stage of the study was conducted by the Center for Inherited Disease Research, using funding from NIH and the Johns Hopkins University in Baltimore.

The research was carried out in conjunction with the work of two other teams: the Diabetes Genetics Initiative, which is a collaboration of the Broad Institute of Harvard and Massachusetts Institute of Technology (MIT), Cambridge, Massachusetts; Lund University, Malmo, Sweden; and Novartis, Basel, Switzerland; and the Wellcome Trust Case Control Consortium/U.K. Type 2 Diabetes Genetics Consortium. The Diabetes Genetics Initiative was led by David Altshuler, M.D., Ph.D., Broad Institute; Leif Groop, M.D., Ph.D., Lund University; and Thomas Hughes, Ph.D., Novartis. The British team was led by Mark McCarthy, M.D., FRCP, Oxford University and Andrew Hattersley, D.M., FRCP, Peninsula Medical School, Plymouth.

"It's been a formidable challenge to identify the complex genetic factors involved in common diseases, such as type 2 diabetes. Now, thanks to the tools and technologies generated by the sequencing of the human genome and subsequent mapping of common human genetic variations, we finally are making significant progress," said NHGRI Director Collins, who led the NIH component of the Human Genome Project.

Type 2 diabetes affects nearly twenty-one million people in the United States and the incidence of the disease has skyrocketed in the United States and many other developed nations over the last thirty years. Diabetes is a major cause of heart disease and stroke, as well as the most common cause in U.S. adults of blindness, kidney failure, and amputations not related to trauma.

NIDDK Director Griffin P. Rodgers, M.D., said, "These genetic findings are exciting news for diabetes research. While more work remains to be done, the newly identified genetic variants may point us in the direction of valuable new drug targets for the prevention or treatment of type 2 diabetes."

Previously known as adult onset or non-insulin-dependent diabetes (NIDDM), type 2 diabetes usually appears after age forty, often in overweight, sedentary individuals. However, an increasing number of younger people and even children are developing the disease, which is characterized by the resistance of target tissues to respond to insulin and a gradual failure of insulin-secreting cells in the pancreas.

In addition to lifestyle factors like obesity, poor diet, and lack of exercise, doctors have long known that heredity plays a significant role in the risk of developing type 2 diabetes. People who have a parent or sibling with type 2 diabetes face a 3.5-times greater risk than people without a family history of the disease. However, researchers have only recently begun to zero in on particular genetic variants that increase or decrease susceptibility to the disease.

To make their discoveries, researchers used a relatively new, comprehensive strategy known as a genome-wide association study. "Genome-wide association studies offer a powerful way to uncover the genetic variations that contribute to diabetes, as well as other common conditions, such as asthma, arthritis, heart disease, cancer, and mental illnesses," Dr. Boehnke said. "Once susceptibility genes are identified, researchers then can use this information to develop better approaches to detecting, treating, and preventing disease."

To conduct a genome-wide association study, researchers use two groups of participants: a large group of people with the disease being studied and a large group of otherwise similar people without the disease. Utilizing DNA purified from blood or cells, researchers quickly survey each participant's complete set of DNA, or genome, for strategically selected markers of genetic variation.

If certain genetic variations are found more frequently in people with the disease compared to healthy people, the variations are said to be associated with the disease. The associated genetic variations can serve as a strong pointer to the region of the genome where the genetic risk factor resides. However, the first variants detected may not themselves directly influence disease susceptibility, and the actual causative variant may lie nearby. This means researchers often need to take additional steps, such as sequencing every DNA base pair in that particular region of the genome, to identify the exact genetic variant that affects disease risk.

In the latest work, researchers began by scanning the genomes of more than 2,300 Finnish people who took part in the Finland-United States Investigation Of NIDDM Genetics (FUSION) and Finrisk 2002 studies. About half of the participants had type 2 diabetes and the other half had normal blood glucose levels.

"We thank all the Finnish citizens who participated in this study. Their generosity has created a lasting legacy that will help to reduce the terrible toll that diabetes is taking on the world's health," said Dr. Tuomilehto of the Diabetes Unit in Finland's National Public Health Institute.

To validate their findings, the researchers compared their initial results with results from genome scans of 3,000 Swedish and Finnish participants in the Diabetes Genetics Initiative and 5,000 British participants in the Wellcome Trust Case Control Consortium, led by Peter Donnelly, D.Phil., Oxford University. After identifying promising leads through this approach, the three research teams jointly replicated their findings using smaller, more focused sets of genetic markers in additional groups totaling more than 22,000 people from Finland, Poland, Sweden, the United Kingdom, and the United States. All told, the genomes of 32,554 people were tested for the study, making it one of the largest genome-wide association efforts conducted to date.

"This is a phenomenal accomplishment, in terms of both the breadth and depth of the research. By pulling together and sharing their data, these three groups were able to achieve far more than any one of them could have done alone," said Eric D. Green, M.D., Ph.D., director of NHGRI's Division of Intramural Research. "This is scientific collaboration at its best."

Ultimately, the researchers identified four new diabetes-associated variations, as well as confirmed previous findings that associated six other genetic variants with increased diabetes risk. The newly identified diabetes-associated variations lie in or near the following:

- **IGF2BP2:** This gene codes for a protein called insulin-like growth factor 2 mRNA binding protein 2. Insulin-like growth factor 2 is thought to play a role in regulating insulin action.

- **CDKAL1:** This gene codes for a protein called CDK5 regulatory subunit associated protein1-like1. The protein may affect the activity of the cyclin dependent kinase 5 (CDK5) protein, which stimulates insulin production and may influence other processes in the pancreas's insulin-producing cells, known as beta cells. In addition, excessive activity of CDK5 in the pancreas may lead to the degeneration of beta cells.

- **CDKN2A and CDKN2B:** The proteins produced by these two genes inhibit the activity of cyclin-dependent protein kinases, including one that has been shown to influence the growth of beta cells in mice. Interestingly, these genes have been heavily studied for their role in cancer, but their contribution to diabetes comes as a complete surprise.

- **Chromosome 11:** One intriguing association is located in a region of chromosome 11 not known to contain any genes. Researchers speculate that the variant sequences may regulate the activity of genes located elsewhere in the genome, but more work is needed to determine the exact relationships to pathways involved in type 2 diabetes.

The genetic variants associated with diabetes that were confidently confirmed by the new research are: TCF7L2, SLC30A8, HHEX, PPARG, KCNJ11, and FTO. A variant in FTO was recently associated with increased risk of obesity. (T. Frayling et al. A Common Variant in the FTO Gene Is Associated with Body Mass Index and Predisposes to Childhood and Adult Obesity. *Science Express*, Published online April 12, 2007.) The latest study found that variations in or near the FTO gene are also associated with greater risk of type 2 diabetes, which is likely related to an increased predisposition to obesity.

When the genomes of the Finnish participants were scanned for all ten diabetes-associated genetic variants, researchers could identify individuals whose genetic profiles placed them at increased risk for type 2 diabetes—including one subset of people who faced a risk four times higher than those at the lowest genetic risk. This "could potentially have value in a personalized preventive medicine program," the researchers wrote.

However, the researchers emphasized that their predictions of disease risk need to be interpreted with caution because the diabetes group in their sample was "enriched" with people who had affected siblings and because the healthy group excluded people who had impaired glucose tolerance or impaired fasting glucose.

Major Collaboration Uncovers Surprising New Genetic Clues to Diabetes

An international team that included scientists from the National Human Genome Research Institute (NHGRI), part of the National Institutes of Health (NIH), reported it has identified six more genetic variants involved in type 2 diabetes, boosting to sixteen the total number of genetic risk factors associated with increased risk of the disease. None of the genetic variants uncovered by the new study had previously been suspected of playing a role in type 2 diabetes. Intriguingly, the new variant most strongly associated with type 2 diabetes also was recently implicated in a very different condition: prostate cancer.

The unprecedented analysis, published in the March 30, 2008, advance online edition of *Nature Genetics*, combined genetic data from more than seventy thousand people. The work was carried out through the collaborative efforts of more than ninety researchers at more than forty centers in Europe and North America.

"None of the genes we have found was previously on the radar screen of diabetes researchers," said one of the paper's senior authors, Mark McCarthy, M.D., of the University of Oxford in England. "Each of these genes, therefore, provides new clues to the processes that go wrong when diabetes develops, and each provides an opportunity for the generation of new approaches for treating or preventing this condition."

When considered individually, the genetic variants discovered to date account for only small differences in the risk of developing type 2 diabetes. But researchers say when all of the variants are analyzed together, some significant differences in risk are likely to emerge. "By combining information from the large number of genes now implicated in diabetes risk, it may be possible to use genetic tools to identify people at unusually high or low risk of diabetes. However, until we know how to use this information to prompt beneficial changes in people's treatment or lifestyle, widespread genetic testing would be premature," said another senior author, David Altshuler, M.D., Ph.D., of Massachusetts General Hospital in Boston and the Broad Institute of Massachusetts Institute of Technology and Harvard in Cambridge, Massachusetts.

Type 2 diabetes affects more than two hundred million people worldwide, including nearly twenty-one million people in the United States. Previously known as adult-onset, or non-insulin-dependent diabetes mellitus (NIDDM), type 2 diabetes usually appears after age forty, often in overweight, sedentary people. However, a growing number of younger people—and even children—are developing the disease.

Diabetes is a major cause of heart disease and stroke in U.S. adults, as well as the most common cause of blindness, kidney failure, and amputations not related to trauma. Type 2 diabetes is characterized by the resistance of target tissues to respond to insulin, which controls glucose levels in the blood; and a gradual failure of insulin-secreting cells in the pancreas.

"These new variants, along with other recent genetic findings, provide a window into disease causation that may be our best hope for the next generation of therapeutics. By pinpointing particular pathways involved in diabetes risk, these discoveries can empower new approaches to understanding environmental influences and to the development of new, more precisely targeted drugs," said NHGRI Director Francis

S. Collins, M.D., Ph.D., who is a co-author of the study. Dr. Collins's laboratory is a participant in the FINRISK 2002 and Finland-United States Investigation of NIDDM Genetics (FUSION), which were among the studies that contributed data to the new analysis. FUSION is funded by NHGRI's Division of Intramural Research and the National Institute of Diabetes and Digestive and Kidney Diseases (NIDDK).

Researchers said more work is needed to understand the impact of their discovery that a genetic variant called JAZF1 appears to be involved in diabetes as well as prostate cancer. One of the study's lead authors, Eleftheria Zeggini, Ph.D., of the University of Oxford, said, "This is now the second example of a gene which affects both type 2 diabetes and prostate cancer. We don't yet know what the connections are, but this may have important implications for the future design of drugs for both of these conditions."

The research was conducted by the DIAbetes Genetics Replication And Meta-analysis (DIAGRAM) consortium, which brought together many groups active in the field of diabetes research. In the *Nature Genetics* paper, DIAGRAM researchers combined the data from three previously published genome-wide association studies in an effort to boost the statistical power of their searches—an approach that scientists refer to as meta-analysis. The strategy paid off, enabling researchers to identify six genetic variants associated with type 2 diabetes that had gone undetected in the smaller, individual studies.

Newly Identified Genes Influence Insulin and Glucose Regulation

An international research consortium has found thirteen new genetic variants that influence blood glucose regulation, insulin resistance, and the function of insulin-secreting beta cells in populations of European descent. Five of the newly discovered variants increase the risk of developing type 2 diabetes, the most common form of diabetes.

The results of two studies, conducted by the Meta-Analyses of Glucose and Insulin Related Traits Consortium (MAGIC), provide important clues about the role of beta cells in the development of type 2 diabetes. The studies, funded in part by the National Institutes of Health, appear online January 17, 2010, in *Nature Genetics*.

"The findings from these ambitious, large-scale studies represent an enormous achievement in international cooperation involving hundreds of researchers and many thousands of individuals who contributed genetic samples for the study. The results give us exciting new directions for future research in the biology of type 2 diabetes, which poses a major and growing public health problem worldwide," said NIH Director Francis S. Collins, M.D., Ph.D., an author of both papers.

In one paper, the MAGIC investigators set out to find genes that influence metabolic traits, including fasting glucose and insulin levels and measures of beta cell function and insulin resistance. About 2.5 million genetic variants were analyzed in twenty-one genome-wide association studies (GWAS) that had enrolled 46,186 individuals who did not have diabetes and had been tested for measures of glucose and insulin regulation. GWAS look for common genetic associations by scanning the deoxyribonucleic acid (DNA) of thousands of individuals. The huge numbers of genetic samples boosts the chances of finding subtle associations of genetic variants with specific diseases or traits. The most common variation is a change in a single nucleotide polymorphism (SNP), or single base pair change, in one of the building blocks of DNA.

The initial analysis yielded twenty-five candidate SNPs that were further tested in genetic samples from about seventy-seven thousand additional individuals. This step led to sixteen SNPs that were clearly associated with fasting glucose and beta cell function and two SNPs associated with fasting insulin and insulin resistance. The investigators then asked whether any of the SNPs raise type 2 diabetes risk by comparing gene variants from thousands of people with and without type 2 diabetes.

Among the five variants that raise type 2 diabetes risk, one of the more intriguing SNPs is in the region of ADCY5, which influences fasting and postprandial glucose levels. Another is in FADS1, which is linked with fasting glucose as well as lipid traits. None of the variants found in the MAGIC studies were associated with type 1 diabetes, an autoimmune disease that has been traced mainly to genes that regulate immune function.

"The hallmarks of type 2 diabetes are insulin resistance and impaired beta cell function. We were intrigued to find that most of the newly found variants influence insulin secretion rather than insulin resistance. Only one variant, near IGF1, is associated with insulin resistance," said lead author Inês Barroso, Ph.D., of the Wellcome Trust Sanger Institute, Cambridge, England.

Beta cell impairment may play a larger role in type 2 diabetes than previously recognized, the authors suggest. Also, the environment may contribute to insulin resistance more than it does to insulin secretion. Learning how the genes influence cell signaling and development, glucose sensing, and hormonal regulation will assist the development of targeted methods to prevent and treat diabetes, they conclude.

"Our study shows that genetic studies of glycemic traits can identify loci for type 2 diabetes risk," says lead co-author Jose Florez, M.D., Ph.D., of Massachusetts General Hospital and Harvard Medical School. "However, not all loci that influence blood glucose regulation are associated with greater risk for type 2 diabetes. Some loci elevate fasting glucose slightly but do not raise diabetes risk. It appears that it's not the mere elevation in glucose, but how glucose is raised, that determines type 2 diabetes risk."

In the second paper, MAGIC researchers evaluated genetic associations with glucose levels two hours after an oral glucose challenge in a subset of 15,234 participants. They found that a genetic variant in the gene GIPR, which codes for the receptor of gastric inhibitory polypeptide, a beta cell regulating hormone, influences blood glucose levels after a glucose challenge, or sugary meal. Individuals with the risk variant have reduced beta cell function.

The discovery highlights the role of incretin hormones, which are released from endocrine cells in the gut. "This finding adds to a growing body of evidence implicating the incretin pathways in type 2 diabetes risk. These pathways, which stimulate insulin secretion in response to digestion of food, may offer a potential avenue for therapeutic intervention," said senior author Richard Watanabe, Ph.D., of the University of Southern California.

The variants were found in populations of European descent, but the researchers expect that some will have similar effects in other populations. Future research will attempt to answer that question. "Even with the discovery of these variants, we've only explained about 10 percent of the genetic contribution to fasting glucose in people who do not have diabetes," Florez cautioned. Yet undiscovered genes may be found by studies that increase sample sizes to detect smaller effects and look for less common variants as well as non-SNP variants—for example, insertions, deletions, and duplications of DNA that haven't been well studied yet.

Chapter 59

Stem Cell Research

Chapter Contents

Section 59.1

Stem Cell Breakthrough Offers Diabetes Hope

Scientists have discovered a new technique for turning embryonic stem cells into insulin-producing pancreatic tissue in what could prove a significant breakthrough in the quest to find new treatments for diabetes.

The University of Manchester team, working with colleagues at the University of Sheffield, were able to genetically manipulate the stem cells so that they produced an important protein known as a "transcription factor."

Stem cells have the ability to become any type of cell, so scientists believe they may hold the key to treating a number of diseases including Alzheimer, Parkinson and diabetes.

However, a major stumbling block to developing new treatments has been the difficulty scientists have faced ensuring the stem cells turn into the type of cell required for any particular condition—in the case of diabetes, pancreatic cells.

"Unprompted, the majority of stem cells turn into simple nerve cells called neurons," explained Dr. Karen Cosgrove, who led the team in Manchester's Faculty of Life Sciences.

"Less than one percent of embryonic stem cells would normally become insulin-producing pancreatic cells, so the challenge has been to find a way of producing much greater quantities of these cells."

The pancreas contains different types of specialized cells—exocrine cells, which produce enzymes to aid digestion, and endocrine cells, including beta cells, which produce the hormone insulin to regulate the blood glucose levels. Diabetes results when there is not enough insulin to meet the body's demands.

There are two forms of the disease: type 1 diabetes is due to not enough insulin being produced by the pancreas, while type 2 or adult-onset diabetes occurs when the body fails to respond properly to the insulin that is produced.

The team found that the transcription factor PAX4 encouraged high numbers of embryonic stem cells—about 20 percent—to become pancreatic beta cells with the potential to produce insulin when transplanted into the body.

Furthermore, the scientists for the first time were able to separate the new beta cells from other types of cell produced using a technique called "fluorescent-activated cell sorting," which uses a special dye to color the pancreatic cells green.

"Research in the United States has shown that transplanting a mixture of differentiated cells and stem cells can cause cancer, so the ability to isolate the pancreatic cells in the lab is a major boost in our bid to develop a successful therapy," said Dr. Cosgrove.

"Scientists have had some success increasing the number of pancreatic cells produced by altering the environment in which the stem cells develop, so the next stage of our research will be to combine both methods to see what proportions we can achieve."

Scientists believe that transplanting functional beta cells into patients, most likely into their liver where there is a strong blood supply, offers the best hope for finding a cure for type 1 diabetes. It could also offer hope to those with type 2 diabetes whose condition requires insulin injections.

But the more immediate benefit of the team's research is likely to be in providing researchers with a ready-made supply of human pancreatic cells on which to study the disease process of diabetes and test new drugs.

The research, which was funded by the Juvenile Diabetes Research Foundation and the Medical Research Council, is published in the journal *Public Library of Science (PLoS) One*.

Section 59.2

Stem Cells Crucial to Diabetes Cure in Mice

© 2009 Baylor College of Medicine. Reprinted with permission.

More than five years ago, Dr. Lawrence C. B. Chan and colleagues in his Baylor College of Medicine (BCM) laboratory cured mice with type 1 diabetes by using a gene to induce liver cells to make insulin.

"Now we know how it works," said Chan, director of the federally designed Diabetes and Endocrinology Research Center at BCM and chief of the division of endocrinology in BCM's department of medicine. "The answer is adult stem cells."

A gene called neurogenin3 proved critical to inducing cells in the liver to produce insulin on a continuing basis, said Chan and Dr. Vijay Yechoor, assistant professor of medicine-endocrinology and first author of the report that appears in the current issue of the journal *Developmental Cell*. The research team used a disarmed virus called a vector to deliver the gene to the livers of diabetic mice by a procedure commonly known as gene therapy—enough to drop sugar levels to normal, said Yechoor.

"The mice responded within a week," said Yechoor. The levels of sugar in their blood plummeted to normal and stayed that way for the rest of their normal lives.

Two-Step Response

The quick response generated more questions as did the length of time that the animals stayed healthy.

They found that there was a two-step response. At first, the neurogenin3 gene goes into the mature liver cells and causes them to make small quantities of insulin.

"This is a transient effect," he said. "Liver cells lose the capacity to make insulin after about six weeks."

However, they found that other cells that made larger quantities of insulin showed up later, clustered around the portal veins (blood vessels that carry blood from the intestines and abdominal organs to the liver).

"They look similar to normal pancreatic islet cells (that make insulin normally)," said Yechoor.

Neurogenin3 Changes Cell Fate

They found that these "islet" cells came from a small population of adult stem cells usually found near the portal vein. Only a few are needed usually because they serve as a safety net in case of liver injury. When that occurs, they quickly activate to form mature liver cells or bile duct cells.

However, neurogenin3 changes their fates, directing them down a path to becoming insulin-producing islet cells located in the liver. The mature liver cell cannot make this change because its fate appears to be fixed before exposure to neurogenin3.

The islet cells in the liver look similar to those made by the pancreas after an injury, said Yechoor.

"If we didn't use neurogenin3, none of this would happen," he said. "Neurogenin3 is necessary and sufficient to produce these changes."

Concept Important

Chan cautioned that much more work is needed before similar results could be seen in humans. The gene therapy they undertook in the animals used a disarmed viral vector that could still have substantial toxic effects in humans.

"The concept is important because we can induce normal adult stem cells to acquire a new cell fate. It might even be applicable to regenerating other organs or tissues using a different gene from other types of adult stem cells," he said.

Finding a way to use the treatment in humans sounds easier than it is, he said. The environment in which cells grow appears to be an important part of the cell fate determination.

However, he and Yechoor plan to continue their work with the eventual goal of providing a workable treatment for people with diabetes.

Others who took part in this research include Victoria Liu, Christie Espiritu, Antoni Paul, Kazuhiro Oka, and Hideto Kojima. (Kojima is now with Shiga University of Medical Science in Otsu, Japan.)

Funding for this work came from the National Institutes of Health, the NIDDK-designated Diabetes and Endocrinology Research Center at BCM, the Betty Rutherford Chair in Diabetes Research (held by Chan), St. Luke's Episcopal Hospital, the Iacocca Foundation, and the T. T. & W. F. Chao Global Foundation.

Chapter 60

Pancreatic Islet Transplantation

What are pancreatic islets?

The pancreas, an organ about the size of a hand, is located behind the lower part of the stomach. It makes insulin and enzymes that help the body digest and use food. Throughout the pancreas are clusters of cells called the islets of Langerhans. Islets are made up of several types of cells, including beta cells that make insulin.

Insulin is a hormone that helps the body use glucose for energy. Diabetes develops when the body doesn't make enough insulin, cannot use insulin properly, or both, causing glucose to build up in the blood. In type 1 diabetes—an autoimmune disease—the beta cells of the pancreas no longer make insulin because the body's immune system has attacked and destroyed them. A person who has type 1 diabetes must take insulin daily to live. Type 2 diabetes usually begins with a condition called insulin resistance, in which the body has difficulty using insulin effectively. Over time, insulin production declines as well, so many people with type 2 diabetes eventually need to take insulin.

What is pancreatic islet transplantation?

In an experimental procedure called islet transplantation, islets are taken from the pancreas of a deceased organ donor. The islets

Reprinted from the National Institute of Diabetes and Digestive and Kidney Diseases, National Institutes of Health, NIH Publication No. 07-4693, March 2007.

are purified, processed, and transferred into another person. Once implanted, the beta cells in these islets begin to make and release insulin. Researchers hope that islet transplantation will help people with type 1 diabetes live without daily injections of insulin.

Research developments. Scientists have made many advances in islet transplantation in recent years. Since reporting their findings in the June 2000 issue of the *New England Journal of Medicine*, researchers at the University of Alberta in Edmonton, Canada, have continued to use and refine a procedure called the Edmonton protocol to transplant pancreatic islets into selected patients with type 1 diabetes that is difficult to control. In 2005, the researchers published five-year follow-up results for sixty-five patients who received transplants at their center and reported that about 10 percent of the patients remained free of the need for insulin injections at five-year follow-up. Most recipients returned to using insulin because the transplanted islets lost their ability to function over time. The researchers noted, however, that many transplant recipients were able to reduce their need for insulin, achieve better glucose stability, and reduce problems with hypoglycemia, also called low blood sugar.

In its 2006 annual report, the Collaborative Islet Transplant Registry, which is funded by the National Institute of Diabetes and Digestive and Kidney Diseases, presented data from twenty-three islet transplant programs on 225 patients who received islet transplants between 1999 and 2005. According to the report, nearly two-thirds of recipients achieved "insulin independence"—defined as being able to stop insulin injections for at least fourteen days—during the year following transplantation. However, other data from the report showed that insulin independence is difficult to maintain over time. Six months after their last infusion of islets, more than half of recipients were free of the need for insulin injections, but at two-year follow-up, the proportion dropped to about one-third of recipients. The report described other benefits of islet transplantation, including reduced need for insulin among recipients who still needed insulin, improved blood glucose control, and greatly reduced risk of episodes of severe hypoglycemia.

In a 2006 report of the Immune Tolerance Network's international islet transplantation study, researchers emphasized the value of transplantation in reversing a condition known as hypoglycemia unawareness. People with hypoglycemia unawareness are vulnerable to dangerous episodes of severe hypoglycemia because they are not able to recognize that their blood glucose levels are too low. The study showed that even partial islet function after transplant can eliminate hypoglycemia unawareness.

Transplant procedure. Researchers use specialized enzymes to remove islets from the pancreas of a deceased donor. Because the islets are fragile, transplantation occurs soon after they are removed. Typically a patient receives at least ten thousand islet "equivalents" per kilogram of body weight, extracted from two donor pancreases. Patients often require two transplants to achieve insulin independence. Some transplants have used fewer islet equivalents taken from a single donated pancreas.

Transplants are often performed by a radiologist, who uses x-rays and ultrasound to guide placement of a catheter—a small plastic tube—through the upper abdomen and into the portal vein of the liver. The islets are then infused slowly through the catheter into the liver. The patient receives a local anesthetic and a sedative. In some cases, a surgeon may perform the transplant through a small incision, using general anesthesia.

Islets begin to release insulin soon after transplantation. However, full islet function and new blood vessel growth associated with the islets take time. The doctor will order many tests to check blood glucose levels after the transplant, and insulin is usually given until the islets are fully functional.

What are the benefits and risks of islet transplantation?

The goal of islet transplantation is to infuse enough islets to control the blood glucose level without insulin injections. Other benefits may include improved glucose control and prevention of potentially dangerous episodes of hypoglycemia. Because good control of blood glucose can slow or prevent the progression of complications associated with diabetes, such as heart disease, kidney disease, and nerve or eye damage, a successful transplant may reduce the risk of these complications.

Risks of islet transplantation include the risks associated with the transplant procedure—particularly bleeding and blood clots—and side effects from the immunosuppressive drugs that transplant recipients must take to stop the immune system from rejecting the transplanted islets.

Immunosuppressive drugs. Rejection is the biggest problem with any transplant. The immune system is programmed to destroy bacteria, viruses, and tissue it recognizes as "foreign," including transplanted islets. In addition, the autoimmune response that destroyed transplant recipients' own islets in the first place can recur and attack the transplanted islets. Immunosuppressive drugs are needed to keep the transplanted islets functioning.

The Edmonton protocol introduced the use of a new combination of immunosuppressive drugs, also called anti-rejection drugs, including daclizumab (Zenapax®), sirolimus (Rapamune®), and tacrolimus (Prograf®). Daclizumab is given intravenously right after the transplant and then discontinued. Sirolimus and tacrolimus, the two main drugs that keep the immune system from destroying the transplanted islets, must be taken for life or for as long as the islets continue to function. These drugs have significant side effects and their long-term effects are still not fully known. Immediate side effects of immunosuppressive drugs may include mouth sores and gastrointestinal problems, such as stomach upset and diarrhea. Patients may also have increased blood cholesterol levels, hypertension, anemia, fatigue, decreased white blood cell counts, decreased kidney function, and increased susceptibility to bacterial and viral infections. Taking immunosuppressive drugs also increases the risk of tumors and cancer.

Researchers continue to develop and study modifications to the Edmonton protocol drug regimen, including the use of new drugs and new combinations of drugs designed to help reduce destruction of transplanted islets and promote their successful implantation. These therapies may help transplant recipients achieve better function and durability of transplanted islets with fewer side effects. The ultimate goal is to achieve immune tolerance of the transplanted islets, where the patient's immune system no longer recognizes the islets as foreign. If achieved, immune tolerance would allow patients to maintain transplanted islets without long-term immunosuppression.

Researchers are also trying to find new approaches that will allow successful transplantation without the use of immunosuppressive drugs. For example, one study is testing the transplantation of islets that are encapsulated with a special coating designed to prevent rejection.

Shortage of islets. A major obstacle to widespread use of islet transplantation is the shortage of islets. Although organs from about seven thousand deceased donors become available each year in the United States, fewer than half of the donated pancreases are suitable for whole organ pancreas transplantation or for harvesting of islets—enough for only a small percentage of those with type 1 diabetes. However, researchers are pursuing various approaches to solve this problem, such as transplanting islets from a single donated pancreas, from a portion of the pancreas of a living donor, or from pigs. Researchers have transplanted pig islets into other animals, including monkeys, by encapsulating the islets or by using drugs to prevent rejection. Another approach is creating islets from other types of cells, such as stem cells. New technologies could then be employed to grow islets in the laboratory.

Chapter 61

Artificial Pancreas

New research suggests that artificial pancreas technology can help diabetics gain greater blood sugar control overnight, even when they have eaten a big meal or had wine for dinner.

The promise of this emerging technology is to free diabetics from the need to constantly monitor their blood sugar levels by letting a computer program do the job—constantly adjusting glucose and insulin levels as needed. Using this technology is still seen as a stopgap, however, while a biological solution to diabetes is sought.

"We have pioneered the development of a closed-loop artificial pancreas because we believe it will significantly impact the lives of individuals with both type 1 and type 2 diabetes, by providing exquisite control of blood sugar," Dr. Richard A. Insel, executive vice president for research at the Juvenile Diabetes Research Foundation (JDRF), said.

For people with type 1 diabetes, controlling their blood sugar levels is a full-time job. Too much insulin can cause low blood sugar (hypoglycemia), which can be life threatening, while too little causes the serious damage of diabetes such as kidney, vision, and circulation problems.

"The promise in the near term of these technologies is not only to help us reduce significantly the risk of long-term diabetic complications, but also to reduce the risk of having a catastrophic hypoglycemic event, and further help people with diabetes live easier," Aaron Kowalski, research director of the JDRF's Artificial Pancreas Project, said.

"This will help keep people healthy while we drive toward a biological approach, which will take longer," he said.

In the first report, Dr. Roman Hovorka, a principal research associate in the department of pediatrics at the University of Cambridge, reported that the technology can significantly improve overnight blood sugar control in adults without the fear of developing hypoglycemia. With the technology, patients maintained their blood sugar levels within the target range for 70 percent of the time, compared to 47 percent of the time among those not using the technology.

Moreover, glucose control was demonstrated in real-life situations such as after a large meal and having a glass of white wine.

"We let them consume about three-quarters of a bottle of wine to simulate what happens after a large meal," Hovorka said. "What has been shown is that drinking alcohol in the evening causes hypoglycemia early in the morning."

These results were similar to findings in children where the system extended the amount of time spent at target blood sugar levels, he added. "We reduced hypoglycemia by half," he said.

"Our plan is to move into home studies, which hopefully will happen later on this year," Hovorka said.

Meanwhile, Marilyn Ritholz, a senior psychologist at the Joslin Diabetes Center and an assistant professor of psychology at the Harvard Medical School, reported on a study on psychological barriers to continuous blood sugar monitoring.

"So far, studies have not shown which factors are associated with successful or unsuccessful continuous glucose monitoring [CGM]," she said.

Ritholz's team found that people who were better at coping with the frustration of using the device were more successful at keeping their blood sugar under control.

Frustrations included warning alarms and problems at the insertion point of the device. "We found that the people who did well used a more problem-solving approach and persisted in trying to learn how to use the CGM," she said.

People who were not successful used "emotion-based coping," Ritholz said. "They easily became overwhelmed and they just gave up."

In addition, successful people had more involvement and support from their spouse or "significant other," she added. All patients felt self-conscious wearing the device, Ritholz noted.

"We know that CGM success or failure is as dependent on the human experience as it is on the perfection of the technology," she said.

Dr. William Tamborlane, chief of pediatric endocrinology at Yale University School of Medicine and co-chair of the Juvenile Diabetes

Research Foundation's Continuous Glucose Monitoring Group, said the system only works if worn almost every day.

Studies have shown that children and adults over twenty-five who used CGM were able to reduce their blood sugar levels. However, teenagers did not see a benefit, probably because they were less likely to wear the device, Tamborlane said.

People who used the device more than six days per week saw improvement, regardless of age, he added.

To get more people to use CGM, "the industry needs to come up with better systems and better devices," he said.

Artificial pancreas technology combines CGM with an insulin pump and a sophisticated computer program that controls when and how much insulin to deliver.

The device delivers two hormones that are deficient in type 1 diabetes—insulin, which keeps blood sugar levels from going too high after a meal, and glucagon, a naturally occurring hormone that prevents blood sugar levels from dropping too low.

However, the complicated computer algorithm for the pump system is still being developed.

Chapter 62

Clinical Trials and Diabetes

Chapter Contents

Section 62.1

What You Need to Know about Clinical Trials

"Understanding Clinical Trials," ClinicalTrials.gov, September 20, 2007.

What is a clinical trial?

Although there are many definitions of clinical trials, they are generally considered to be biomedical or health-related research studies in human beings that follow a pre-defined protocol. There are both interventional and observational types of studies. Interventional studies are those in which the research subjects are assigned by the investigator to a treatment or other intervention, and their outcomes are measured. Observational studies are those in which individuals are observed and their outcomes are measured by the investigators.

Why participate in a clinical trial?

Participants in clinical trials can play a more active role in their own healthcare, gain access to new research treatments before they are widely available, and help others by contributing to medical research.

Who can participate in a clinical trial?

All clinical trials have guidelines about who can participate. Using inclusion/exclusion criteria is an important principle of medical research that helps to produce reliable results. The factors that allow someone to participate in a clinical trial are called "inclusion criteria" and those that disallow someone from participating are called "exclusion criteria". These criteria are based on such factors as age, gender, the type and stage of a disease, previous treatment history, and other medical conditions. Before joining a clinical trial, a participant must qualify for the study. Some research studies seek participants with illnesses or conditions to be studied in the clinical trial, while others need healthy participants. It is important to note that inclusion and exclusion criteria are not used to reject people personally. Instead, the criteria are used to identify appropriate participants and keep them safe. The criteria help ensure that researchers will be able to answer the questions they plan to study.

What happens during a clinical trial?

The clinical trial process depends on the kind of trial being conducted. The clinical trial team includes doctors and nurses as well as social workers and other healthcare professionals. They check the health of the participant at the beginning of the trial, give specific instructions for participating in the trial, monitor the participant carefully during the trial, and stay in touch after the trial is completed.

Some clinical trials involve more tests and doctor visits than the participant would normally have for an illness or condition. For all types of trials, the participant works with a research team. Clinical trial participation is most successful when the protocol is carefully followed and there is frequent contact with the research staff.

What is informed consent?

Informed consent is the process of learning the key facts about a clinical trial before deciding whether or not to participate. It is also a continuing process throughout the study to provide information for participants. To help someone decide whether or not to participate, the doctors and nurses involved in the trial explain the details of the study. If the participant's native language is not English, translation assistance can be provided. Then the research team provides an informed consent document that includes details about the study, such as its purpose, duration, required procedures, and key contacts. Risks and potential benefits are explained in the informed consent document. The participant then decides whether or not to sign the document. Informed consent is not a contract, and the participant may withdraw from the trial at any time.

What are the benefits and risks of participating in a clinical trial?

Benefits. Clinical trials that are well designed and well executed are the best approach for eligible participants to play an active role in their own healthcare, gain access to new research treatments before they are widely available, obtain expert medical care at leading healthcare facilities during the trial, and help others by contributing to medical research.

Risks. There are risks to clinical trials. There may be unpleasant, serious, or even life-threatening side effects to experimental treatment. The experimental treatment may not be effective for the participant. The protocol may require more of their time and attention than would a nonprotocol treatment, including trips to the study site, more treatments, hospital stays or complex dosage requirements.

What are side effects and adverse reactions?

Side effects are any undesired actions or effects of the experimental drug or treatment. Negative or adverse effects may include headache, nausea, hair loss, skin irritation, or other physical problems. Experimental treatments must be evaluated for both immediate and long-term side effects.

How is the safety of the participant protected?

The ethical and legal codes that govern medical practice also apply to clinical trials. In addition, most clinical research is federally regulated with built-in safeguards to protect the participants. The trial follows a carefully controlled protocol, a study plan that details what researchers will do in the study. As a clinical trial progresses, researchers report the results of the trial at scientific meetings, to medical journals, and to various government agencies. Individual participants' names will remain secret and will not be mentioned in these reports.

What should people consider before participating in a trial?

People should know as much as possible about the clinical trial and feel comfortable asking the members of the healthcare team questions about it, the care expected while in a trial, and the cost of the trial. The following questions might be helpful for the participant to discuss with the healthcare team. Some of the answers to these questions are found in the informed consent document:

- What is the purpose of the study?
- Who is going to be in the study?
- Why do researchers believe the experimental treatment being tested may be effective? Has it been tested before?
- What kinds of tests and experimental treatments are involved?
- How do the possible risks, side effects, and benefits in the study compare with my current treatment?

- How might this trial affect my daily life?
- How long will the trial last?
- Will hospitalization be required?
- Who will pay for the experimental treatment?
- Will I be reimbursed for other expenses?
- What type of long-term follow-up care is part of this study?
- How will I know that the experimental treatment is working? Will results of the trials be provided to me?
- Who will be in charge of my care?

What kind of preparation should a potential participant make for the meeting with the research coordinator or doctor?

- Plan ahead and write down possible questions to ask.
- Ask a friend or relative to come along for support and to hear the responses to the questions.
- Bring a tape recorder to record the discussion to replay later.

Every clinical trial in the United States must be approved and monitored by an Institutional Review Board (IRB) to make sure the risks are as low as possible and are worth any potential benefits. An IRB is an independent committee of physicians, statisticians, community advocates, and others that ensures that a clinical trial is ethical and the rights of study participants are protected. All institutions that conduct or support biomedical research involving people must, by federal regulation, have an IRB that initially approves and periodically reviews the research.

Does a participant continue to work with a primary healthcare provider while in a trial?

Yes. Most clinical trials provide short-term treatments related to a designated illness or condition, but do not provide extended or complete primary healthcare. In addition, by having the healthcare provider work with the research team, the participant can ensure that other medications or treatments will not conflict with the protocol.

Can a participant leave a clinical trial after it has begun?

Yes. A participant can leave a clinical trial, at any time. When withdrawing from the trial, the participant should let the research team know about it, and the reasons for leaving the study.

Where do the ideas for trials come from?

Ideas for clinical trials usually come from researchers. After researchers test new therapies or procedures in the laboratory and in animal studies, the experimental treatments with the most promising laboratory results are moved into clinical trials. During a trial, more and more information is gained about an experimental treatment, its risks, and how well it may or may not work.

Who sponsors clinical trials?

Clinical trials are sponsored or funded by a variety of organizations or individuals such as physicians, medical institutions, foundations, voluntary groups, and pharmaceutical companies, in addition to federal agencies such as the National Institutes of Health (NIH), the Department of Defense (DOD), and the Department of Veteran's Affairs (VA). Trials can take place in a variety of locations, such as hospitals, universities, doctors' offices, or community clinics.

What is a protocol?

A protocol is a study plan on which all clinical trials are based. The plan is carefully designed to safeguard the health of the participants as well as answer specific research questions. A protocol describes what types of people may participate in the trial; the schedule of tests, procedures, medications, and dosages; and the length of the study. While in a clinical trial, participants following a protocol are seen regularly by the research staff to monitor their health and to determine the safety and effectiveness of their treatment.

What is a placebo?

A placebo is an inactive pill, liquid, or powder that has no treatment value. In clinical trials, experimental treatments are often compared with placebos to assess the experimental treatment's effectiveness. In some studies, the participants in the control group will receive a placebo instead of an active drug or experimental treatment.

What is a control or control group?

A control is the standard by which experimental observations are evaluated. In many clinical trials, one group of patients will be given an experimental drug or treatment, while the control group is given either a standard treatment for the illness or a placebo.

What are the different types of clinical trials?

Treatment trials test experimental treatments, new combinations of drugs, or new approaches to surgery or radiation therapy.

Prevention trials look for better ways to prevent disease in people who have never had the disease or to prevent a disease from returning. These approaches may include medicines, vaccines, vitamins, minerals, or lifestyle changes.

Diagnostic trials are conducted to find better tests or procedures for diagnosing a particular disease or condition.

Screening trials test the best way to detect certain diseases or health conditions.

Quality of life trials (or supportive care trials) explore ways to improve comfort and the quality of life for individuals with a chronic illness.

What are the phases of clinical trials?

Clinical trials are conducted in phases. The trials at each phase have a different purpose and help scientists answer different questions.

In Phase I trials, researchers test an experimental drug or treatment in a small group of people (twenty to eighty people) for the first time to evaluate its safety, determine a safe dosage range, and identify side effects.

In Phase II trials, the experimental study drug or treatment is given to a larger group of people (one hundred to three hundred people) to see if it is effective and to further evaluate its safety.

In Phase III trials, the experimental study drug or treatment is given to large groups of people (one thousand to three thousand people) to confirm its effectiveness, monitor side effects, compare it to commonly used treatments, and collect information that will allow the experimental drug or treatment to be used safely.

In Phase IV trials, post-marketing studies delineate additional information including the drug's risks, benefits, and optimal use.

What is "expanded access"?

Expanded access is a means by which manufacturers make investigational new drugs available, under certain circumstances, to treat a patient(s) with a serious disease or condition who cannot participate in a controlled clinical trial.

Most human use of investigational new drugs takes place in controlled clinical trials conducted to assess the safety and efficacy of new drugs. Data from these trials are used to determine whether a drug is safe and effective, and serve as the basis for the drug marketing application. Sometimes, patients do not qualify for these controlled trials because of other health problems, age, or other factors, or are otherwise unable to enroll in such trials (e.g., a patient may not live sufficiently close to a clinical trial site).

For patients who cannot participate in a clinical trial of an investigational drug, but have a serious disease or condition that may benefit from treatment with the drug, U.S. Food and Drug Association (FDA) regulations enable manufacturers of such drugs to provide those patients access to the drug under certain situations, known as "expanded access." For example, the drug cannot expose patients to unreasonable risks given the severity of the disease to be treated and the patient does not have any other satisfactory therapeutic options (e.g., an approved drug that could be used to treat the patient's disease or condition). The manufacturer must be willing to make the drug available for expanded access use. The primary intent of expanded access is to provide treatment for a patient's disease or condition, rather than to collect data about the study drug.

Some investigational drugs are available for treatment use from pharmaceutical manufacturers through expanded access programs listed in ClinicalTrials.gov. If you or a loved one is interested in treatment with an investigational drug under an expanded access protocol listed in ClinicalTrials.gov, review the protocol eligibility criteria and inquire at the Contact Information number. If there is not an expanded access protocol listed in ClinicalTrials.gov, you or your healthcare provider may contact a manufacturer of an investigational drug directly to ask about expanded access programs.

Section 62.2

Clinical Research in Diabetes

Many people think of clinical trials when they hear the term "clinical research," but in fact trials are only one aspect of what the term means. Clinical research describes many different elements of scientific investigation. Simply put, it involves human subjects and helps translate basic research (done in labs) into new treatments and information to benefit patients. In addition to clinical trials, some research in epidemiology, physiology and pathophysiology, health services, education, outcomes, and mental health can all fall under the clinical research umbrella.

Clinical Research and Diabetes

There is still a lot that researchers do not know about type 1 diabetes and type 2 diabetes. Much research begins in animal models such as worms, zebra fish, and mice, but clinical research is necessary in order to determine how much of this research also applies to humans. It advances the basic research from the lab bench to the bedside, in order to benefit people living with or at risk for diabetes. Clinical research is desirable for study participants because through participation they can benefit from the newest, most cutting-edge diabetes approaches and products.

Clinical research helps explain:

- how and why diabetes develops;
- genetic and environmental factors that may play a role;
- the success of education programs and health services programs to improve diabetes care and self-management;
- possible avenues to prevent diabetes;
- what new products and medications are most beneficial;
- how to prevent or reverse diabetes complications.

Researchers Are Searching for Answers

- Why does diabetes run in families? What factors cause some people to develop diabetes while others do not?

- What physical differences exist between people with diabetes and those without?

- How do diabetes complications develop and how effective are attempts to prevent them through medication, education, or health services?

- How can patients achieve better long-term diabetes management success through new education programs?

- Does brain chemistry change when someone develops diabetes? Do these changes result in mood disorders or make self-management more difficult?

Part Eight

Additional Help and Information

Chapter 63

Glossary of Terms Related to Diabetes

acanthosis nigricans: A skin condition characterized by darkened skin patches; common in those with insulin resistance.

angiotensin-converting enzyme (ACE) inhibitor: An oral medicine that lowers blood pressure. It also helps slow down kidney damage in diabetics.

albumin: The main protein in blood. People who are developing diabetic kidney disease leak small amounts of albumin into the urine. As the amount of albumin in the urine increases, the kidneys' ability to filter the blood decreases.

albuminuria: A condition in which the urine has more than normal amounts of a protein called albumin.

alpha cell: A type of cell in the pancreas that makes and releases a hormone called glucagons, which tells the liver to release glucose into the blood for energy.

alpha-glucosidase inhibitor: A class of oral medicine for type 2 diabetes that slows down the digestion of foods high in carbohydrate. The result is a slower and lower rise in blood glucose after meals.

Excerpted from "The Diabetes Dictionary," National Institute of Diabetes and Digestive and Kidney Diseases, National Institutes of Health, NIH Publication No. 10-3016, December 2009.

amylin: A hormone formed by beta cells in the pancreas that regulates the timing of glucose release into the bloodstream after eating by slowing the emptying of the stomach.

amylin mimetic: A type of injectable medicine for diabetes that mimics the effect of the hormone amylin.

amyotrophy: A type of neuropathy resulting in pain, weakness, or wasting in the muscles.

A1C: A test that measures a person's average blood glucose level over the past two to three months.

angiotensin receptor blocker (ARB): An oral medicine that lowers blood pressure. It also helps slow down kidney damage in diabetics.

autoimmune disease: A disorder of the body's immune system in which the immune system mistakenly attacks and destroys body tissue that it believes to be foreign.

autonomic neuropathy: A type of neuropathy affecting the lungs, heart, stomach, intestines, bladder, or genitals.

beta cell: A cell that makes insulin. Beta cells are located in the islets of the pancreas.

biguanide: A class of oral medicine used to treat type 2 diabetes that lowers blood glucose by reducing the amount of glucose produced by the liver. Also used to treat insulin resistance.

blood glucose: The main sugar found in the blood and the body's main source of energy. Also called blood sugar.

blood glucose level: The amount of glucose in a given amount of blood. In the United States, blood glucose levels are noted in milligrams per deciliter, or mg/dL.

blood glucose meter: A small, portable machine used by people with diabetes to check their blood glucose levels.

blood urea nitrogen (BUN): A waste product in the blood from the breakdown of protein. As kidney function decreases, the BUN level increases.

body mass index (BMI): A measure used to evaluate body weight relative to a person's height. BMI is used to find out if a person is underweight, normal weight, overweight, or obese.

bolus: An extra amount of insulin taken to cover an expected rise in blood glucose, often related to a meal or snack.

brittle diabetes: A term used when a person's blood glucose level moves often from low to high and from high to low.

carbohydrate: One of the three main nutrients in food. Foods that provide carbohydrate are starches, vegetables, fruits, dairy products, and sugars.

carbohydrate counting: A method of meal planning for people with diabetes based on counting the number of grams of carbohydrate in food.

combination diabetes pill: A pill that includes two or more different medicines.

combination therapy: The use of different medicines together to manage blood glucose levels.

continuous glucose monitoring system (CGMS): A small sensor inserted below the skin that measures blood glucose levels approximately twelve times per hour.

creatinine: A waste product from meat protein in the diet and from the muscles of the body. As kidney disease progresses, the level of creatinine in the blood increases.

creatinine clearance: A test that measures how efficiently the kidneys remove creatinine and other wastes from the blood.

dawn phenomenon: The early-morning (4 a.m. to 8 a.m.) rise in blood glucose.

dextrose: Simple sugar found in blood that serves as the body's main source of energy. Also called glucose.

diabetes insipidus: A condition characterized by frequent and heavy urination, excessive thirst, and an overall feeling of weakness. This condition may be caused by a defect in the pituitary gland or in the kidney. In diabetes insipidus, blood glucose levels are normal.

diabetic ketoacidosis: An emergency condition in which extremely high blood glucose levels, along with a severe lack of insulin, result in the breakdown of body fat for energy and an accumulation of ketones in the blood and urine. Untreated DKA can lead to coma and death.

diabetic myelopathy: Damage to the spinal cord found in some people with diabetes.

diabetic retinopathy: Damage to the small blood vessels in the retina. Loss of vision may result. Also called diabetic eye disease.

dialysis: The process of cleaning wastes from the blood artificially. The two major forms of dialysis are hemodialysis and peritoneal dialysis.

exchange lists: One of several approaches for diabetes meal planning. Foods are categorized into three groups based on their nutritional content. Lists provide the serving sizes for carbohydrates, meat and meat substitutes, and fats. These lists allow for substitution for different groups to keep the nutritional content fixed.

fasting blood glucose test: A check of a person's blood glucose level after the person has not eaten for eight to twelve hours—usually overnight.

fructosamine test: A test that measures the number of blood glucose molecules linked to protein molecules in the blood and provides information about a person's average blood glucose level for the previous three weeks.

gastroparesis: A form of neuropathy that affects the stomach. Digestion of food may be incomplete or delayed, resulting in nausea, vomiting, or bloating, making blood glucose control difficult.

gestational diabetes mellitus: A type of diabetes that develops only during pregnancy and usually disappears upon delivery, but increases the mother's risk of developing diabetes later in life.

glaucoma: An increase in fluid pressure inside the eye that may lead to vision loss.

glomerular filtration rate (GFR): The rate at which the kidneys filter wastes and extra fluid from the blood, measured in milliliters per minute.

glucagon: A hormone produced by the alpha cells in the pancreas that raises blood glucose.

glucose: One of the simplest forms of sugar.

glucose gel: Pure glucose in gel form used for treating hypoglycemia.

glucose tablets: Chewable tablets made of pure glucose used for treating hypoglycemia.

glycemic index: A ranking of carbohydrate-containing foods, based on the food's effect on blood glucose compared with a standard reference food.

glycemic load: A ranking of a carbohydrate-containing food, based on the food's glycemic index and the amount of carbohydrate in a typical serving.

glycogen: The form of glucose found in the liver and muscles; the main source of stored fuel in the body.

glycosuria: The presence of glucose in the urine.

hyperglycemia: Higher than normal blood glucose.

hyperinsulinemia: A condition in which the level of insulin in the blood is higher than normal.

hyperlipidemia: Higher than normal fat and cholesterol levels in the blood.

hyperosmolar hyperglycemic nonketotic syndrome (HHNS): An emergency condition in which one's blood glucose level is very high and ketones are not present in the blood or urine. If HHNS is not treated, it can lead to coma or death.

hypertension: A condition present when blood flows through the blood vessels with a force greater than normal. Also called high blood pressure.

hypoglycemia: Also called low blood glucose, a condition that occurs when one's blood glucose is lower than normal, usually below 70 mg/dL. If left untreated, hypoglycemia may lead to unconsciousness.

hypoglycemia unawareness: A state in which a person does not feel or recognize the symptoms of hypoglycemia.

hypotension: Low blood pressure or a sudden drop in blood pressure.

immunosuppressant: A drug given to stop the natural responses of the body's immune system, used in people who have received organ transplants and patients with autoimmune diseases.

impaired fasting glucose (IFG): A condition in which a fasting blood glucose test shows a level of glucose higher than normal but not high enough for a diagnosis of diabetes. IFG, also called pre-diabetes, is a level of 100 to 125 mg/dL.

impaired glucose tolerance (IGT): A condition in which blood glucose levels are higher than normal but are not high enough for a diagnosis of diabetes. IGT, also called pre-diabetes, is a level of 140 to 199 mg/dL two hours after the start of an oral glucose tolerance test.

implantable insulin pump: A small pump placed inside the body to deliver insulin in response to remote-control commands from the user.

inhaled insulin: A type of insulin under development taken with a special device that enables the user to breathe in insulin through the mouth.

insulin: A hormone that helps the body use glucose for energy. The beta cells of the pancreas make insulin. When the body cannot make enough insulin, insulin is taken by injection or other means.

insulin infuser: A device for taking insulin in which a small tube is inserted just below the skin and remains in place for several days. Insulin is injected into the end of the tube.

insulin pen: A device for injecting insulin that looks like a fountain pen and holds replaceable cartridges of insulin.

insulin pump: An insulin-delivering device about the size of a deck of cards that can be worn on a belt or kept in a pocket. An insulin pump connects to narrow, flexible plastic tubing that ends with a needle inserted just under the skin. Users set the pump to give a steady trickle or basal amount of insulin continuously throughout the day. Pumps release bolus doses of insulin at meals and at times when blood glucose is too high, based on doses set by the user.

insulin resistance: The body's inability to respond to and use the insulin it produces.

intensive therapy: A treatment for diabetes in which blood glucose is kept as close to normal as possible.

intermediate-acting insulin: A type of insulin with an onset of one to three hours, a peak at eight hours, and a duration of twelve to sixteen hours.

islets: Groups of cells located in the pancreas that make hormones that help the body break down and use food.

islet transplantation: Moving the islets from a donor pancreas into a person whose pancreas has stopped producing insulin.

jet injector: A device that uses high pressure instead of a needle to propel insulin through the skin and into the body.

ketone: A chemical produced when there is a shortage of insulin in the blood and the body breaks down body fat for energy. High levels of ketones can lead to diabetic ketoacidosis and coma.

ketonuria: A condition occurring when ketones are present in the urine, a warning sign of diabetic ketoacidosis.

ketosis: A ketone buildup in the body that may lead to diabetic ketoacidosis.

lactic acidosis: A serious condition in which there is a buildup of lactic acid in the body.

lancet: A spring-loaded device used to prick the skin with a small needle to obtain a drop of blood for blood glucose monitoring.

long-acting insulin: A type of insulin with an onset of one hour, no peak, and a duration of twenty to twenty-six hours.

maturity-onset diabetes of the young (MODY): A monogenic form of diabetes that usually first occurs during adolescence or early adulthood.

metabolic syndrome: A grouping of health conditions associated with an increased risk for heart disease and type 2 diabetes. Conditions include hypertension, a large waist, high triglyceride levels, low high-density lipoprotein (HDL) cholesterol levels, and above-normal blood glucose levels. Metabolic syndrome was previously called Syndrome X.

mixed dose: A combination of two types of insulin in one injection. Usually a rapid- or short-acting insulin is combined with a longer-acting insulin to provide both short- and long-term control of blood glucose levels.

neonatal diabetes mellitus: A rare, monogenic form of diabetes that occurs in the first six months of life.

nephropathy: Disease of the kidneys.

neuropathy: Disease of the nervous system. The three major forms in people with diabetes are peripheral neuropathy, autonomic neuropathy, and mononeuropathy.

oral glucose tolerance test (OGTT): A test to diagnose prediabetes and diabetes, given after an overnight fast. Test results show how the body uses glucose over time.

oral hypoglycemic agents: Medicines taken by mouth by people with type 2 diabetes to keep blood glucose levels as close to normal as possible.

pancreas: An organ that makes insulin and enzymes for digestion. The pancreas is located behind the lower part of the stomach and is about the size of a hand.

pancreas transplantation: A surgical procedure to take a healthy whole or partial pancreas from a donor and place it into a person with diabetes.

pen injector: A pen-like device for injecting insulin; contains a needle and a cartridge of insulin.

peripheral neuropathy: Nerve damage that affects the feet, legs, or hands. Peripheral neuropathy causes pain, numbness, or a tingling feeling.

polydipsia: Excessive thirst; may be a sign of diabetes.

polyphagia: Excessive hunger; may be a sign of diabetes.

polyuria: Excessive urination; may be a sign of diabetes.

postprandial blood glucose: The blood glucose level one to two hours after eating.

prediabetes: A condition in which blood glucose levels are higher than normal but are not high enough for a diagnosis of diabetes.

preprandial blood glucose: The blood glucose level before eating.

proteinuria: A condition in which the urine contains large amounts of protein, a sign that the kidneys are not working properly.

rapid-acting insulin: A type of insulin with an onset of fifteen minutes, a peak at thirty to ninety minutes, and a duration of three to five hours.

renal threshold of glucose: The blood glucose concentration at which the kidneys start to excrete glucose into the urine.

secondary diabetes: A type of diabetes caused by another disease or certain drugs or chemicals.

short-acting insulin: A type of insulin with an onset of thirty to sixty minutes, a peak at two to four hours, and a duration of five to eight hours.

Somogyi effect: When the blood glucose level swings high following low blood glucose, or hypoglycemia.

sulfonylurea: A class of oral medicine for type 2 diabetes that lowers blood glucose by helping the pancreas make more insulin and by helping the body better use the insulin it makes.

type 1 diabetes: A condition characterized by high blood glucose levels caused by a total lack of insulin. Occurs when the body's immune system attacks the insulin-producing beta cells in the pancreas and destroys them.

type 2 diabetes: A condition characterized by high blood glucose levels caused by either a lack of insulin or the body's inability to use insulin efficiently.

Chapter 64

Recipes for People with Diabetes and Their Families

What Is Diabetes?

Diabetes means that your blood glucose (blood sugar) is too high. Glucose comes from the food we eat. An organ called the pancreas makes insulin. Insulin helps glucose get from your blood into your cells. Cells take the glucose and turn it into energy.

When you have diabetes, your body has a problem making or properly using insulin. As a result, glucose builds up in your blood and cannot get into your cells. If the blood glucose stays too high, it can damage your body.

What Are the Symptoms of Diabetes?

Common symptoms of diabetes include the following:

• Having to urinate often

• Being very thirsty

• Feeling very hungry or tired

• Losing weight without trying

But many people with diabetes have no symptoms at all.

Excerpted from "Tasty Recipes for People with Diabetes and Their Families," National Diabetes Education Program, September 2008.

Why Should I Be Concerned about Diabetes?

Diabetes is a very serious disease. Do not be misled by phrases that suggest diabetes is not a serious disease, such as "a touch of sugar," "borderline diabetes," or "my blood glucose is a little bit high."

Diabetes can lead to other serious health problems. When high levels of glucose in the blood are not controlled, they can slowly damage your eyes, heart, kidneys, nerves, and feet.

What Are the Types of Diabetes?

There are three main types of diabetes:

- **Type 1 diabetes:** In this type of diabetes, the body does not make insulin. People with type 1 diabetes need to take insulin every day.

- **Type 2 diabetes:** In this type of diabetes, the body does not make enough insulin or use insulin well. Some people with type 2 diabetes have to take diabetes pills, insulin, or both. Type 2 diabetes is the most common form of diabetes.

- **Gestational diabetes:** This type of diabetes can occur when a woman is pregnant. It raises the risk that both she and her child might develop diabetes later in life.

You Can Control Diabetes

Diabetes can be managed. You can successfully manage diabetes and avoid the serious health problems it can cause if you follow these steps:

- Ask your doctor how you can learn more about your diabetes to help you feel better today and in the future.

- Make healthy food choices and be physically active most days. Following this advice will help you keep off extra pounds and will also help keep your blood glucose under control.

- Check your blood glucose as your doctor tells you to.

- If you are taking diabetes medications, take them even if you feel well.

- To avoid problems with your diabetes, see your healthcare team at least twice a year. Finding and treating any problems early will prevent them from getting worse. Ask how diabetes can affect your eyes, heart, kidneys, nerves, legs, and feet.

- Be actively involved in your diabetes care. Work with your healthcare team to come up with a plan for making healthy food choices and being active—a plan that you can stick to.

Creating a Healthy Meal Plan

This chapter is a place to start creating healthy meals. Ask your doctor to refer you to a registered dietitian or a diabetes educator who can help you create a meal plan for you and your family. The dietitian will work with you to come up with a meal plan tailored to your needs. Your meal plan will take into account things like the following:

- Your blood glucose levels
- Your weight
- Medicines you take
- Other health problems you have
- How physically active you are

Making Healthy Food Choices

Eat smaller portions. Learn what a serving size is for different foods and how many servings you need in a meal.

Eat less fat. Choose fewer high-fat foods and use less fat for cooking. You especially want to limit foods that are high in saturated fats or trans fat, such as the following:

- Fatty cuts of meat
- Whole milk and dairy products made from whole milk
- Cakes, candy, cookies, crackers, and pies
- Fried foods
- Salad dressings
- Lard, shortening, stick margarine, and nondairy creamers

Eat more fiber by eating more whole-grain foods. Whole grains can be found in the following foods:

- Breakfast cereals made with 100 percent whole grains

- Oatmeal

- Whole grain rice

- Whole-wheat bread, bagels, pita bread, and tortillas

Eat a variety of fruits and vegetables every day. Choose fresh, frozen, canned, or dried fruit and 100 percent fruit juices most of the time. Eat plenty of veggies like these:

- Dark green veggies (e.g., broccoli, spinach, brussels sprouts)

- Orange veggies (e.g., carrots, sweet potatoes, pumpkin, winter squash)

- Beans and peas (e.g., black beans, garbanzo beans, kidney beans, pinto beans, split peas, lentils)

Eat fewer foods that are high in sugar, such as the following:

- Fruit-flavored drinks

- Sodas

- Tea or coffee sweetened with sugar

Use less salt in cooking and at the table. Eat fewer foods that are high in salt, such as the following:

- Canned and package soups

- Canned vegetables

- Pickles

- Processed meats

Never skip meals. Stick to your meal plan as best you can.
Limit the amount of alcohol you drink.
Make changes slowly. It takes time to achieve lasting goals.
Following a meal plan that is made for you will help you feel better, keep your blood glucose levels in your target range, take in the right amount of calories, and get enough nutrients.
Note: There are several ways to make a diabetes meal plan. One popular and flexible approach is the Exchange Program method, which provides a quick way to estimate energy, carbohydrates, protein, and fat content in any food or meal. Food from each exchange (starch, meat and meat substitute, fruit, vegetable, milk, and fat) is defined so that

one serving of each food contains the same amount of carbohydrate, protein, fat, and energy (calories). Another method is carbohydrate counting. Using this method, you focus on eating a specific number of carbohydrates at specific times of the day.

Spanish Omelet / Tortilla española

This tasty dish provides a healthy array of vegetables and can be used for breakfast, brunch, or any meal! Serve with fresh fruit salad and a whole-grain dinner roll.

Ingredients

5 small potatoes, peeled and sliced

Vegetable cooking spray

1/2 medium onion, minced

1 small zucchini, sliced

1 1/2 cups green/red peppers, sliced thin

5 medium mushrooms, sliced

3 whole eggs, beaten

5 egg whites, beaten

Pepper and garlic salt with herbs, to taste

3 ounces shredded part-skim mozzarella cheese

1 Tbsp. low-fat parmesan cheese

Directions

- Preheat oven to 375° F.
- Cook potatoes in boiling water until tender.
- In a nonstick pan, add vegetable spray and warm at medium heat.
- Add onion and sauté until brown. Add vegetables and sauté until tender but not brown.
- In a medium mixing bowl, slightly beat eggs and egg whites, pepper, garlic salt, and low-fat mozzarella cheese. Stir egg-cheese mixture into the cooked vegetables.

- In a ten-inch pie pan or ovenproof skillet, add vegetable spray and transfer potatoes and egg mixture to pan. Sprinkle with low-fat parmesan cheese and bake until firm and brown on top, about twenty to thirty minutes.

- Remove omelet from oven, cool for ten minutes, and cut into five pieces.

Exchanges

Meat 2

Bread 2

Vegetable 2/3

Fat 2

Note: Diabetic exchanges are calculated based on the American Diabetes Association Exchange System.

Nutrition Facts	
Spanish Omelet	
Serving Size $\frac{1}{5}$ of omelet	
Amount Per Serving	
Calories	Calories from Fat
260	90
% Daily Value (DV)*	
Total Fat 10g	**15%**
Saturated Fat 3.5g	**18%**
Trans Fat 0g	
Cholesterol 135mg	**45%**
Sodium 240mg	**10%**
Total Carbohydrate 30g	**10%**
Dietary Fiber 3g	**12%**
Sugars 3g	
Protein 16g	
Vitamin A	8%
Vitamin C	60%
Calcium	15%
Iron	8%
* Percent Daily Values are based on a 2,000 calorie diet.	

Figure 64.1. Nutrition Facts Label, Spanish Omelet

Beef or Turkey Stew / Carne de res o de pavo guisada

This dish goes nicely with a green leaf lettuce and cucumber salad and a dinner roll. Plantains or corn can be used in place of the potatoes.

Ingredients

1 pound lean beef or turkey breast, cut into cubes

2 Tbsp. whole-wheat flour

1/4 tsp. salt (optional)

1/4 tsp. pepper

1/4 tsp. cumin

1 1/2 Tbsp. olive oil

2 cloves garlic, minced

2 medium onions, sliced

2 stalks celery, sliced

1 medium red/green bell pepper, sliced

1 medium tomato, finely minced

5 cups beef or turkey broth, fat removed

5 small potatoes, peeled and cubed

12 small carrots, cut into large chunks

1 1/4 cups green peas

Directions

- Preheat oven to 375° F.
- Mix the whole-wheat flour with salt, pepper, and cumin. Roll the beef or turkey cubes in the mixture. Shake off excess flour.
- In a large skillet, heat olive oil over medium-high heat. Add beef or turkey cubes and sauté until nicely brown, about seven to ten minutes.
- Place beef or turkey in an ovenproof casserole dish.
- Add minced garlic, onions, celery, and peppers to skillet and cook until vegetables are tender, about five minutes.

- Stir in tomato and broth. Bring to a boil and pour over turkey or beef in casserole dish. Cover dish tightly and bake for one hour at 375° F.

- Remove from oven and stir in potatoes, carrots, and peas. Bake for another twenty to twenty-five minutes or until tender.

Exchanges

Lean Meat 3

Vegetable 2 1/3

Bread 2 2/3

Fat 1

Note: Diabetic exchanges are calculated based on the American Diabetes Association Exchange System.

Nutrition Facts	
Beef or Turkey Stew	
Serving Size 1½ cup	
Amount Per Serving	
Calories	Calories from Fat
320	60
% Daily Value (DV)*	
Total Fat 7g	**11%**
Saturated Fat 1.5g	**8%**
Trans Fat 0g	
Cholesterol 40mg	**13%**
Sodium 520mg	**22%**
Total Carbohydrate 41g	**14%**
Dietary Fiber 8g	**32%**
Sugars 9g	
Protein 24g	
Vitamin A	340%
Vitamin C	80%
Calcium	6%
Iron	15%
* Percent Daily Values are based on a 2,000 calorie diet.	

Figure 64.2. *Nutrition Facts Label, Beef or Turkey Stew*

Caribbean Red Snapper / *Pargo rojo caribeño*

This fish can be served on top of vegetables along with whole-grain rice and garnished with parsley. Salmon or chicken breast can be used in place of red snapper.

Ingredients

2 Tbsp. olive oil

1 medium onion, chopped

1/2 cup red pepper, chopped

1/2 cup carrots, cut into strips

1 clove garlic, minced

1/2 cup dry white wine

3/4 pound red snapper fillet

1 large tomato, chopped

2 Tbsp. pitted ripe olives, chopped

2 Tbsp. crumbled low-fat feta or low-fat ricotta cheese

Directions

- In a large skillet, heat olive oil over medium heat. Add onion, red pepper, carrots, and garlic. Sauté mixture for ten minutes. Add wine and bring to boil. Push vegetables to one side of the pan.

- Arrange fillets in a single layer in center of skillet. Cover and cook for five minutes.

- Add tomato and olives. Top with cheese. Cover and cook for three minutes or until fish is firm but moist.

- Transfer fish to serving platter. Garnish with vegetables and pan juices.

- Serving Suggestion: Serve with whole grain rice. One-half cup cooked rice equals one serving of rice.

Exchanges

Meat 2 1/3

Vegetable 1 1/4

Bread 1/2

Fat 2

Note: Diabetic exchanges are calculated based on the American Diabetes Association Exchange System.

Nutrition Facts	
Caribbean Red Snapper	
Serving Size ¼ red snapper with ½ cup vegetables (233g)	
Amount Per Serving	
Calories 220	Calories from Fat 80
	% Daily Value (DV)*
Total Fat 10g	**15%**
Saturated Fat 2g	**10%**
Trans Fat 0g	
Cholesterol 35mg	**12%**
Sodium 160mg	**7%**
Total Carbohydrate 8g	**3%**
Dietary Fiber 2g	**8%**
Sugars 4g	
Protein 19g	
Vitamin A	80%
Vitamin C	70%
Calcium	8%
Iron	4%
* Percent Daily Values are based on a 2,000 calorie diet.	

Figure 64.3. *Nutrition Facts Label, Caribbean Red Snapper*

Two Cheese Pizza / Pizza de dos quesos

Serve your pizza with fresh fruit and a mixed green salad garnished with red beans to balance your meal.

Ingredients

2 Tbsp. whole wheat flour

1 can (10 ounces) refrigerated pizza crust

Vegetable cooking spray

2 Tbsp. olive oil

1/2 cup low-fat ricotta cheese

1/2 tsp. dried basil

1 small onion, minced

2 cloves garlic, minced

1/4 tsp. salt (optional)

4 ounces shredded part-skim mozzarella cheese

2 cups mushrooms, chopped

1 large red pepper, cut into strips

Directions

- Preheat oven to 425° F.

- Spread whole wheat flour over working surface. Roll out dough with rolling pin to desired crust thickness.

- Coat cookie sheet with vegetable cooking spray. Transfer pizza crust to cookie sheet. Brush olive oil over crust.

- Mix low-fat ricotta cheese with dried basil, onion, garlic, and salt. Spread this mixture over crust.

- Sprinkle crust with part-skim mozzarella cheese. Top cheese with mushrooms and red pepper.

- Bake at 425° F for thirteen to fifteen minutes or until cheese melts and crust is deep golden brown.

Nutrition Facts	
Two Cheese Pizza	
Serving Size 2 slices (¼ of pie)	
Amount Per Serving	
Calories 420	Calories from Fat 170
% Daily Value (DV)*	
Total Fat 19g	**29%**
Saturated Fat 7g	**35%**
Trans Fat 0g	
Cholesterol 25mg	**8%**
Sodium 580mg	**24%**
Total Carbohydrate 44g	**15%**
Dietary Fiber 3g	**12%**
Sugars 5g	
Protein 20g	
Vitamin A	30%
Vitamin C	90%
Calcium	40%
Iron	15%
* Percent Daily Values are based on a 2,000 calorie diet.	

Figure 64.4. *Nutrition Facts Label, Two Cheese Pizza*

- Cut into eight slices.

Exchanges

Meat 2 1/2

Bread 3

Vegetable 1

Fat 3 3/4

Note: Diabetic exchanges are calculated based on the American Diabetes Association Exchange System.

Rice with Chicken, Spanish Style / Arroz con pollo

This is a good way to get vegetables into the meal plan. Serve with a mixed green salad and some whole wheat bread.

Ingredients

2 Tbsp. olive oil

2 medium onions, chopped

6 cloves garlic, minced

2 stalks celery, diced

2 medium red/green peppers, cut into strips

1 cup mushrooms, chopped

2 cups uncooked whole-grain rice

3 pounds boneless chicken breast, cut into bite-sized pieces, skin removed

1 1/2 tsp. salt (optional)

2 1/2 cups low-fat chicken broth

Saffron or Sazón® for color

3 medium tomatoes, chopped

1 cup frozen peas

1 cup frozen corn

1 cup frozen green beans

Olives or capers for garnish (optional)

Directions

- Heat olive oil over medium heat in a nonstick pot. Add onion, garlic, celery, red/green pepper, and mushrooms. Cook over medium heat, stirring often, for three minutes or until tender.

- Add whole-grain rice and sauté for two to three minutes, stirring constantly to mix all ingredients.

- Add chicken, salt, chicken broth, water, Saffron/Sazón, and tomatoes. Bring water to a boil.

- Reduce heat to medium-low, cover, and let the casserole simmer until water is absorbed and rice is tender, about twenty minutes.

- Stir in peas, corn, and beans and cook for eight to ten minutes. When everything is hot, the casserole is ready to serve. Garnish with olives or capers, if desired.

Exchanges

Meat 5 1/3

Bread 3

Vegetable 1

Fat 1 1/3

Nutrition Facts	
Rice with Chicken, Spanish Style	
Serving Size 1½ cup	
Amount Per Serving	
Calories	Calories from Fat
400	60
% Daily Value (DV)*	
Total Fat 7g	**11%**
Saturated Fat 1.5g	**8%**
Trans Fat 0g	
Cholesterol 85mg	**28%**
Sodium 530mg	**22%**
Total Carbohydrate 46g	**15%**
Dietary Fiber 3g	**12%**
Sugars 5g	
Protein 37g	
Vitamin A	30%
Vitamin C	70%
Calcium	4%
Iron	20%
* Percent Daily Values are based on a 2,000 calorie diet.	

Figure 64.5. *Nutrition Facts Label, Rice with Chicken, Spanish Style*

Pozole

Only a small amount of oil is needed to sauté meat.

Ingredients

2 pounds lean beef, cubed

1 Tbsp. olive oil

1 large onion, chopped

1 clove garlic, finely chopped

1/4 tsp. salt

1/8 tsp. pepper

1/4 cup fresh cilantro, chopped

1 can (15 ounces) stewed tomatoes

2 ounces tomato paste

1 can (1 pound 13 ounces) hominy

Directions

- In a large pot, heat olive oil. Add beef and sauté.
- Add onion, garlic, salt, pepper, cilantro, and enough water to cover meat. Stir to mix ingredients evenly. Cover pot and cook over low heat until meat is tender.
- Add tomatoes and tomato paste. Continue cooking for about twenty minutes.
- Add hominy and continue cooking another fifteen minutes, stirring occasionally. If too thick, add water for desired consistency.
- Option: Skinless, boneless chicken breasts can be used instead of beef cubes.

Exchanges

Meat 3

Bread 1

Vegetable 1/2

Fat 1 1/3

Note: Diabetic exchanges are calculated based on the American Diabetes Association Exchange System.

Nutrition Facts	
Pozole	
Serving Size 1 cup	
Amount Per Serving	
Calories 220	Calories from Fat 70
	% Daily Value (DV)*
Total Fat 7g	**11%**
Saturated Fat 2g	**10%**
Trans Fat 0g	
Cholesterol 70mg	**23%**
Sodium 390mg	**16%**
Total Carbohydrate 17g	**6%**
Dietary Fiber 3g	**12%**
Sugars 5g	
Protein 21g	
Vitamin A	4%
Vitamin C	10%
Calcium	4%
Iron	15%
* Percent Daily Values are based on a 2,000 calorie diet.	

Figure 64.6. Nutrition Facts Label, Pozole

Avocado Tacos / Tacos de aguacate

Ingredients

1 medium onion, cut into thin strips

2 large green peppers, cut into thin strips

2 large red peppers, cut into thin strips

1 cup fresh cilantro, finely chopped

1 ripe avocado, peeled and seeded, cut into 12 slices

1 1/2 cups fresh tomato salsa (see ingredients below)

581

12 flour tortillas

Vegetable cooking spray

Fresh Tomato Salsa Ingredients

1 cup tomatoes, diced

1/3 cup onions, diced

1/2 clove garlic, minced

2 tsp. cilantro

1/3 tsp. jalapeño peppers, chopped

1/2 tsp. lime juice

Pinch of cumin

Directions

- Mix together all salsa ingredients and refrigerate in advance.

- Coat skillet with vegetable spray.

- Lightly sauté onion and green and red peppers.

- Warm tortillas in oven and fill with peppers, onions, avocado, and salsa. Fold tortillas and serve. Top with cilantro.

Exchanges

Bread 3

Vegetable 1

Fat 1 1/2

Note: Diabetic exchanges are calculated based on the American Diabetes Association Exchange System.

Nutrition Facts	
Avocado Tacos	
Serving Size 1 taco	
Amount Per Serving	
Calories	Calories from Fat
270	80
	% Daily Value (DV)*
Total Fat 8g	**12%**
Saturated Fat 2g	**10%**
Trans Fat 0g	
Cholesterol 0mg	**0%**
Sodium 460mg	**19%**
Total Carbohydrate 43g	**14%**
Dietary Fiber 5g	**20%**
Sugars 4g	
Protein 7g	
Vitamin A	25%
Vitamin C	100%
Calcium	10%
Iron	15%
* Percent Daily Values are based on a 2,000 calorie diet.	

Figure 64.7. Nutrition Facts Label, Avocado Tacos

Tropical Fruits Fantasia /
Fantasía de frutas tropicales

Ingredients

8 ounces fat-free, sugar-free orange yogurt

5 medium strawberries, cut into halves

3 ounces honeydew melon, cut into slices (or 1/2 cup cut into cubes)

3 ounces cantaloupe melon, cut into slices (or 1/2 cup cut into cubes)

1 mango, peeled and seeded, cut into cubes

1 papaya, peeled and seeded, cut into cubes

3 ounces watermelon, seeded and cut into slices (or 1/2 cup cut into cubes)

2 oranges, seeded and cut into slices

1/2 cup unsweetened orange juice

Directions

- Add yogurt and all fruits to a bowl and carefully mix together

- Pour orange juice over fruit mixture.

- Mix well and serve 1/2 cup as your dessert.

Exchanges

Fruit 2 3/4

Milk 1/3

Note: Diabetic exchanges are calculated based on the American Diabetes Association Exchange System.

Nutrition Facts	
Tropical Fruits Fantasia	
Serving Size ½ cup	
Amount Per Serving	
Calories 170	Calories from Fat 5
	% Daily Value (DV)*
Total Fat 0.5g	**1%**
Saturated Fat 0g	**0%**
Trans Fat 0g	
Cholesterol 0mg	**0%**
Sodium 40mg	**2%**
Total Carbohydrate 41g	**14%**
Dietary Fiber 5g	**20%**
Sugars 30g	
Protein 4g	
Vitamin A	50%
Vitamin C	230%
Calcium	15%
Iron	2%
* Percent Daily Values are based on a 2,000 calorie diet.	

Figure 64.8. *Nutrition Facts Label, Tropical Fruits Fantasia*

References

American Diabetes Association. Reading Food Labels. American Diabetes Association Website. Available at www.diabetes.org/food-and -fitness/food/what-can-i-eat/taking-a-closer-look-at-labels.html.

American Diabetes Association. Virtual Grocery Store. American Diabetes Association Website. Available at www.diabetes.org/food-and -fitness/.

Bestfoods CPC International, Inc. *Live Healthy America, A Guide from Mazola*. Coventry, CT: Mazola; 1991.

Centers for Disease Control and Prevention. *Take Charge of Your Diabetes. 3rd edition*. Atlanta: U.S. Department of Health and Human Services; 2003. Available at www.cdc.gov/diabetes/pubs/pdf/tctd.pdf.

Centers for Disease Control and Prevention. Fruits & Veggies—More Matters. Centers for Disease Control and Prevention Website. Available at www.fruitsandveggiesmatter.gov.

Gardner L. *Health and the Hispanic Kitchen / La Salud y la Cocina Latina*. Potomac, MD: Precepts, Inc.; 1996.

National Cattlemen's Beef Association. *Eating Smart Even When You Are Pressed for Time*. Chicago: National Cattleman's Beef Association; 1996.

National Cancer Institute. *Celebre la Cocina Hispana, Healthy Hispanic Recipes*. Washington, DC: U.S. Department of Health and Human Services; 1995. NIH Publication Number 95-3906(s).

Pockenpaugh N, Poleman C. *Nutrition: Essential and Diet Therapy. 8th edition*. Philadelphia: WB Saunders; 1996.

Sizer F, Whitney E. *Nutrition: Concepts and Controversies. 8th edition*. Belmont, CA: Wadsworth Publishing; 2000.

U.S. Department of Agriculture. Nutrition Value of Foods. *Home and Garden Bulletin* Number 72. Department of Agriculture Website. Available at www.nal.usda.gov/fnic/foodcomp/Data/HG72/hg72_2002.pdf.

U.S. Department of Health and Human Services. A Healthier You. Department of Health and Human Services Website. Available at www .health.gov/dietaryguidelines/dga2005/healthieryou/contents.htm.

U.S. Department of Health and Human Services and U.S. Department of Agriculture. *Dietary Guidelines for Americans. 6th edition*.

Washington, DC: U.S. Government Printing Office; 2005. Available at www.health.gov/dietaryguidelines.

U.S. Food and Drug Administration. How to Understand and Use the Nutrition Facts Label. Food and Drug Administration Website. Available at www.cfsan.fda.gov/~dms/foodlab.html. Available in Spanish at www.cfsan.fda.gov/~dms/stransfa.html.

Warshaw H. *Diabetes Meal Planning Made Easy: How to Put the Food Pyramid to Work for Your Busy Lifestyle*. Alexandria, VA: American Diabetes Association; 2000.

Chapter 65

Financial Help for Diabetes Care

Diabetes treatment is expensive. According to the American Diabetes Association, people with diabetes spend an average of $11,744 a year on healthcare expenses—more than twice the amount spent by people without diabetes.

Many people who have diabetes need help paying for their care. For those who qualify, a variety of governmental and nongovernmental programs can help cover health care expenses. This chapter is meant to help people with diabetes and their family members find and access such resources.

Medicare

Medicare is federal health insurance for the following groups:

- People sixty-five or older

- People younger than sixty-five with certain disabilities or amyotrophic lateral sclerosis (ALS) also called Lou Gehrig disease

- People of any age with end-stage renal disease—permanent kidney failure requiring dialysis or a kidney transplant

Excerpted from "Financial Help for Diabetes Care," National Institute of Diabetes and Digestive and Kidney Diseases, National Institutes of Health, NIH Publication No. 09-4638, May 2009.

Medicare Health Plans

People with Medicare can choose how to get their health and prescription drug coverage. The following options are available:

- Original Medicare

- Medicare Advantage Plans—such as health maintenance organizations (HMOs) or preferred provider organizations (PPOs)

- Other Medicare health plans

Original Medicare. Original Medicare, managed by the federal government, has two parts: Medicare Part A is hospital insurance and Medicare Part B is medical insurance. People in this plan usually pay a fee for each healthcare service or supply they receive.

People who are in Original Medicare can add prescription drug coverage—Medicare Part D—by joining a Medicare Prescription Drug Plan. These plans are run by insurance companies and other private companies approved by Medicare.

People can also choose to buy insurance to help fill the gaps in Part A and Part B coverage. This insurance is known as Medigap or Medicare Supplement Insurance.

Medicare Advantage Plans. Medicare Advantage Plans are health plan options, like an HMO or PPO, approved by Medicare and offered by private companies. These plans are part of Medicare and are sometimes called Part C or MA Plans. Medicare Advantage Plans provide Medicare Part A and Part B coverage and usually Medicare Part D coverage. The companies that run these plans must follow rules set by Medicare. Not all Medicare Advantage Plans work the same way. People considering one of these plans should find out the plan's rules before joining.

Other Medicare health plans. Other Medicare health plans include Medicare Cost Plans, Demonstrations/Pilot Programs, and Programs of All-Inclusive Care for the Elderly (PACE). These plans provide hospital and medical insurance coverage, and some also provide prescription drug coverage.

Medicare Covers Diabetes Services and Supplies

Original Medicare helps pay for the diabetes services, supplies, and equipment listed below. Coinsurance or deductibles may apply. In addition, Medicare covers some preventive services for people who are at risk for diabetes. A person must have Medicare Part B or Medicare Part D to receive these covered services and supplies.

Medicare Part B helps pay for the following:

- Diabetes screening tests for people at risk of developing diabetes
- Diabetes self-management training
- Diabetes supplies such as glucose monitors, test strips, and lancets
- Insulin pumps and insulin if used with an insulin pump
- Flu and pneumonia shots
- Foot exams and treatment for people with diabetes
- Eye exams to check for glaucoma and diabetic retinopathy
- Medical nutrition therapy services for people with diabetes or kidney disease, when referred by a doctor
- Therapeutic shoes or inserts, in some cases

Medicare Part D helps pay for the following:

- diabetes medicines;
- insulin, but not insulin used with an insulin pump
- diabetes supplies like needles and syringes for injecting insulin

People who are in a Medicare Advantage Plan or other Medicare health plan should check their plan's membership materials and call for details about how the plan provides the diabetes services, supplies, and medicines covered by Medicare.

More Information about Medicare

More information about Medicare is available at www.medicare.gov, the official U.S. government website for people with Medicare. The website has a full range of information about Medicare. Through the Medicare website, people can also do the following things:

- Find out if they are eligible for Medicare and when they can enroll
- Learn about their Medicare health plan options
- Find out what Medicare covers
- Find a Medicare Prescription Drug Plan
- Compare Medicare health plan options in their area

- Find a doctor who participates in Medicare

- get information about the quality of care provided by nursing homes, hospitals, home health agencies, and dialysis facilities

Medicare information can also be obtained from the following agencies or programs:

- Each state has a State Health Insurance Assistance Program (SHIP) that provides free health insurance counseling. A state's SHIP may have a unique name. SHIP counselors can help people choose a Medicare health plan or a Medicare Prescription Drug Plan. The phone number for the SHIP in each state is available by calling Medicare or visiting www.medicare.gov.

- The Social Security Administration can provide information about eligibility for Medicare. People can contact the agency at 800-772-1213, visit its website at www.socialsecurity.gov, or check with their local Social Security office to learn if they are eligible for Medicare.

- State Medical Assistance (Medicaid) offices in each state can provide information about help for people with Medicare who have limited income and resources. The phone number for each state's Medicaid office can be obtained by visiting www.medicare. gov or calling Medicare.

Help for People with Medicare Who Have Limited Income and Resources

People who have Medicare and have limited income and resources may qualify for help paying for some healthcare and prescription drug costs from one of the following programs:

- **Extra help paying for Medicare prescription drug coverage:** Those who meet certain income requirements may qualify for extra help from Medicare to pay prescription drug costs. People can apply for this help by calling Social Security; visiting www.socialsecurity.gov to apply online; visiting their local Social Security office; or by contacting their State Medical Assistance (Medicaid) office. Each state's SHIP can provide information and answer questions about this program.

- **State pharmacy assistance programs (SPAPs):** Several states have SPAPs that help certain people pay for prescription drugs. Each SPAP makes its own rules about how to provide drug coverage to its members. Information about each state's SPAP can be obtained by calling Medicare or the state's SHIP.

- **Medicaid programs for people with Medicare:** State Medicaid programs help pay medical costs for some people with Medicare who have limited income and resources. People who qualify for both Medicare and Medicaid may get coverage for services that aren't fully covered by Medicare, such as nursing home and home health care. States also have programs called Medicare Savings Programs that pay Medicare premiums and, in some cases, may also pay Medicare Part A and Part B deductibles and coinsurance. More information is available at www.medicare.gov. The phone number for the State Medical Assistance (Medicaid) office for each state can be obtained by calling Medicare. Each state's SHIP can also provide more information.

Medicaid

Medicaid, also called Medical Assistance, is a joint federal and state government program that helps pay medical costs for some people with limited income and resources. Medicaid programs and income limits for Medicaid vary from state to state. The State Medical Assistance (Medicaid) office can help people find out whether they qualify for Medicaid or provide more information about Medicaid programs. To contact a state Medicaid office, people can do the following things:

- Search for Medicaid information for a state at www.GovBenefits.gov

- Visit www.medicare.gov and select "Find Helpful Phone Numbers and Websites" under "Search Tools," or call 800-MEDICARE (800-633-4227) and say "Medicaid."

- Check the government pages of the phone book for the local department of human services or department of social services, which can provide the needed information

State Children's Health Insurance Program (SCHIP)

SCHIP is a federal and state government partnership to expand health coverage to uninsured children from families with income that is too low to afford private or employer-sponsored health insurance but too high to qualify for Medicaid. The free or low-cost coverage is available to eligible children younger than nineteen.

SCHIP provides an extensive package of benefits including doctor visits, hospital care, and more. Information about the program is available at www.insurekidsnow.gov or by calling 877-KIDS-NOW (877-543-7669). Callers to the toll-free, confidential hotline are automatically connected to their state's program.

Health Insurance for Those Not Eligible for Medicare or Medicaid

People who are not eligible for Medicare or Medicaid may be able to purchase private health insurance. Many insurers consider diabetes that has already been diagnosed a pre-existing condition, so finding coverage may be difficult for people with diabetes. Insurance companies often have a specific waiting period during which they do not cover diabetes-related expenses for new enrollees, although they will cover other medical expenses that arise during this time.

Certain state and federal laws may help. Many states now require insurance companies to cover diabetes supplies and education. The Health Insurance Portability and Accountability Act (HIPAA), passed by Congress in 1996, limits insurance companies from denying coverage because of a pre-existing condition.

More information about these laws is available from each state's insurance regulatory office. Some state offices may be called the state insurance department or commission. This office can also help identify an insurance company that offers individual coverage.

The Georgetown University Health Policy Institute offers consumer guides on health insurance topics, including guides for each state about getting and keeping health insurance. The guides are available at www.healthinsuranceinfo.net.

Health Insurance after Leaving a Job

When leaving a job, a person may be able to continue the group health insurance provided by the employer for up to eighteen months under a federal law called the Consolidated Omnibus Budget Reconciliation Act, or COBRA. People pay more for group health insurance through COBRA than they did as employees, but group coverage is cheaper than individual coverage. People who have a disability before becoming eligible for COBRA or who are determined by the Social Security Administration to be disabled within the first sixty days of COBRA coverage may be able to extend COBRA coverage an additional eleven months, for up to twenty-nine months of coverage. COBRA may also cover young people who were insured under a parent's policy but have reached the age limit and are trying to obtain their own insurance.

If a person doesn't qualify for coverage or if COBRA coverage has expired, other options may be available:

- Some states require employers to offer conversion policies, in which people stay with their insurance company but buy individual coverage.

- Some professional and alumni organizations offer group coverage for members.

- Most states have a high-risk health insurance pool or other means for covering people otherwise unable to get health insurance. Information about high-risk pools is available at www .nahu.org/consumer/hrpguide.cfm.

- Some insurance companies also offer stopgap policies designed for people who are between jobs.

Each state insurance regulatory office can provide more information about these and other options.

Health Care Services

The Bureau of Primary Health Care, a service of the Health Resources and Services Administration, offers primary and preventive health care to medically underserved populations through community health centers. For people with no insurance, fees for care are based on family size and income. Information about local health centers is available by visiting the Bureau's website at www.bphc.hrsa.gov.

The Department of Veterans Affairs (VA) runs hospitals and clinics that serve veterans who have service-related health problems or who simply need financial aid. Veterans who would like to find out more about VA health care can call 800-827-1000 or visit www1.va.gov/health.

Many local governments have public health departments that can help people who need medical care. The local county or city government's health and human services office can provide further information.

Hospital Care

People who are uninsured and need hospital care may be able to get help from a program known as the Hill-Burton Act. Although the program originally provided hospitals with federal grants for modernization, today it provides free or reduced-fee medical services to people with low incomes. The Department of Health and Human Services administers the program.

Kidney Disease: Resources for Dialysis and Transplantation

Kidney failure, also called end-stage renal disease, is a complication of diabetes. People of any age with kidney failure can get Medicare Part A—hospital insurance—if they meet certain criteria. To qualify for Medicare on the basis of kidney failure, a person must need regular dialysis or have had a kidney transplant, and must have worked long enough—or be the dependent child or spouse of someone who has worked long enough—under Social Security, the Railroad Retirement Board, or as a government employee or be receiving—or be the spouse or dependent child of a person who is receiving—Social Security, Railroad Retirement, or Office of Personnel Management benefits.

People with Medicare Part A can also get Medicare Part B. Enrolling in Part B is optional. However, a person needs to have both Part A and Part B for Medicare to cover certain dialysis and kidney transplant services.

Those who don't qualify for Medicare may be able to get help from their state to pay for their dialysis treatments.

Information about financing an organ transplant is available from the United Network for Organ Sharing (UNOS), www.unos.org.

Prescription Drugs and Medical Supplies

Healthcare providers may be able to assist people who need help paying for their medicines and supplies by directing them to local programs or even providing free samples.

A free nylon filament—similar to a bristle on a hairbrush—is available to check feet for nerve damage. The filament, with instructions for use, can be obtained by calling 1-888-ASK-HRSA (1-888-275-4772) or by accessing www.hrsa.gov/leap.

Prescription drug coverage for those eligible for Medicare is available through Medicare's Prescription Drug Plans and many Medicare Advantage Plans. More information is available at the Medicare website at www.medicare.gov.

Drug companies that sell insulin or diabetes medications usually have patient assistance programs. Such programs are available only through a physician. The Pharmaceutical Research and Manufacturers of America and its member companies sponsor an interactive website with information about drug assistance programs at www.PPARx.org.

Also, because programs for the homeless sometimes provide aid, people can contact a local shelter for more information about how to obtain free medications and medical supplies. The number of the nearest shelter may be listed in the phone book under Human Service Organizations or Social Service Organizations.

Prosthetic Care

People who have had an amputation may be concerned about paying their rehabilitation expenses. The following organizations provide financial assistance or information about locating financial resources for people who need prosthetic care:

- Amputee Coalition of America, www.amputee-coalition.org

- Easter Seals, www.easterseals.com

Classroom Services

Public agencies and other organizations that provide services and assistance, such as providing special equipment, to children with diabetes and other disabilities and to their families are listed on the State Resource Sheets published by the National Dissemination Center for Children with Disabilities (NICHCY). Each state's resource sheet lists the names and addresses of agencies in the state. The free resource sheets are available at www.nichcy.org/states.

College-aged students who have diabetes-related disabilities may be faced not only with the costs of tuition, but also with additional expenses generally not incurred by other students. These costs may include special equipment and disability-related medical expenses not covered by insurance. Some special equipment and support services may be available at the educational institution, through community organizations, through the state vocational rehabilitation agency, or through specific disability organizations. The names and addresses of these and other agencies are also listed in the State Resource Sheets available from the NICHCY.

The HEATH Resource Center, an online clearinghouse on postsecondary education for individuals with disabilities, offers information about sources of financial aid and the education of students with a disability. Contact the clearinghouse at www.heath.gwu.edu.

Technological Assistance

Assistive technology, which can help people with disabilities function more effectively at home, at work, and in the community, can include computers, adaptive equipment, wheelchairs, bathroom modifications, and medical or corrective services. The following organizations provide information, awareness, and training in the use of technology to aid people with disabilities:

- Alliance for Technology Access (ATA), www.ATAccess.org

- United Cerebral Palsy (UCP), www.ucp.org/ucp_channelsub.cfm/ 1/14/86

Food and Nutrition Assistance for Women with Diabetes or Gestational Diabetes

Food, nutrition education, and access to healthcare services are available through the U.S. Department of Agriculture's Women, Infants, and Children (WIC) program. The WIC program provides assistance to women during pregnancy or the period following childbirth and to infants and children up to age five. Applicants must meet residential, financial need, and nutrition risk criteria to be eligible for assistance. Having diabetes or gestational diabetes is considered a medically based nutrition risk and would qualify a woman for assistance through the WIC program if she meets the financial need requirements and has lived in a particular state the required amount of time. The WIC website provides a page of contact information for each state and Indian tribe. Contact the WIC's national headquarters at www.fns.usda.gov/wic.

Social Security Disability Insurance (SSDI) and Supplemental Security Income (SSI) Benefits

The Social Security Administration pays disability benefits through the SSDI and SSI programs. These benefits are not the same as Social Security benefits. To receive SSDI benefits, a person must be unable to work and must have earned the required number of work credits. SSI is a monthly amount paid to people with limited income and resources who are disabled, blind, or age sixty-five or older and meet certain other conditions.

More information is available by contacting the local Social Security office for more information.

Local Resources

Local resources such as the following charitable groups may offer financial help for some of the many expenses related to diabetes:

- Lions Clubs International can help with vision care. Visit www .lionsclubs.org.

- Elks clubs provide charitable activities that benefit youth and veterans. Visit www.elks.org.

- Shriners of North America offer free treatment for children at Shriners hospitals throughout the country. Visit www.shrinershq .org.

- Kiwanis International clubs conduct service projects to help children and communities. Visit www.kiwanis.org.

In many areas, nonprofit or special interest groups such as those listed above can sometimes provide financial assistance or help with fund-raising. Religious organizations also may offer assistance. In addition, some local governments may have special trusts set up to help people in need. The local library or local city or county government's health and human services office may provide more information about such groups.

Chapter 66

Directory of Diabetes-Related Resources

American Association of Clinical Endocrinologists
245 Riverside Avenue
Suite 200
Jacksonville, FL 32202
Phone: 904-353-7878
Website: http://www.aace.com

American Association of Diabetes Educators
200 W. Madison Street
Suite 800
Chicago, IL 60606
Toll-Free: 800-338-3633
Website:
http://www.diabeteseducator.org
E-mail: aade@aadenet.org

American Diabetes Association
National Service Center
1701 North Beauregard Street
Alexandria, VA 22311
Toll-Free: 800-DIABETES
(342-2383)
Website: http://www.diabetes.org
E-mail: AskADA@diabetes.org

Canadian Diabetes Association
1400-522 University Avenue
Toronto ON M5G 2R5
CANADA
Toll-Free: 800-BANTING
(226-8464)
Website: http://www.diabetes.ca
Email: info@diabetes.ca

Resources in this chapter were compiled from several sources deemed reliable. All contact information was verified and updated in February 2011.

Centers for Disease Control and Prevention
1600 Clifton Road
Atlanta, GA 30333
Toll-Free: 800-CDC-INFO
(232-4636)
TTY: 888-232-6348
Website: http://www.cdc.gov
E-mail: cdcinfo@cdc.gov

Diabetes Action Research and Education Foundation
426 "C" Street, NE
Washington, DC 20002
Phone: 202-333-4520
Fax: 202-558-5240
Website: http://www
.diabetesaction.org

Diabetes Insipidus Foundation
1232 24th Street
Ames, IA 50010
Website:
http://www.diabetesinsipidus.org

Diabetes Teaching Center
University of California, San Francisco
400 Parnassus Avenue
5th Floor
Box 1222
San Francisco, CA 94143-1222
Phone: 415-353-2266
Fax: 415-353-2392
Website:
http://www.deo.ucsf.edu
E-mail:
diabetesteachingcenter
@ucsfmedctr.org

Johns Hopkins Diabetes Center
Website: http://www
.hopkinsmedicine.org/diabetes

Joslin Diabetes Center
One Joslin Place
Boston, MA 02215
Website: http://www.joslin.org

National Center for Complementary and Alternative Medicine
NCCAM
National Institutes of Health
9000 Rockville Pike
Bethesda, Maryland 20892
NCCAM Clearinghouse
P.O. Box 7923
Gaithersburg, MD 20898
Toll-Free: 888-644-6226
Fax: 866-464-3616
TTY: 866-464-3615
Website: http://nccam.nih.gov
E-mail: info@nccam.nih.gov

National Diabetes Education Program
1 Diabetes Way
Bethesda, MD 20814-9692
Toll-Free: 888-693-NDEP
(6337)
TTY: 866-569-1162
Website:
http://www.ndep.nih.gov
E-mail: ndep@mail.nih.gov

National Diabetes Information Clearinghouse
1 Information Way
Bethesda, MD 20892-2560
Toll-Free; 800-860-8747
Phone: 301-654-3327
Website: http://www.diabetes
.niddk.nih.gov
E-mail: ndic@info.niddk.nih.gov

National Institute on Aging
Building 31, Room 5C27
31 Center Drive, MSC 2292
Bethesda, MD 20892
Phone: 301-496-1752
Fax: 301-496-1072
TTY: 800-222-4225
Website: http://www.nia.nih.gov

Diabetic Eye Disease

EyeCare America
P.O. Box 429098
San Francisco, CA 94142
Phone: 877-887-6327
Fax: 415-561-8567
Website:
http://www.eyecareamerica.org

National Eye Institute (NEI)
31 Center Drive MSC 2510
Bethesda, MD 20892-2510
Phone: 301-496-5248
Website: http://www.nei.nih.gov
E-mail: 2020@nei.nih.gov

Prevent Blindness America
211 West Wacker Drive
#1700
Chicago, IL 60606
Toll-Free: 800-331-2020
Phone: 312-363-6001
Website:
http://www.preventblindness.org
E-mail:
info@preventblindness.org

Diabetic Kidney Disease

American Association of Kidney Patients
3505 E. Frontage Road,
Suite 315
Tampa, FL 33607
Toll-Free: 800-749-2257
Fax: 813-636-8122
Website: http://www.aakp.org
E-mail: info@aakp.org

National Kidney Disease Education Program
3 Kidney Information Way
Bethesda, MD 20892
Toll-Free: 866-4-KIDNEY
(454-3639)
Fax: 301-402-8182
Website: http://www.nkdep.nih.gov
E-mail: nkdep@info.niddk.nih.gov

National Kidney Foundation
30 East 33rd Street
New York, NY 10016
Toll-Free: 800-622-9010
Website: http://www.kidney.org

Juvenile Diabetes

Children With Diabetes
Website: www
.childrenwithdiabetes.com

Nemours Foundation
Website:
http://www.kidshealth.org

Juvenile Diabetes Research Foundation International
26 Broadway, 14th Floor
New York, NY 10004
Toll-Free: 800-533-CURE
(2873)
Website: http://www.jdrf.org
E-mail: info@jdrf.org

Index

Index

Health Reference Series